AF751894

KAPLAN

# MCAT®

# Organic Chemistry Review

# 2027–2028

Edited by Alexander Stone Macnow, MD

**ACKNOWLEDGMENTS**

**Editor-in-Chief, 2027–2028 Edition**
M. Dominic Eggert

**Contributing Editors, 2027–2028 Edition**
Ae-Ri Kim, PhD; Elizabeth Minten, MD PhD; Gregory J. Riviello, MA; Christopher Vestuto

**Prior Edition Editorial Staff:** Elisabeth Fassas, MD MSc



Published by Kaplan North America, LLC
1515 West Cypress Creek Road
Fort Lauderdale, Florida 33309

Printed in India.



ISBN: 979-8-3497-0126-9

10 9 8 7 6 5 4 3 2 1

Kaplan Publishing print books are available at special quantity discounts to use for sales promotions, employee premiums, or educational purposes. For more information or to purchase books, please call the Simon & Schuster special sales department at 866-506-1949.

# TABLE OF CONTENTS

# THE *KAPLAN MCAT REVIEW* TEAM


**Alexander Stone Macnow, MD**
Editor-in-Chief

**Kelly Kyker-Snowman, MS**
Kaplan MCAT Faculty

**M. Dominic Eggert**
Editor



Reviewers and Editors: Elmar R. Aliyev; James Burns; Jonathan Cornfield; Alisha Maureen Crowley; Brandon Deason, MD; Nikolai Dorofeev, MD; Benjamin Downer, MS; Colin Doyle; Christopher Durland; Marilyn Engle; Eleni M. Eren; Raef Ali Fadel; Elizabeth Flagge; Adam Grey; Tyra Hall-Pogar, PhD; Scott Huff; Samer T. Ismail; Elizabeth A. Kudlaty; Ningfei Li; John P. Mahon; Matthew A. Meier; Nainika Nanda; Caroline Nkemdilim Opene; Kaitlyn E. Prenger; Uneeb Qureshi; Derek Rusnak, MA; Kristen L. Russell, ME; Bela G. Starkman, PhD; Michael Paul Tomani, MS; Lauren K. White; Nicholas M. White; Allison Ann Wilkes, MS; Kerranna Williamson, MBA; and Tony Yu

Thanks to Kevin Anderson; Rebecca Anderson; Jeff Batzli; Jurre Blom; Hari Priya Chandran; Eric Chiu; James Coleman; Deepika Devan; Tim Eich; Samantha Fallon; Tyler Fara; Owen Farcy; Dan Frey; Robin Garmise; Rita Garthaffner; Joanna Graham; Allison Gudenau; Allison Harm; Beth Hoffberg; Aaron Lemon-Strauss; Keith Lubeley; Diane McGarvey; Leonard Mendoza; Petros Minasi; Elizabeth Minten, MD, PhD; Beena P V; John Polstein; Deeangelee Pooran-Kublall, MD, MPH; Andrea Repole; Rochelle Rothstein, MD; Larry Rudman; Tor Sanden; Srividhya Sankar; Sylvia Tidwell Scheuring; Carly Schnur; Aiswarya Sivanand; Todd Tedesco; Karin Tucker; Bonnie Wang; Lee Weiss; Christina Wheeler; Kristen Workman; Amy Zarkos; and the countless others who made this book possible.

# GETTING STARTED CHECKLIST

## Getting Started Checklist

- [ ] Register for your free online assets: if you bought this book new as part of a set, scan the QR code on the front of the book set's slipcase and enter the unique code there; if you bought this book separately, instead go to **www.kaptest.com/moreonline**.
- [ ] Create a study calendar that ensures you complete content review and sufficient practice by Test Day!
- [ ] As you finish a chapter and the online practice for that chapter, check it off on the table of contents.
- [ ] Register to take the MCAT at **www.aamc.org/mcat.**
- [ ] Set aside time during your prep to make sure the rest of your application—personal statement, recommendations, and other materials—is ready to go!
- [ ] Take a moment to admire your completed checklist, then get back to the business of prepping for this exam!

# PREFACE

And now it starts: your long, yet fruitful journey toward wearing a white coat. Proudly wearing that white coat, though, is hopefully only part of your motivation. You are reading this book because you want to be a healer.

If you're serious about going to medical school, then you are likely already familiar with the importance of the MCAT in medical school admissions. While the holistic review process puts additional weight on your experiences, extracurricular activities, and personal attributes, the fact remains: along with your GPA, your MCAT score remains one of the two most important components of your application portfolio—at least early in the admissions process. Each additional point you score on the MCAT pushes you in front of thousands of other students and makes you an even more attractive applicant. But the MCAT is not simply an obstacle to overcome; it is an opportunity to show schools that you will be a strong student and a future leader in medicine.

We at Kaplan take our jobs very seriously and aim to help students see success not only on the MCAT, but as future physicians. We work with our learning science experts to ensure that we're using the most up-to-date teaching techniques in our resources. Multiple members of our team hold advanced degrees in medicine or associated biomedical sciences, and are committed to the highest level of medical education. Kaplan has been working with the MCAT for over 50 years and our commitment to premed students is unflagging; in fact, Stanley Kaplan created this company when he had difficulty being accepted to medical school due to unfair quota systems that existed at the time.

We stand now at the beginning of a new era in medical education. As citizens of this 21st-century world of healthcare, we are charged with creating a patient-oriented, culturally competent, cost-conscious, universally available, technically advanced, and research-focused healthcare system, run by compassionate providers. Suffice it to say, this is no easy task. Problem-based learning, integrated curricula, and classes in interpersonal skills are some of the responses to this demand for an excellent workforce—a workforce of which you'll soon be a part.

We're thrilled that you've chosen us to help you on this journey. Please reach out to us to share your challenges, concerns, and successes. Together, we will shape the future of medicine in the United States and abroad; we look forward to helping you become the doctor you deserve to be.

Good luck!

Alexander Stone Macnow, MD
Editor-in-Chief
Department of Pathology and Laboratory Medicine
Hospital of the University of Pennsylvania

BA, Musicology—Boston University, 2008
MD—Perelman School of Medicine at the University of Pennsylvania, 2013

# ABOUT THE MCAT

## Anatomy of the MCAT

Here is a general overview of the structure of Test Day:

| Section | Number of Questions | Time Allotted |
|---|---|---|
| Test-Day Certification | | 4 minutes |
| Tutorial (optional) | | 10 minutes |
| Chemical and Physical Foundations of Biological Systems | 59 | 95 minutes |
| Break (optional) | | 10 minutes |
| Critical Analysis and Reasoning Skills (CARS) | 53 | 90 minutes |
| Lunch Break (optional) | | 30 minutes |
| Biological and Biochemical Foundations of Living Systems | 59 | 95 minutes |
| Break (optional) | | 10 minutes |
| Psychological, Social, and Biological Foundations of Behavior | 59 | 95 minutes |
| Void Question | | 3 minutes |
| Satisfaction Survey (optional) | | 5 minutes |

The structure of the four sections of the MCAT is shown below.

| Chemical and Physical Foundations of Biological Systems | |
|---|---|
| **Time** | 95 minutes |
| **Format** | • 59 questions<br>• 10 passages<br>• 44 questions are passage-based, and 15 are discrete (stand-alone) questions.<br>• Score between 118 and 132 |
| **What It Tests** | • Biochemistry: 25%<br>• Biology: 5%<br>• General Chemistry: 30%<br>• Organic Chemistry: 15%<br>• Physics: 25% |

| Critical Analysis and Reasoning Skills (CARS) | |
|---|---|
| **Time** | 90 minutes |
| **Format** | • 53 questions<br>• 9 passages<br>• All questions are passage-based. There are no discrete (stand-alone) questions.<br>• Score between 118 and 132 |
| **What It Tests** | Disciplines:<br>• Humanities: 50%<br>• Social Sciences: 50%<br>Skills:<br>• *Foundations of Comprehension: 30%*<br>• *Reasoning Within the Text: 30%*<br>• *Reasoning Beyond the Text: 40%* |
| **Biological and Biochemical Foundations of Living Systems** | |
| **Time** | 95 minutes |
| **Format** | • 59 questions<br>• 10 passages<br>• 44 questions are passage-based, and 15 are discrete (stand-alone) questions.<br>• Score between 118 and 132 |
| **What It Tests** | • Biochemistry: 25%<br>• Biology: 65%<br>• General Chemistry: 5%<br>• Organic Chemistry: 5% |
| **Psychological, Social, and Biological Foundations of Behavior** | |
| **Time** | 95 minutes |
| **Format** | • 59 questions<br>• 10 passages<br>• 44 questions are passage-based, and 15 are discrete (stand-alone) questions.<br>• Score between 118 and 132 |
| **What It Tests** | • Biology: 5%<br>• Psychology: 65%<br>• Sociology: 30% |
| **Total** | |
| **Testing Time** | 375 minutes (6 hours, 15 minutes) |
| **Total Seat Time** | 447 minutes (7 hours, 27 minutes) |
| **Questions** | 230 |
| **Score** | 472 to 528 |

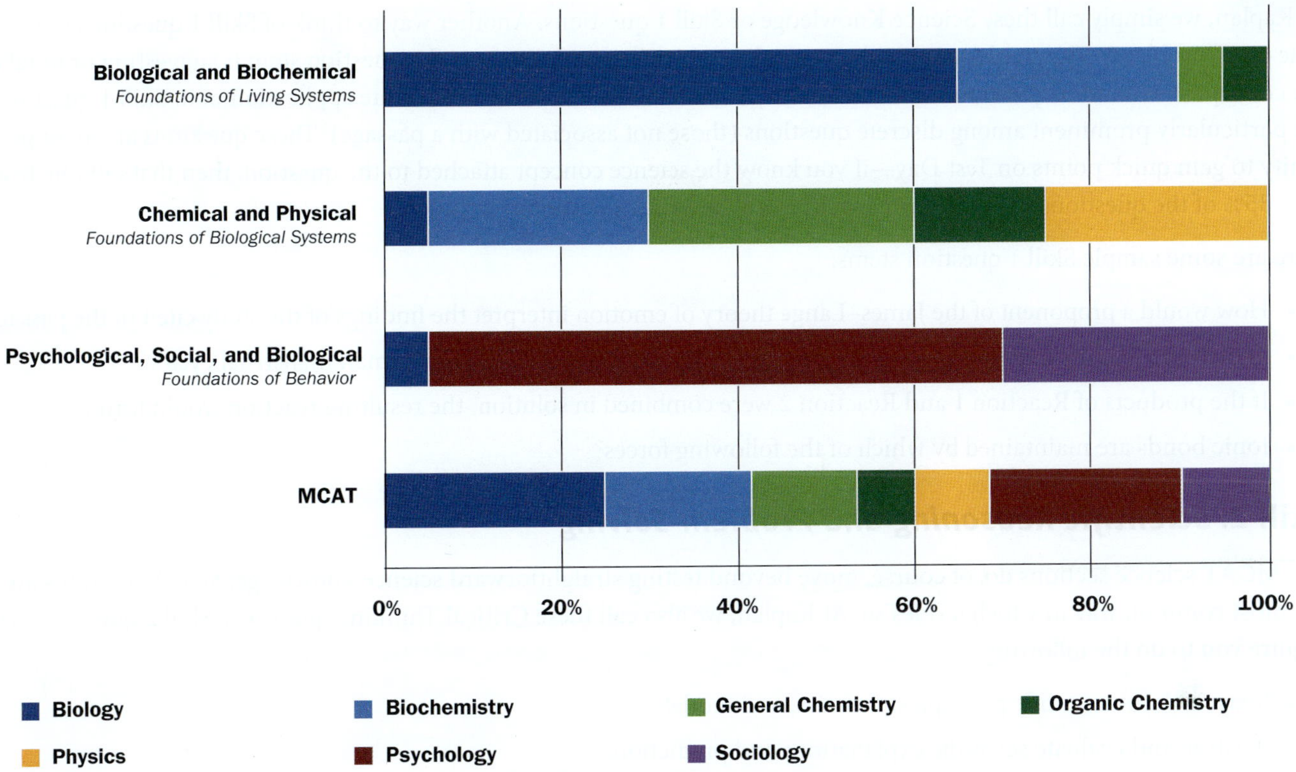


## *Scientific Inquiry and Reasoning Skills* (SIRS)

The AAMC has defined four *Scientific Inquiry and Reasoning Skills* (SIRS) that will be tested in the three science sections of the MCAT:

1. *Knowledge of Scientific Concepts and Principles* (35% of questions)
2. *Scientific Reasoning and Problem-Solving* (45% of questions)
3. *Reasoning About the Design and Execution of Research* (10% of questions)
4. *Data-Based and Statistical Reasoning* (10% of questions)

Let's see how each one breaks down into more specific Test Day behaviors. Note that the bullet points of specific objectives for each of the SIRS are taken directly from the *Official Guide to the MCAT Exam*; the descriptions of what these behaviors mean and sample question stems, however, are written by Kaplan.

## Skill 1: *Knowledge of Scientific Concepts and Principles*

This is probably the least surprising of the four SIRS; the testing of science knowledge is, after all, one of the signature qualities of the MCAT. Skill 1 questions will require you to do the following:

- Recognize correct scientific principles
- Identify the relationships among closely related concepts
- Identify the relationships between different representations of concepts (verbal, symbolic, graphic)
- Identify examples of observations that illustrate scientific principles
- Use mathematical equations to solve problems

At Kaplan, we simply call these Science Knowledge or Skill 1 questions. Another way to think of Skill 1 questions is as "one-step" problems. The single step is either to realize which scientific concept the question stem is suggesting or to take the concept stated in the question stem and identify which answer choice is an accurate application of it. Skill 1 questions are particularly prominent among discrete questions (those not associated with a passage). These questions are an opportunity to gain quick points on Test Day—if you know the science concept attached to the question, then that's it! On Test Day, 35% of the questions in each science section will be Skill 1 questions.

Here are some sample Skill 1 question stems:

- How would a proponent of the James–Lange theory of emotion interpret the findings of the study cited in the passage?
- Which of the following most accurately describes the function of FSH in the human menstrual cycle?
- If the products of Reaction 1 and Reaction 2 were combined in solution, the resulting reaction would form:
- Ionic bonds are maintained by which of the following forces?

## Skill 2: *Scientific Reasoning and Problem-Solving*

The MCAT science sections do, of course, move beyond testing straightforward science knowledge; Skill 2 questions are the most common way in which it does so. At Kaplan, we also call these Critical Thinking questions. Skill 2 questions will require you to do the following:

- Reason about scientific principles, theories, and models
- Analyze and evaluate scientific explanations and predictions
- Evaluate arguments about causes and consequences
- Bring together theory, observations, and evidence to draw conclusions
- Recognize scientific findings that challenge or invalidate a scientific theory or model
- Determine and use scientific formulas to solve problems

Just as Skill 1 questions can be thought of as "one-step" problems, many Skill 2 questions are "two-step" problems, and more difficult Skill 2 questions may require three or more steps. These questions can require a wide spectrum of reasoning skills, including integration of multiple facts from a passage, combination of multiple science content areas, and prediction of an experiment's results. Skill 2 questions also tend to ask about science content without actually mentioning it by name. For example, a question might describe the results of one experiment and ask you to predict the results of a second experiment without actually telling you what underlying scientific principles are at work—part of the question's difficulty will be figuring out which principles to apply in order to get the correct answer. On Test Day, 45% of the questions in each science section will be Skill 2 questions.

Here are some sample Skill 2 question stems:

- Which of the following experimental conditions would most likely yield results similar to those in Figure 2?
- All of the following conclusions are supported by the information in the passage EXCEPT:
- The most likely cause of the anomalous results found by the experimenter is:
- An impact to a person's chest quickly reduces the volume of one of the lungs to 70% of its initial value while not allowing any air to escape from the mouth. By what percentage is the force of outward air pressure increased on a 2 $cm^2$ portion of the inner surface of the compressed lung?

## Skill 3: *Reasoning About the Design and Execution of Research*

The MCAT is interested in your ability to critically appraise and analyze research, as this is an important day-to-day task of a physician. We call these questions Experimental and Research Design questions or Skill 3 for short. Skill 3 questions will require you to do the following:

- Identify the role of theory, past findings, and observations in scientific questioning
- Identify testable research questions and hypotheses
- Distinguish between samples and populations and distinguish results that support generalizations about populations
- Identify independent and dependent variables
- Reason about the features of research studies that suggest associations between variables or causal relationships between them (such as temporality and random assignment)
- Identify conclusions that are supported by research results
- Determine the implications of results for real-world situations
- Reason about ethical issues in scientific research

Over the years, the AAMC has received input from medical schools to require more practical research skills of MCAT test takers, and Skill 3 questions are the response to these demands. This skill is unique in that the outside knowledge you need to answer Skill 3 questions is not taught in any one undergraduate course; instead, the research design principles needed to answer these questions are learned gradually throughout your science classes and especially through any laboratory work you have completed. It should be noted that Skill 3 comprises 10% of the questions in each science section on Test Day.

Here are some sample Skill 3 question stems:

- What is the dependent variable in the study described in the passage?
- The major flaw in the method used to measure disease susceptibility in Experiment 1 is:
- Which of the following procedures is most important for the experimenters to follow in order for their study to maintain a proper, randomized sample of research subjects?
- A researcher would like to test the hypothesis that individuals who move to an urban area during adulthood are more likely to own a car than are those who have lived in an urban area since birth. Which of the following studies would best test this hypothesis?

## Skill 4: *Data-Based and Statistical Reasoning*

Lastly, the science sections of the MCAT test your ability to analyze the visual and numerical results of experiments and studies. We call these Data and Statistical Analysis questions. Skill 4 questions will require you to do the following:

- Use, analyze, and interpret data in figures, graphs, and tables
- Evaluate whether representations make sense for particular scientific observations and data
- Use measures of central tendency (mean, median, and mode) and measures of dispersion (range, interquartile range, and standard deviation) to describe data
- Reason about random and systematic error

- Reason about statistical significance and uncertainty (interpreting statistical significance levels and interpreting a confidence interval)
- Use data to explain relationships between variables or make predictions
- Use data to answer research questions and draw conclusions

Skill 4 is included in the MCAT because physicians and researchers spend much of their time examining the results of their own studies and the studies of others, and it's very important for them to make legitimate conclusions and sound judgments based on that data. The MCAT tests Skill 4 on all three science sections with graphical representations of data (charts and bar graphs), as well as numerical ones (tables, lists, and results summarized in sentence or paragraph form). On Test Day, 10% of the questions in each science section will be Skill 4 questions.

Here are some sample Skill 4 question stems:

- According to the information in the passage, there is an inverse correlation between:
- What conclusion is best supported by the findings displayed in Figure 2?
- A medical test for a rare type of heavy metal poisoning returns a positive result for 98% of affected individuals and 13% of unaffected individuals. Which of the following types of error is most prevalent in this test?
- If a fourth trial of Experiment 1 was run and yielded a result of 54% compliance, which of the following would be true?

## SIRS Summary

Discussing the SIRS tested on the MCAT is a daunting prospect given that the very nature of the skills tends to make the conversation rather abstract. Nevertheless, with enough practice, you'll be able to identify each of the four skills quickly, and you'll also be able to apply the proper strategies to solve those problems on Test Day. If you need a quick reference to remind you of the four SIRS, these guidelines may help:

**Skill 1** (**Science Knowledge**) questions ask:

- Do you remember this science content?

**Skill 2** (**Critical Thinking**) questions ask:

- Do you remember this science content? And if you do, could you please apply it to this novel situation?
- Could you answer this question that cleverly combines multiple content areas at the same time?

**Skill 3** (**Experimental and Research Design**) questions ask:

- Let's forget about the science content for a while. Could you give some insight into the experimental or research methods involved in this situation?

**Skill 4** (**Data and Statistical Analysis**) questions ask:

- Let's forget about the science content for a while. Could you accurately read some graphs and tables for a moment? Could you make some conclusions or extrapolations based on the information presented?

## *Critical Analysis and Reasoning Skills* (CARS)

The *Critical Analysis and Reasoning Skills* (CARS) section of the MCAT tests three discrete families of textual reasoning skills; each of these families requires a higher level of reasoning than the last. Those three skills are as follows:

1. *Foundations of Comprehension* (30% of questions)
2. *Reasoning Within the Text* (30% of questions)
3. *Reasoning Beyond the Text* (40% of questions)

These three categories of skills are tested through nine humanities- and social sciences-themed passages, with approximately 5 to 7 questions per passage. Let's take a more in-depth look into these three types. Again, the bullet points of specific objectives for each of the CARS are taken directly from the *Official Guide to the MCAT Exam*; the descriptions of what these behaviors mean and sample question stems, however, are written by Kaplan.

## *Foundations of Comprehension*

Questions in this category will ask for basic facts and simple inferences about the passage; the questions themselves will be similar to those seen on reading comprehension sections of other standardized exams like the SAT® and ACT®. *Foundations of Comprehension* questions will require you to do the following:

- Understand the basic components of the text
- Infer meaning from rhetorical devices, word choice, and text structure

This covers a wide range of question skills (Summarize Text, Recognize Opinion, Paraphrase Detail, and Interpret Meaning), but finding the correct answer to all *Foundations of Comprehension* questions will follow from a basic understanding of the passage and the point of view of its author (and occasionally that of other voices in the passage). Because these questions tend to avoid digging too deeply into the passage, Kaplan calls these *surface* questions.

Here are some sample *Foundations of Comprehension* question stems:

- **Summarize Text**—The author's primary thesis in this passage is:
- **Recognize Opinion**—Based on the information in the second paragraph, which of the following is the most accurate summary of the opinion held by Schubert's critics?
- **Paraphrase Detail**—According to the passage, which of the following is FALSE about literary reviews in the 1920s?
- **Interpret Meaning**—The word "obscure" (paragraph 3), when used in reference to the historian's actions, most nearly means:

## *Reasoning Within the Text*

While *Foundations of Comprehension* questions will usually depend on interpreting a single piece of information in the passage or understanding the passage as a whole, *Reasoning Within the Text* questions require more thought because they will ask you to identify the purpose of a particular piece of information in the context of the passage, or ask how one piece of information relates to another. *Reasoning Within the Text* questions will require you to:

- Integrate different components of the text to draw relevant conclusions

In other words, questions in this type often ask either *How do these two details relate to one another?* or *What else must be true that the author didn't say?* The CARS section will also ask you to judge certain parts of the passage or even judge the author. These questions, which fall under the *Reasoning Within the Text* skill, can ask you to identify authorial bias, evaluate the credibility of cited sources, determine the logical soundness of an argument, identify the importance of a particular fact or statement in the context of the passage, or search for relevant evidence in the passage to support a given conclusion. This category, which Kaplan refers to as *deep* questions because of their tendency to venture into the deep reasoning of the passage, encompasses the following skills: Describe Purpose, Evaluate Reasoning, and Make Deduction.

Here are some sample *Reasoning Within the Text* question stems:

- **Describe Purpose**—The author's discussion of the effect of socioeconomic status on social mobility primarily serves which of the following functions?
- **Evaluate Reasoning**—Which of the following facts is used in the passage as the most prominent piece of evidence in favor of the author's conclusions?
- **Make Deduction**—In putting together the argument in the passage, the author most likely assumes:

## *Reasoning Beyond the Text*

The distinguishing factor of *Reasoning Beyond the Text* questions is in the title of the category: the word *Beyond*. Questions of this type, which make up a larger share of the CARS section than questions from either of the other two types, will always introduce a completely new situation that was not present in the passage itself; these questions will ask you to determine how one influences the other. *Reasoning Beyond the Text* questions will require you to:

- Apply or extrapolate ideas from the passage to new contexts
- Assess the impact of introducing new factors, information, or conditions to ideas from the passage

Because they always introduce ideas not discussed in the passage, Kaplan refers to these as *new info* questions. They test the following skills: Anticipate Response, Predict Outcome/Explanation, Imagine Example/Analogy, and Strengthen/Weaken Argument.

Here are some sample *Reasoning Beyond the Text* question stems:

- **Anticipate Response**—If a document were located that demonstrated Berlioz intended to include a chorus of at least 700 in his *Grande Messe des Morts*, how would the author likely respond?
- **Imagine Example/Analogy**—Which of the following is the best example of a "virtuous rebellion," as it is defined in the passage?
- **Predict Outcome/Explanation**—Extending the author's discussion of ancient Greek history, a conflict between a democracy and an oligarchy would most likely result in:
- **Strengthen/Weaken Argument**—Which of the following sentences, if added to the end of the passage, would most WEAKEN the author's conclusions in the last paragraph?

## CARS Summary

Through the *Foundations of Comprehension* category of skills, the CARS section tests many of the reading skills you have been building on since grade school, albeit in the context of very challenging doctorate-level passages. But through the two other categories (*Reasoning Within the Text* and *Reasoning Beyond the Text*), the MCAT demands that you understand the deep structure of passages and the arguments within them at an advanced level. And, of course, all of this is tested under very tight timing restrictions: only 102 seconds per question—and that doesn't even include the time spent reading the passages.

Here's a quick reference guide to the three categories and 11 skills tested in CARS:

***Foundations of Comprehension*** skills:

- Interpret Meaning: Use context to determine what a word/phrase from the passage is intended to communicate.
- Recognize Opinion: Identify what the author or someone else feels about a passage idea based on word choice or other context clues.
- Paraphrase Detail: Recognize a specific piece of information that is stated or strongly implied at one location in the passage.
- Summarize Text: Articulate the main idea of the passage or of a part of it.

***Reasoning Within the Text*** skills:

- Describe Purpose: Identify why the author wrote the passage or a part of it.
- Evaluate Reasoning: Characterize logical connections between ideas in the passage.
- Make Deduction: Infer a claim that follows from multiple parts of the passage, such as an assumption in an argument.

***Reasoning Beyond the Text*** skills:

- Anticipate Response: Identify what the author or someone else would feel/say/do about a new situation based on its similarities to passage ideas.
- Predict Outcome/Explanation: Apply causal reasoning or another connection from the passage to a new situation.
- Strengthen/Weaken Argument: Characterize the logical relationship between a new claim and arguments from the passage.
- Imagine Example/Analogy: Identify new examples of categories defined in the passage or analogies of passage concepts.

## Scoring

Each of the four sections of the MCAT is scored between 118 and 132, with the median at approximately 125. This means the total score ranges from 472 to 528, with the median at about 500. Why such peculiar numbers? The AAMC stresses that this scale emphasizes the importance of the central portion of the score distribution, where most students score (around 125 per section, or 500 total), rather than putting undue focus on the high end of the scale.

Note that there is no wrong answer penalty on the MCAT, so you should select an answer for every question—even if it is only a guess.

The AAMC has released the 2022–2024 correlation between scaled score and percentile, as shown on the following page. It should be noted that the percentile scale is adjusted and renormalized over time and thus can shift slightly from year to year. Percentile rank updates are released by the AAMC around May 1 of each year.

| Total Score | Percentile | Total Score | Percentile |
|---|---|---|---|
| 528 | 100 | 499 | 46 |
| 527 | 100 | 498 | 42 |
| 526 | 100 | 497 | 39 |
| 525 | 100 | 496 | 36 |
| 524 | 100 | 495 | 34 |
| 523 | 99 | 494 | 31 |
| 522 | 99 | 493 | 28 |
| 521 | 98 | 492 | 25 |
| 520 | 97 | 491 | 23 |
| 519 | 96 | 490 | 21 |
| 518 | 95 | 489 | 18 |
| 517 | 94 | 488 | 16 |
| 516 | 92 | 487 | 14 |
| 515 | 91 | 486 | 12 |
| 514 | 89 | 485 | 11 |
| 513 | 87 | 484 | 9 |
| 512 | 84 | 483 | 8 |
| 511 | 82 | 482 | 6 |
| 510 | 79 | 481 | 5 |
| 509 | 77 | 480 | 4 |
| 508 | 74 | 479 | 3 |
| 507 | 71 | 478 | 2 |
| 506 | 68 | 477 | 2 |
| 505 | 65 | 476 | 1 |
| 504 | 62 | 475 | 1 |
| 503 | 58 | 474 | <1 |
| 502 | 55 | 473 | <1 |
| 501 | 52 | 472 | <1 |
| 500 | 49 | | |

Source: AAMC. 2025. *Summary of MCAT Total and Section Scores*. Accessed October 2025.
**https://students-residents.aamc.org/mcat-research-and-data/percentile-ranks-mcat-exam**

Further information on score reporting is included at the end of the next section (see *After Your Test*).

## MCAT Policies and Procedures

We strongly encourage you to download the latest copy of *MCAT® Essentials*, available on the AAMC's website, to ensure that you have the latest information about registration and Test Day policies and procedures; this document is updated annually. A brief summary of some of the most important rules is provided here.

## MCAT Registration

The only way to register for the MCAT is online. You can access AAMC's registration system at **www.aamc.org/mcat**.

The AAMC posts the schedule of testing, registration, and score release dates in the fall before the MCAT testing year, which runs from January into September. See the AAMC's website for the exact dates that registration opens each year. There is one standard registration fee, but the fee for changing your test date or test center increases the closer you get to your MCAT.

## Fees and the Fee Assistance Program (FAP)

Payment for test registration must be made by American Express, Discover, MasterCard, or VISA. As described earlier, the fee for rescheduling your exam or changing your testing center increases as one approaches Test Day. In addition, it is not uncommon for test centers to fill up well in advance of the registration deadline. For these reasons, we recommend identifying your preferred Test Day as soon as possible and registering. There are ancillary benefits to having a set Test Day, as well: when you know the date you're working toward, you'll study harder and are less likely to keep pushing back the exam. The AAMC offers a Fee Assistance Program (FAP) for students with financial hardship to help reduce the cost of taking the MCAT, as well as for the American Medical College Application Service (AMCAS®) application. Further information on the FAP can be found at **www.aamc.org/students/applying/fap**.

## Testing Security

On Test Day, you will be required to present a qualifying form of ID. Generally, a current driver's license or United States passport will be sufficient (consult the AAMC website for the full list of qualifying criteria). When registering, take care to spell your first and last names (middle names, suffixes, and prefixes are not required and will not be verified on Test Day) precisely the same as they appear on this ID; failure to provide this ID at the test center or differences in spelling between your registration and ID will be considered a "no-show," and you will not receive a refund for the exam.

During Test Day registration, other identity data collected may include: a digital palm vein scan, a Test Day photo, a digitization of your valid ID, and signatures. Some testing centers may use a metal detection wand to ensure that no prohibited items are brought into the testing room. Prohibited items include all electronic devices, including watches and timers, calculators, cell phones, and any and all forms of recording equipment; food, drinks (including water), and cigarettes or other smoking paraphernalia; hats and scarves (except for religious purposes); and books, notes, or other study materials. If you require a medical device, such as an insulin pump or pacemaker, you must apply for accommodated testing. During breaks, you are allowed access to food and drink, but not to electronic devices, including cell phones.

Testing centers are under video surveillance and the AAMC does not take potential violations of testing security lightly. The bottom line: *know the rules and don't break them.*

## Accommodations

Students with disabilities or medical conditions can apply for accommodated testing. Documentation of the disability or condition is required, and requests may take two months—or more—to be approved. For this reason, it is recommended that you begin the process of applying for accommodated testing as early as possible. More information on applying for accommodated testing can be found at **www.aamc.org/students/applying/mcat/accommodations**.

## After Your Test

When your MCAT is all over, no matter how you feel you did, be good to yourself when you leave the test center. Celebrate! Take a nap. Watch a movie. Get some exercise. Plan a trip or outing. Call up all of your neglected friends or message them on social media. Go out for snacks or drinks with people you like. Whatever you do, make sure that it has absolutely nothing to do with thinking too hard—you deserve some rest and relaxation.

Perhaps most importantly, do not discuss specific details about the test with anyone. For one, it is important to let go of the stress of Test Day, and reliving your exam only inhibits you from being able to do so. But more significantly, the Examinee Agreement you sign at the beginning of your exam specifically prohibits you from discussing or disclosing exam content. The AAMC is known to seek out individuals who violate this agreement and retains the right to prosecute these individuals at their discretion. This means that you should not, under any circumstances, discuss the exam in person or over the phone with other individuals—including us at Kaplan—or post information or questions about exam content to Facebook, Student Doctor Network, or other online social media. You are permitted to comment on your "general exam experience," including how you felt about the exam overall or an individual section, but this is a fine line. In summary: *if you're not certain whether you can discuss an aspect of the test or not, just don't do it!* Do not let a silly Facebook post stop you from becoming the doctor you deserve to be.

Scores are typically released approximately one month after Test Day. The release is staggered during the afternoon and evening, ending at 5 p.m. Eastern Standard Time. This means that not all examinees receive their scores at exactly the same time. Your score report will include a scaled score for each section between 118 and 132, as well as your total combined score between 472 and 528. These scores are given as confidence intervals. For each section, the confidence interval is approximately the given score $\pm 1$; for the total score, it is approximately the given score $\pm 2$. You will also be given the corresponding percentile rank for each of these section scores and the total score.

## AAMC Contact Information

For further questions, contact the MCAT team at the Association of American Medical Colleges:

**MCAT Resource Center**
**Association of American Medical Colleges**
**www.aamc.org/mcat**
(202) 828-0600
**www.aamc.org/contactmcat**

# HOW THIS BOOK WAS CREATED

The *Kaplan MCAT Review* project began shortly after the release of the *Preview Guide for the MCAT 2015 Exam*, 2nd edition. Through thorough analysis by our staff psychometricians, we were able to analyze the relative yield of the different topics on the MCAT, and we began constructing tables of contents for the books of the *Kaplan MCAT Review* series. A dedicated staff of 30 writers, 7 editors, and 32 proofreaders worked over 5,000 combined hours to produce these books. The format of the books was heavily influenced by weekly meetings with Kaplan's learning science team.

In the years since this book was created, a number of opportunities for expansion and improvement have occurred. This edition is the product of our largest revision since the series' creation more than a decade ago.

To better accommodate students who prefer learning visually, our six science titles have added more than 500 new images and updated more than a hundred existing figures. All of these new images were chosen by an expert team of MCAT faculty members, led by veteran teachers and tutors with advanced science or medical degrees. Our objective with these new images was not to add visual flair but to enhance student learning outcomes. Toward that end, our team of medical illustrators partnered with our MCAT experts to ensure scientific accuracy and relevance for the exam.

On top of this extensive science image expansion, we completely rewrote *Critical Analysis and Reasoning Skills Review* based on what we've learned from more than ten years of helping students improve on the CARS section in our classrooms. In addition to this collective experience, internal data suggests that our new approach is more effective at helping students get higher CARS scores. Our streamlined and simplified CARS strategies accompany an extended focus on the critical thinking skills tested on the exam, best embodied by our new Skillbuilder activities that enable targeted skill practice in a lower pressure setting.

**These books were submitted for publication in January 2026. For any updates after this date, please visit www.kaptest.com/retail-book-corrections-and-updates.**

If you have any questions about the content presented here, email KaplanMCATfeedback@kaplan.com. For other questions not related to content, email booksupport@kaplan.com.

Each book has been vetted through at least ten rounds of review. To that end, the information presented in these books is true and accurate to the best of our knowledge. Still, your feedback helps us improve our prep materials. Please notify us of any inaccuracies or errors in the books by sending an email to KaplanMCATfeedback@kaplan.com.

# USING THIS BOOK

*Kaplan MCAT Organic Chemistry Review*, and the other six books in the *Kaplan MCAT Review* series, bring the Kaplan classroom experience to you—right in your home, at your convenience. This book offers the same Kaplan content review, strategies, and practice that make Kaplan the #1 choice for MCAT prep.

This book is designed to help you review the organic chemistry topics covered on the MCAT. Please understand that content review—no matter how thorough—is not sufficient preparation for the MCAT! The MCAT tests not only your science knowledge but also your critical reading, reasoning, and problem-solving skills. Do not assume that simply memorizing the contents of this book will earn you high scores on Test Day; to maximize your scores, you must also improve your reading and test-taking skills through MCAT-style questions and practice tests.

## Learning Objectives

At the beginning of each section, you'll find a short list of objectives describing the skills covered within that section. Learning objectives for these texts were developed in conjunction with Kaplan's learning science team, and have been designed specifically to focus your attention on tasks and concepts that are likely to show up on your MCAT. These learning objectives will function as a means to guide your study, and indicate what information and relationships you should be focused on within each section. Before starting each section, read these learning objectives carefully. They will not only allow you to assess your existing familiarity with the content, but also provide a goal-oriented focus for your studying experience of the section.

## MCAT Concept Checks

At the end of each section, you'll find a few open-ended questions that you can use to assess your mastery of the material. These MCAT Concept Checks were introduced after numerous conversations with Kaplan's learning science team. Research has demonstrated repeatedly that introspection and self-analysis improve mastery, retention, and recall of material. Complete these MCAT Concept Checks to ensure that you've got the key points from each section before moving on!

## Science Mastery Assessments

At the beginning of each chapter, you'll find 15 concept-focused multiple-choice questions. These are designed to help you assess your understanding of the chapter before you begin reading the chapter. Using the guidance provided with the assessment, you can determine the best way to review each chapter based on your personal strengths and weaknesses. Most of the questions in the Science Mastery Assessments focus on the first of the *Scientific Inquiry and Reasoning Skills* (*Knowledge of Scientific Concepts and Principles*), although there are occasional questions that fall into the second or fourth SIRS (*Scientific Reasoning and Problem-Solving* and *Data-Based and Statistical Reasoning*, respectively). You can complete each chapter's assessment in a testing interface in your online resources, where you'll also find a test-like passage set covering the same content you just studied to ensure you can also apply your knowledge the way the MCAT will expect you to!

## Sidebars

The following is a guide to the five types of sidebars you'll find in *Kaplan MCAT Organic Chemistry Review*:

- **Bridge:** These sidebars create connections between science topics that appear in multiple chapters throughout the *Kaplan MCAT Review* series.
- **Key Concept:** These sidebars draw attention to the most important takeaways in a given topic, and they sometimes offer synopses or overviews of complex information. If you understand nothing else, make sure you grasp the Key Concepts for any given subject.
- **MCAT Expertise:** These sidebars point out how information may be tested on the MCAT or offer key strategy points and test-taking tips that you should apply on Test Day.
- **Mnemonic:** These sidebars present memory devices to help recall certain facts.
- **Real World:** These sidebars illustrate how a concept in the text relates to the practice of medicine or the world at large. While this is not information you need to know for Test Day, many of the topics in Real World sidebars are excellent examples of how a concept may appear in a passage or discrete (stand-alone) question on the MCAT.

## What This Book Covers

The information presented in the *Kaplan MCAT Review* series covers everything listed on the official MCAT content lists. Every topic in these lists is covered in the same level of detail as is common to the undergraduate and postbaccalaureate classes that are considered prerequisites for the MCAT. Note that your premedical classes may include topics not discussed in these books, or they may go into more depth than these books do. Additional exposure to science content is never a bad thing, but all of the content knowledge you are expected to have walking in on Test Day is covered in these books.

Chapter profiles, on the first page of each chapter, represent a holistic look at the content within the chapter, and will include a pie chart as well as text information. The pie chart analysis is based directly on data released by the AAMC, and will give a rough estimate of the importance of the chapter in relation to the book as a whole. Further, the text portion of the Chapter Profiles includes which AAMC content categories are covered within the chapter. These are referenced directly from the AAMC MCAT exam content listing, available on the testmaker's website.

You'll also see High-Yield badges scattered throughout the sections of this book:

## In This Chapter



## 1.1 Amino Acids Found in Proteins High Yield

**LEARNING OBJECTIVES**

After Chapter 1.1, you will be able to:

These badges represent the top 100 topics most tested by the AAMC. In other words, according to the testmaker and all our experience with their resources, a High-Yield badge means more questions on Test Day.

This book also contains a thorough glossary and index for easy navigation of the text.

In the end, this is your book, so write in the margins, draw diagrams, highlight the key points—do whatever is necessary to help you get that higher score. We look forward to working with you as you achieve your dreams and become the doctor you deserve to be!

## Studying with This Book

In addition to providing you with the best practice questions and test strategies, Kaplan's team of learning scientists are dedicated to researching and testing the best methods for getting the most out of your study time. Here are their top four tips for improving retention:

**Review multiple topics in one study session.** This may seem counterintuitive—we're used to practicing one skill at a time in order to improve each skill. But research shows that weaving topics together leads to increased learning. Beyond that consideration, the MCAT often includes more than one topic in a single question. Studying in an integrated manner is the most effective way to prepare for this test.

**Customize the content.** Drawing attention to difficult or critical content can ensure you don't overlook it as you read and re-read sections. The best way to do this is to make it more visual—highlight, make tabs, use stickies, whatever works. We recommend highlighting only the most important or difficult sections of text. Selective highlighting of up to about 10 percent of text in a given chapter is great for emphasizing parts of the text, but over-highlighting can have the opposite effect.

**Repeat topics over time.** Many people try to memorize concepts by repeating them over and over again in succession. Our research shows that retention is improved by spacing out the repeats over time and mixing up the order in which you study content. For example, try reading chapters in a different order the second (or third!) time around. Revisit practice questions that you answered incorrectly in a new sequence. Perhaps information you reviewed more recently will help you better understand those questions and solutions you struggled with in the past.

**Take a moment to reflect.** When you finish reading a section for the first time, stop and think about what you just read. Jot down a few thoughts in the margins or in your notes about why the content is important or what topics came to mind when you read it. Associating learning with a memory is a fantastic way to retain information! This also works when answering questions. After answering a question, take a moment to think through each step you took to arrive at a solution. What led you to the answer you chose? Understanding the steps you took will help you make good decisions when answering future questions.

## Online Resources

In addition to the resources located within this text, you also have online resources awaiting you. If you purchased this book as part of a 7-book set, scan the QR code that appears on your slipcase (the illustrated box that originally contained the books) and enter your unique access code, which appears on a sticker on the front of that slipcase. If you purchased this book separately, book-specific resources are available at **www.kaptest.com/booksonline**. Make sure to log on and take advantage of free practice and additional resources!

Please note that access to the online resources is limited to the original owner of this book.

# STUDYING FOR THE MCAT

The first year of medical school is a frenzied experience for most students. To meet the requirements of a rigorous work schedule, students either learn to prioritize their time or else fall hopelessly behind. It's no surprise, then, that the MCAT, the test specifically designed to predict success in medical school, is a high-speed, time-intensive test. The MCAT demands excellent time-management skills, endurance, and grace under pressure both during the test as well as while preparing for it. Having a solid plan of attack and sticking with it are key to giving you the confidence and structure you need to succeed.

## Creating a Study Plan

The best time to create a study plan is at the beginning of your MCAT preparation. If you don't already use a calendar, you will want to start. You can purchase a planner, print out a free calendar from the Internet, use a built-in calendar or app on one of your smart devices, or keep track using an interactive online calendar. Pick the option that is most practical for you and that you are most likely to use consistently. If you purchased this book new as part of a set, your online resources come with a study plan to space out your readings, chapter quizzes, full-length practice tests, and other study materials (see the previous page for how to log on).

Once you have a calendar, you'll be able to start planning your study schedule with the following steps:

1. **Fill in your obligations and choose a day off.**

   Write in all your school, extracurricular, and work obligations first: class sessions, work shifts, and meetings that you must attend. Then add in your personal obligations: appointments, lunch dates, family and social time, etc. Making an appointment in your calendar for hanging out with friends or going to the movies may seem strange at first, but planning social activities in advance will help you achieve a balance between personal and professional obligations even as life gets busy. Having a happy balance allows you to be more focused and productive when it comes time to study, so stay well-rounded and don't neglect anything that is important to you.

   In addition to scheduling your personal and professional obligations, you should also plan your time off. Taking some time off is just as important as studying. Kaplan recommends taking at least one full day off per week, ideally from all your study obligations but at minimum from studying for the MCAT.

2. **Add in study blocks around your obligations.**

   Once you have established your calendar's framework, add in study blocks around your obligations, keeping your study schedule as consistent as possible across days and across weeks. Studying at the same time of day as your official test is ideal for promoting recall, but if that's not possible, then fit in study blocks wherever you can.

   To make your studying as efficient as possible, block out short, frequent periods of study time throughout the week. From a learning perspective, studying one hour per day for six days per week is much more valuable than studying for six hours all at once one day per week. Specifically, Kaplan recommends studying for no longer than three hours in one sitting. Within those three-hour blocks, also plan to take ten-minute breaks every hour. Use these breaks to get up from your seat, do some quick stretches, get a snack and drink, and clear your mind. Although ten minutes of break for every 50 minutes of studying may sound like a lot, these breaks will allow you to deal with distractions and rest your brain so that, during the 50-minute study blocks, you can remain fully engaged and completely focused.

3. **Add in your full-length practice tests.**

   Next, you'll want to add in full-length practice tests. You'll want to take one test very early in your prep and then spread your remaining full-length practice tests evenly between now and your test date. Staggering tests in this way allows you to form a baseline for comparison and to determine which areas to focus on right away, while also providing realistic feedback throughout your prep as to how you will perform on Test Day.

When planning your calendar, aim to finish your full-length practice tests and the majority of your studying by one week before Test Day, which will allow you to spend that final week completing a brief review of what you already know. In your online resources, you'll find a sample study calendar to use as a starting point. This sample calendar may include more focus than you need in some areas, and less in others, and it may not fit your timeline to Test Day. You will need to customize your study calendar to your needs using the steps above.

The total amount of time you spend studying each week will depend on your schedule, your personal prep needs, and your time to Test Day, but it is recommended that you spend somewhere in the range of 300–350 hours preparing before taking the official MCAT. One way you could break this down is to study for three hours per day, six days per week, for four months, but this is just one approach. You might study six days per week for more than three hours per day. You might study over a longer period of time if you don't have much time to study each week. No matter what your plan is, ensure you complete enough practice to feel completely comfortable with the MCAT and its content. A good sign you're ready for Test Day is when you begin to earn your goal score consistently in practice.

## How to Study

The MCAT covers a large amount of material, so studying for Test Day can initially seem daunting. To combat this, we have some tips for how to take control of your studying and make the most of your time.

## Goal Setting

To take control of the amount of content and practice required to do well on the MCAT, break the content down into specific goals for each week instead of attempting to approach the test as a whole. A goal of "I want to increase my overall score by 5 points" is too big, abstract, and difficult to measure on the small scale. More reasonable goals are "I will read two chapters each day this week." Goals like this are much less overwhelming and help break studying into manageable pieces.

## Active Reading

As you go through this book, much of the information will be familiar to you. After all, you have probably seen most of the content before. However, be very careful: Familiarity with a subject does not necessarily translate to knowledge or mastery of that subject. Do not assume that if you recognize a concept you actually know it and can apply it quickly at an appropriate level. Don't just passively read this book. Instead, read actively. Highlighting can be an excellent tool, but use it sparingly: highlighting every sentence isn't active reading, it's coloring. Frequently stop and ask yourself questions while you read (e.g., *What is the main point? How does this fit into the overall scheme of things? Could I thoroughly explain this to someone else?*). By making connections and focusing on the grander scheme, not only will you ensure you know the essential content, but you also prepare yourself for the level of critical thinking required by the MCAT.

## Focus on Areas of Greatest Opportunity

If you are limited by only having a minimal amount of time to prepare before Test Day, focus on your biggest areas of opportunity first. Areas of opportunity are topic areas that are highly tested and that you have not yet mastered. You likely won't have time to take detailed notes for every page of these books; instead, use your results from practice materials to determine which areas are your biggest opportunities and seek those out. After you've taken a full-length test, make sure you are using your performance report to best identify areas of opportunity. Skim over content matter for which you are already demonstrating proficiency, pausing to read more thoroughly when something looks unfamiliar or particularly difficult. Begin with the Science Mastery Assessment at the beginning of each chapter. If you can get all of those questions correct within a reasonable amount of time, you may be able to quickly skim through that chapter, but if the questions prove to be more difficult, then you may need to spend time reading the chapter or certain subsections of the chapter more thoroughly.

## Practice, Review, and Tracking

Leave time to review your practice questions and full-length tests. You may be tempted, after practicing, to push ahead and cover new material as quickly as possible, but failing to schedule ample time for review will actually throw away your greatest opportunity to improve your performance. The brain rarely remembers anything it sees or does only once. When you carefully review the questions you've solved (and the explanations for them), the process of retrieving that information reopens and reinforces the connections you've built in your brain. This builds long-term retention and repeatable skill sets—exactly what you need to beat the MCAT!

One useful tool for making the most of your review is the How I'll Fix It (HIFI) sheet. You can create a HIFI sheet, such as the sample below, to track questions throughout your prep that you miss or have to guess on. For each such question, figure out why you missed it and supply at least one action step for how you can avoid similar mistakes in the future. As you move through your MCAT prep, adjust your study plan based on your available study time and the results of your review. Your strengths and weaknesses are likely to change over the course of your prep. Keep addressing the areas that are most important to your score, shifting your focus as those areas change.

| Section | Q # | Topic or skill | Why I missed it | How I'll fix it |
|---|---|---|---|---|
| *Chem/Phys* | *42* | *Nuclear chem.* | *Confused electron absorption and emission* | *Reread Physics Chapter 9.2* |
| *Chem/Phys* | *47* | $K_{eq}$ | *Didn't know right equation* | *Memorize equation for* $K_{eq}$ |
| *CARS* | *2* | *Paraphrase Detail* | *Didn't read "not" in answer choice* | *Slow down when finding match* |
| *CARS* | *4* | *Make Deduction* | *Forgot to research answer* | *Reread passage and predict first* |

## Where to Study

One often-overlooked aspect of studying is the environment where the learning actually occurs. Although studying at home is many students' first choice, several problems can arise in this environment, chief of which are distractions. Studying can be a mentally draining process, so as time passes, these distractions become ever more tempting as escape routes. Although you may have considerable willpower, there's no reason to make staying focused harder than it needs to be. Instead of studying at home, head to a library, quiet coffee shop, or another new location whenever possible. This will eliminate many of the usual distractions and also promote efficient studying; instead of studying off and on at home over the course of an entire day, you can stay at the library for three hours of effective studying and enjoy the rest of the day off from the MCAT.

No matter where you study, make your practice as much like Test Day as possible. Just as is required during the official test, don't have snacks or chew gum during your study blocks. Turn off your music, television, and phone. Practice on the computer with your online resources to simulate the computer-based test environment. When completing practice questions, do your work on scratch paper or noteboard sheets rather than writing directly on any printed materials since you won't have that option on Test Day. Because memory is tied to all of your senses, the more test-like you can make your studying environment, the easier it will be on Test Day to recall the information you're putting in so much work to learn.

CHAPTER 1

# NOMENCLATURE

# SCIENCE MASTERY ASSESSMENT

Every pre-med knows this feeling: there is so much content I have to know for the MCAT! How do I know what to do first or what's important?

While the high-yield badges throughout this book will help you identify the most important topics, this Science Mastery Assessment is another tool in your MCAT prep arsenal. This quiz (which can also be taken in your online resources) and the guidance below will help ensure that you are spending the appropriate amount of time on this chapter based on your personal strengths and weaknesses. Don't worry though—skipping something now does not mean you'll never study it. Later on in your prep, as you complete full-length tests, you'll uncover specific pieces of content that you need to review and can come back to these chapters as appropriate.

## How to Use This Assessment

### If you answer 0–7 questions correctly:

Spend about 1 hour to read this chapter in full and take limited notes throughout. Follow up by reviewing **all** quiz questions to ensure that you now understand how to solve each one.

### If you answer 8–11 questions correctly:

Spend 20–40 minutes reviewing the quiz questions. Beginning with the questions you missed, read and take notes on the corresponding subchapters. For questions you answered correctly, ensure your thinking matches that of the explanation and you understand why each choice was correct or incorrect.

### If you answer 12–15 questions correctly:

Spend less than 20 minutes reviewing all questions from the quiz. If you missed any, then include a quick read-through of the corresponding subchapters, or even just the relevant content within a subchapter, as part of your question review. For questions you got correct, ensure your thinking matches that of the explanation and review the Concept Summary at the end of the chapter.

1. Which of the following lists the correct common names for ethanal, methanal, and ethanol, respectively?
   - A. Acetaldehyde, formaldehyde, ethyl alcohol
   - B. Ethyl alcohol, propionaldehyde, isopropyl alcohol
   - C. Ethyl alcohol, formaldehyde, acetaldehyde
   - D. Isopropyl alcohol, ethyl alcohol, formaldehyde

2. Which of the following are considered terminal functional groups?
   - I. Aldehydes
   - II. Ketones
   - III. Carboxylic acids
   - A. I only
   - B. III only
   - C. I and III only
   - D. I, II, and III

3. If all prefixes were dropped, what would be the name of the parent root of this molecule?

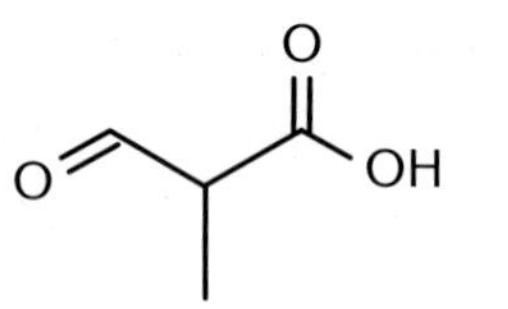


   - A. Propanoate
   - B. Propanol
   - C. Propanoic acid
   - D. Propanoic anhydride

4. What is the highest-priority functional group in this molecule?

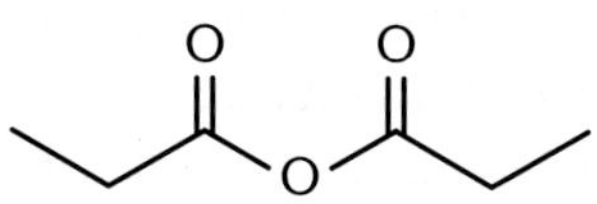


   - A. Anhydride
   - B. Carbonyl
   - C. Ketone
   - D. Alkyl chain

5. The IUPAC name for the following structure ends in what suffix?

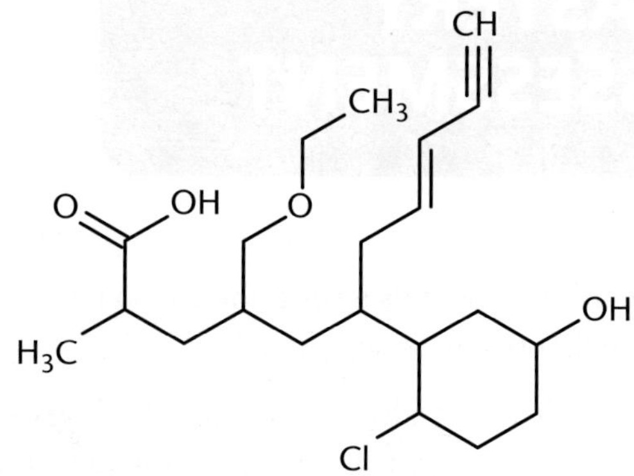


   - A. -ol
   - B. -one
   - C. -oic acid
   - D. -yne

6. Which of the two possibilities below correctly numbers the carbon backbone of this molecule?

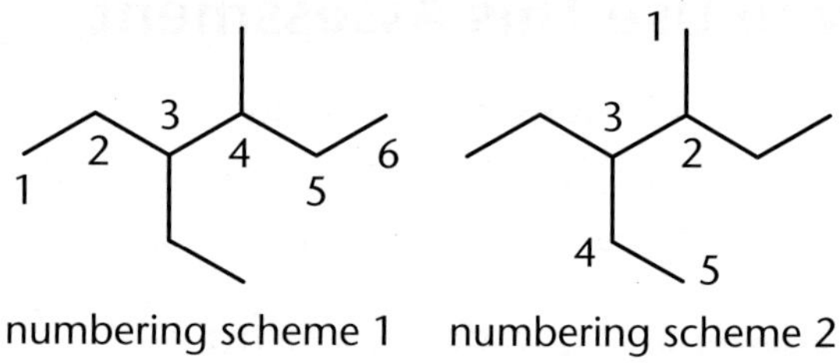


   - A. Numbering scheme 1
   - B. Numbering scheme 2
   - C. Numbering schemes 1 and 2 are equivalent and correct.
   - D. Numbering schemes 1 and 2 are equivalent and incorrect.

7. What is the proper structure for 2,3-dihydroxybutanedioic acid (tartaric acid)?

A.

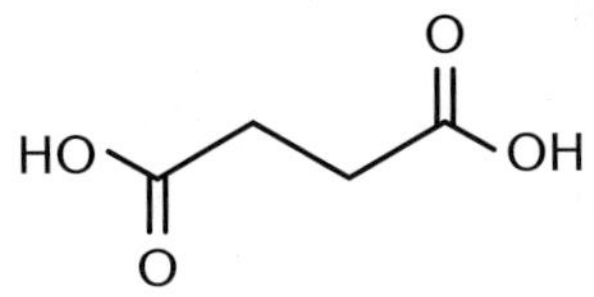


B.

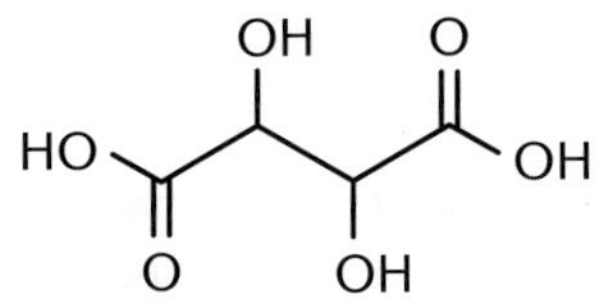


C.

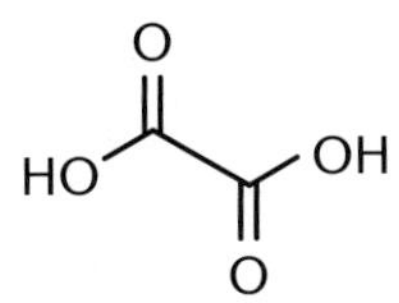


D.

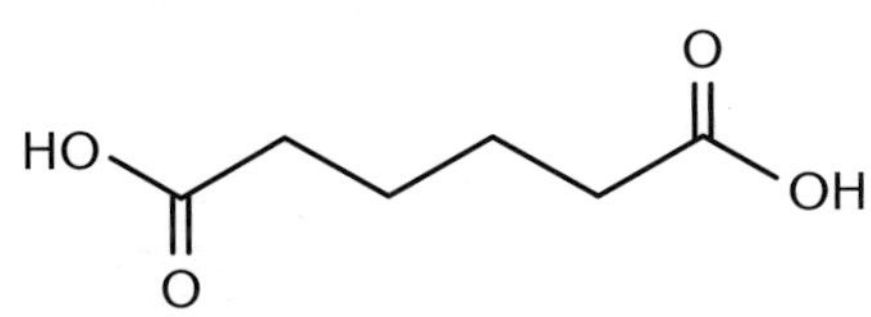


8. The common names for the aldehydes and carboxylic acids that contain only one carbon start with which prefix?
   - A. Para–
   - B. Form–
   - C. Meth–
   - D. Acet–

9. What is the IUPAC name for the following structure?

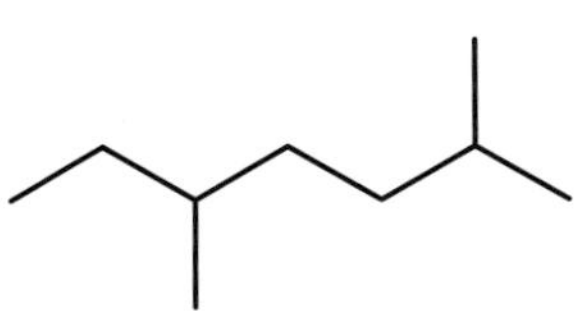

   - A. 2,5-dimethylheptane
   - B. 2-ethyl-5-methylhexane
   - C. 3,6-dimethylheptane
   - D. 5-ethyl-2-methylhexane

10. What is the IUPAC name for the following structure?

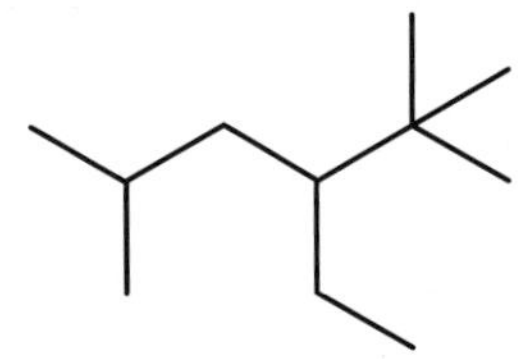

   - A. 4-isopropyl-2-methylhexane
   - B. 3-isopropyl-5-methylhexane
   - C. 2,2,5-trimethyl-3-ethylhexane
   - D. 3-ethyl-2,2,5-trimethylhexane

11. The IUPAC name for the following structure starts with what prefix?

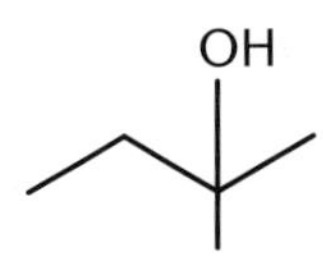


   - A. 3-methyl-
   - B. 2-methyl-
   - C. 2-hydroxy-
   - D. 3-hydroxy-

12. NADH is a coenzyme that releases high-energy electrons into the electron transport chain. It is known as nicotinamide adenine dinucleotide or diphosphopyridine nucleotide. What functional groups exist in this molecule?
   - I. Phosphate
   - II. Amide
   - III. Anhydride
   - A. I only
   - B. II only
   - C. I and II only
   - D. I, II, and III

**13.** Pyruvic acid, one of the end products of glycolysis, is commonly called acetylformic acid. Based on its common name, the structure of pyruvic acid must be:

**A.**

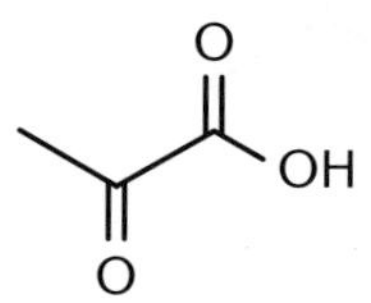


**B.**

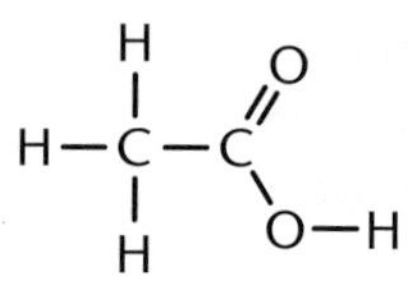


**C.**

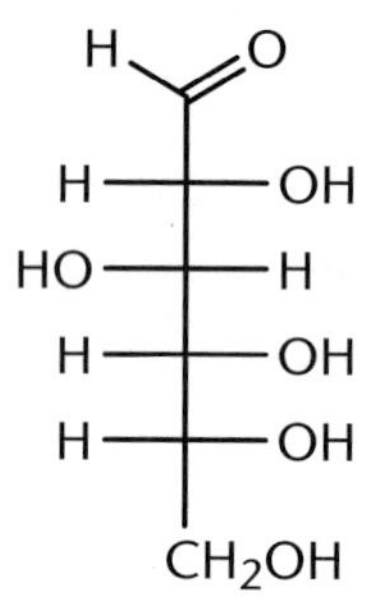


**D.**

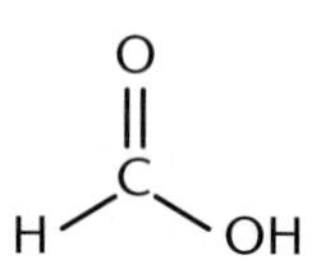


**14.** Which of the following are common names for carboxylic acid derivatives?

**I.** Acetic anhydride

**II.** Formic acid

**III.** Methyl formate

**A.** I and II only
**B.** I and III only
**C.** II and III only
**D.** I, II, and III

**15.** Consider the name 2,3-diethylpentane. Based on the structure implied by this name, the correct IUPAC name for this molecule is:

**A.** 2,3-diethylpentane.
**B.** 1,2-diethylbutane.
**C.** 3-ethyl-4-methylhexane.
**D.** 3-methyl-4-ethylhexane.

**Answer Key follows on next page.**

## Answer Key

1. **A** (See section 1.3)
2. **C** (See section 1.1)
3. **C** (See section 1.4)
4. **A** (See section 1.5)
5. **C** (See section 1.1)
6. **A** (See section 1.2)
7. **B** (See section 1.4)
8. **B** (See section 1.3)
9. **A** (See section 1.2)
10. **D** (See section 1.1)
11. **B** (See section 1.2)
12. **C** (See section 1.5)
13. **A** (See section 1.4)
14. **B** (See section 1.4)
15. **C** (See section 1.2)

*The relevant section of the chapter to review for each question is given in parentheses after the correct answer. Detailed explanations can be found at the end of the chapter.*

CHAPTER 1

# NOMENCLATURE

## In This Chapter



## Introduction

You walk into the pharmacy looking for something to take for a headache and find an entire aisle of drugs just for that purpose: Advil, Aleve, Motrin, Tylenol, ibuprofen, naproxen, acetaminophen, and aspirin. In this list, however, there are only four distinct drugs. In the United States, it is not uncommon for drugs to be known by both generic and brand names—and sometimes, multiple brands market the same medications. As a medical student, you'll have to know both: while a doctor may order *atorvastatin 40 mg qd*, patients will tell you they're taking *Lipitor daily*.

For doctors, a generic name is sufficiently unambiguous to specify a given compound, but this is not true within the pharmaceutical industry. Medications are usually large organic compounds with many functional groups and numerous chiral centers. Chemists needed to be able to describe such compounds, as well as innumerable others. Thus, within chemistry, a specific set of rules for naming and describing compounds was designed. In this chapter, we'll examine the steps for naming a compound and then practice applying them to example compounds. By the end of the chapter, we'll have discussed the most common functional groups for Test Day and how they relate to each other in the nomenclature hierarchy. Note that you may have learned nomenclature for a number of other compounds, including ethers, epoxides, amines, imines, sulfonic acids, and others in your organic chemistry courses; we have restricted the content of this chapter to only the functional groups you are expected to identify on Test Day.

### CHAPTER PROFILE

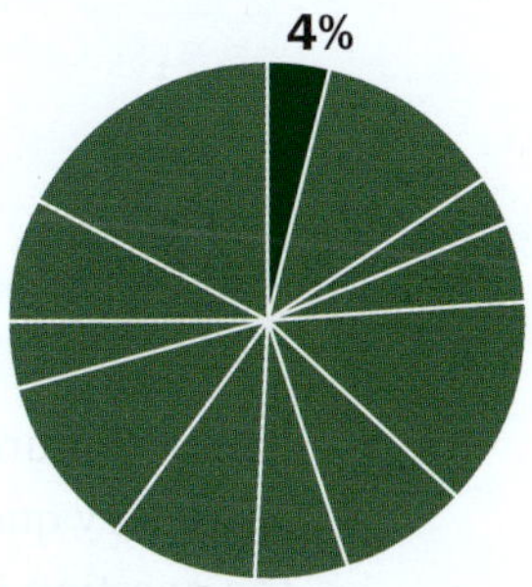


The content in this chapter should be relevant to about 4% of all questions about organic chemistry on the MCAT.

This chapter covers material from the following AAMC content category:

**5D:** Structure, function, and reactivity of biologically-relevant molecules

### MCAT EXPERTISE

According to the AAMC, the MCAT will not include standalone, nomenclature-only organic chemistry questions (such as "name this compound" questions). But as you probably remember from your own classes, nomenclature is the very foundation of the entire subject of organic chemistry, and you will lose points on Test Day if you don't have nomenclature down cold.

# 1.1 IUPAC Naming Conventions

**LEARNING OBJECTIVES**

After Chapter 1.1, you will be able to:

- Identify the parent carbon chain in a complex molecule
- Describe how numbers are integrated into chemical nomenclature
- Apply the five steps of IUPAC nomenclature and name a molecule:

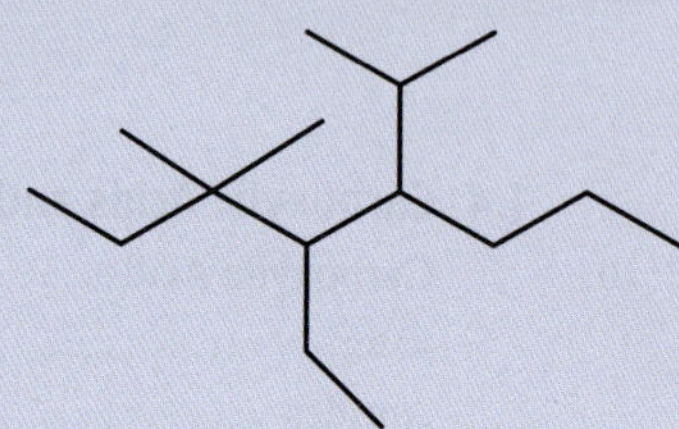

Nomenclature is one of the most important prerequisites for answering organic chemistry questions on Test Day; if you don't know which chemical compound the question is asking about, it's hard to get the answer right! That's why it's so important to understand both IUPAC and common nomenclature. Once you have a handle on these naming systems, you can easily translate question stems and focus on finding the correct answer. Let's begin by examining IUPAC naming conventions before we highlight specific compounds and functional groups.

**MCAT EXPERTISE**

Nomenclature is often tested on the MCAT by providing the question stem and the answer choices in different formats. For example, the question stem may give you the IUPAC name of the reactant, and the answer choices may show product structures—leaving you to figure out both the structure of the reactant and the reaction taking place.

## Naming Steps

The primary goal of the **International Union of Pure and Applied Chemistry (IUPAC)** naming system is to create an unambiguous relationship between the name and structure of a compound. With the conventions established by IUPAC, no two distinct compounds have the same name. The IUPAC naming system greatly simplifies chemical naming. Once we understand the rules, we can match names to structures with ease.

### 1. Identify the Longest Carbon Chain Containing the Highest-Order Functional Group

This will be called the **parent chain** and will be used to determine the root of the name. Keep in mind that if there are double or triple bonds between carbons, they must be considered when identifying the highest-order functional group. We'll examine priorities of functional groups throughout this chapter, but keep in mind that the highest-priority functional group (with the most oxidized carbon) will provide the suffix. This step may sound easy, but be careful! The molecule may be drawn in such a way that the longest carbon chain is not immediately obvious. If there are two or more chains of equal length, then the more substituted chain gets priority as the parent chain. Figure 1.1 shows a hydrocarbon with the longest chain labeled in green next to an example of a chain within the same molecule (highlighted in red) that would be incorrectly identified as the longest.

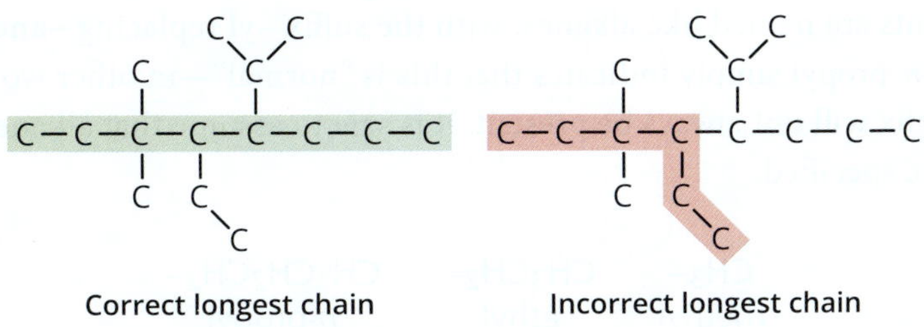


**Figure 1.1** Finding the Longest Carbon Chain

## 2. Number the Chain

In order to appropriately name a compound, we need to number the carbon chain, as shown in Figure 1.2. As a convention, the carbon numbered 1 will be the one closest to the highest-priority functional group. If the functional groups all have the same priority, numbering the chain should make the numbers of the substituted carbons as low as possible.

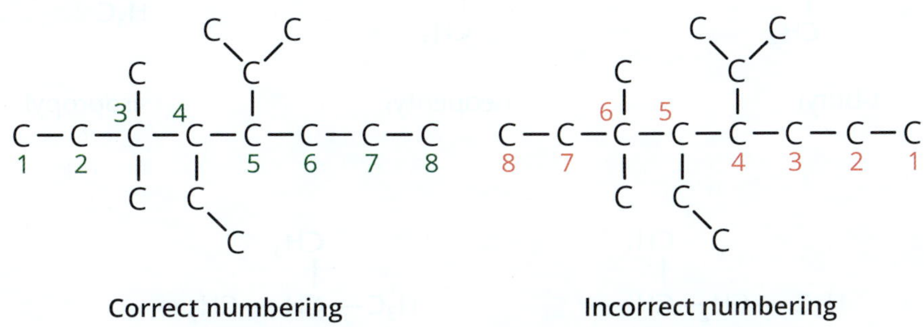


**Figure 1.2** Numbering the Longest Carbon Chain
*The highest-priority functional group should have the lowest possible number; if all substituents have the same priority, make their numbers as low as possible: 3/4/5 is lower than 4/5/6.*

After we have discussed the functional groups most commonly tested on the MCAT, we'll review a table of those functional groups in order of priority. For now, keep in mind that the more oxidized the carbon is, the higher priority it has in the molecule. Oxidation state increases with more bonds to **heteroatoms** (atoms besides carbon and hydrogen, like oxygen, nitrogen, phosphorus, or halogens) and decreases with more bonds to hydrogen.

Just like straight chains, rings are numbered starting at the point of greatest substitution, continuing in the direction that gives the lowest numbers to the highest-priority functional groups. Somewhat counterintuitively, if there is a tie between assigning priority in a molecule with double and triple bonds, the double bond takes precedence.

## 3. Name the Substituents

**Substituents** are functional groups that are not part of the parent chain. A substituent's name will be placed at the beginning of the compound name as a prefix, followed by the name of the longest chain. Remember that only the highest-priority functional group will determine the suffix for the compound and must be part of the parent chain.

Carbon chain substituents are named like alkanes, with the suffix **–yl** replacing **–ane**. The prefix ***n***– that we see in Figure 1.3 on *n*-propyl simply indicates that this is "normal"—in other words, a straight-chain alkane. Because this prefix will not always be present, it is safe to assume that alkane substituents will be normal unless otherwise specified.

| $CH_3–$ | $CH_3CH_2–$ | $CH_3CH_2CH_2–$ |
|---|---|---|
| methyl | ethyl | *n*-propyl |

**Figure 1.3** Common Normal Alkyl Substituents
*The bond on the right side of each substituent connects to the parent molecule.*

In Figure 1.4, we see some examples of what alternative alkyl substituents may look like.

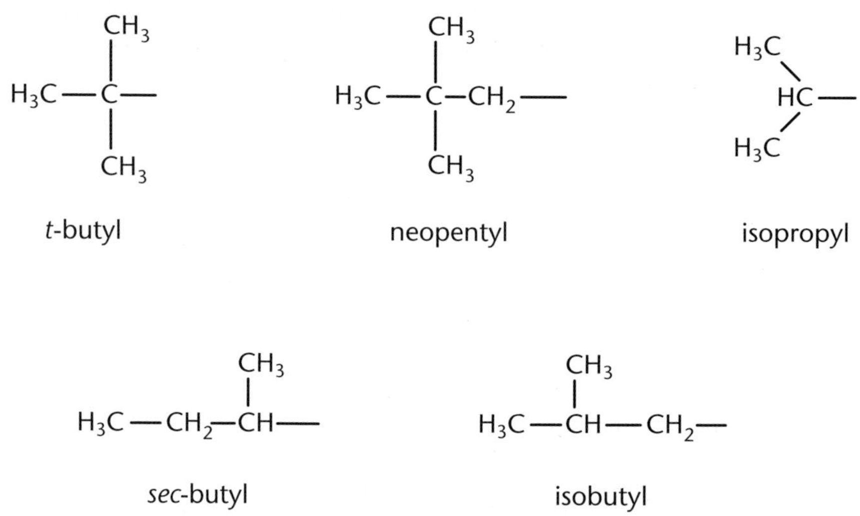


**Figure 1.4** Common Alternative Alkyl Substituents
*The bond on the right side of each substituent connects to the parent molecule.*

If there are multiple substituents of the same type, we use the prefixes **di**–, **tri**–, **tetra**–, and so on to indicate this fact. These prefixes are included directly before the substituent's name.

#### 4. Assign a Number to Each Substituent

Pair the substituents that you have named to the corresponding numbers in the parent chain. Multiple substituents of the same type will get both the di–, tri–, and tetra– prefixes that we have previously noted and also a carbon number designation—even if they are on the same carbon.

#### 5. Complete the Name

Names always begin with the names of the substituents in alphabetical order, with each substituent preceded by its number. Note, however, that prefixes like di–, tri–, and tetra–, as well as the hyphenated prefixes like ***n***–, **sec**– (or **s**–), and ***tert***– (or ***t***–), are ignored while alphabetizing. Nonhyphenated roots that *are* part of the name, however, are included; these are modifiers like **iso**–, **neo**–, or **cyclo**–. These prefixes describe the substituent's structure: iso– refers to a forked structure, neo– to a structure with a quaternary carbon, cyclo– to a ring structure, and *sec*– and *tert*– refer to attachment at a secondary or tertiary carbon, respectively. Then the numbers are separated from each other with commas, and from words with hyphens. Finally, we finish the name with the name of the backbone chain, including the suffix for the functional group of highest priority. Figure 1.5 shows an example of an entire hydrocarbon named with IUPAC nomenclature.

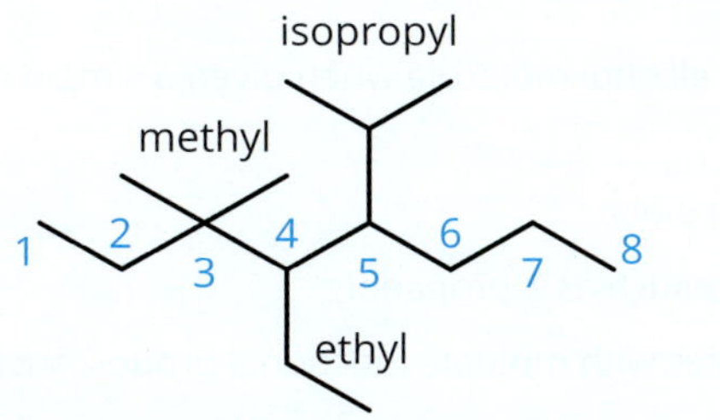


**4-ethyl-5-isopropyl-3, 3-dimethyloctane**

**Figure 1.5** An Example of a Complete IUPAC Name

## MCAT CONCEPT CHECK 1.1

Before you move on, assess your understanding of the material with these questions.

1. List the steps of IUPAC nomenclature:

   1. ______________________________
   2. ______________________________
   3. ______________________________
   4. ______________________________
   5. ______________________________

2. Circle or highlight the parent chain in each of the following compounds:

$$\begin{array}{l} \quad CH_2CH_3 \\ \quad\ | \\ CH_3CH—CH_2—COOH \end{array}$$

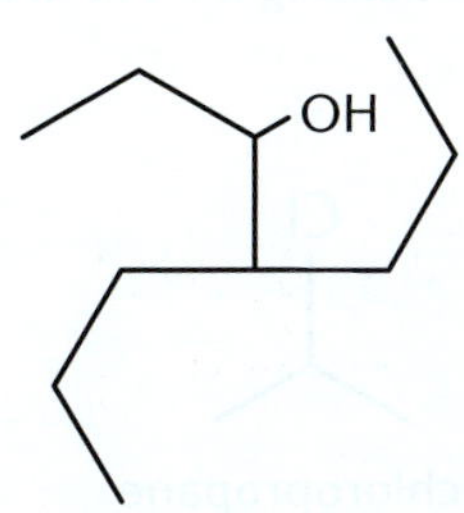


$H_3C—CH_3$

3. Circle and name the substituents in the following molecule, then name the molecule.

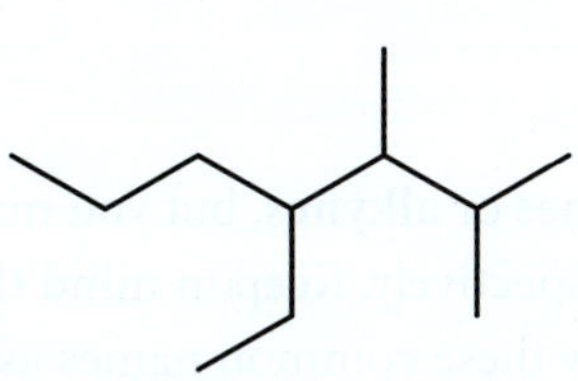

**BRIDGE**

Solutions to concept checks for a given chapter in *MCAT Organic Chemistry Review* can be found near the end of the chapter in which the concept check is located, following the Concept Summary for that chapter.

## 1.2 Hydrocarbons and Alcohols

**LEARNING OBJECTIVES**

After Chapter 1.2, you will be able to:

- Predict the structure of a hydrocarbon or alcohol molecule when given a simple molecular formula, such as $C_9H_{20}$
- Differentiate between geminal and vicinal diols
- Recall common names of key compounds, such as 2-propanol
- Apply priority rules when naming molecules with multiple functional groups, such as:

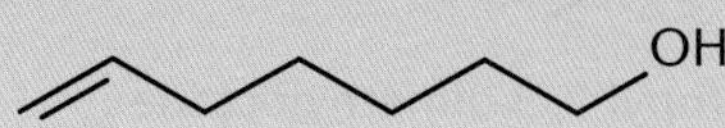

Hydrocarbons are compounds that contain only carbon and hydrogen atoms. Alcohols, on the other hand, contain at least one –OH group, which lends them additional reactivity. In this section, we'll explore the naming of hydrocarbons and alcohols.

### Alkanes

**Alkanes** are simple hydrocarbon molecules with the formula $C_nH_{(2n+2)}$. The names for the first four of these compounds are **meth**ane (one carbon), **eth**ane (two carbons), **prop**ane (three carbons), and **but**ane (four carbons). Alkanes with more than four carbons have a simpler naming pattern in which the name is a root from an ancient language (mostly Greek, but some Latin) describing the number of carbons followed by **–ane**. From 5 to 12, these Greek/Latin roots are: **pent–**, **hex–**, **hept–**, **oct–**, **non–**, **dec–**, **undec–**, and **dodec–**. Some examples of alkanes are shown in Table 1.1.

Halogens are common substituents on alkanes. Alkyl halides are indicated by a prefix: **fluoro–**, **chloro–**, **bromo–**, or **iodo–**. An example of proper IUPAC naming for a molecule that contains an alkyl halide is shown in Figure 1.6.

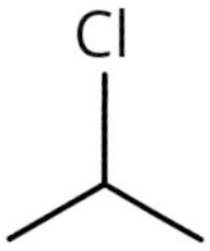

2-chloropropane

**Figure 1.6** Alkyl Halide IUPAC Naming

### Alkenes and Alkynes

The MCAT does not explicitly test reactions of **alkenes** or **alkynes**, but you may still see the suffixes **–ene** and **–yne**, which signify double and triple bonds, respectively. Keep in mind that many of these compounds will also have common names, and it is vital to know these common names as well. On Test Day, you are most likely to encounter double bonds in the context of unsaturated fatty acids or other biochemical compounds. The double or triple bond is named like a substituent and is indicated by the lower-numbered carbon involved in the bond. The number may precede the molecule name, as in 2-butene, or it may be placed near the suffix, as in but-2-ene; both are correct. If there are *multiple* multiple bonds, the numbering is generally separated from the suffix, as in 1,3-butadiene.

| Number of Carbons | Name | Structure |
|---|---|---|
| 1 | Methane | $CH_4$ |
| 2 | Ethane | $H_3C—CH_3$ |
| 3 | Propane | 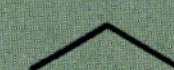 |
| 4 | Butane | 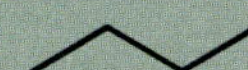 |
| 5 | Pentane | 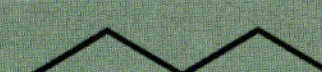 |
| 6 | Hexane | 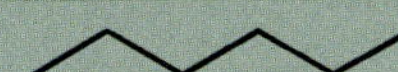 |
| 7 | Heptane | 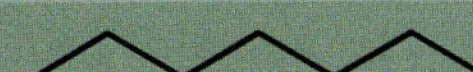 |
| 8 | Octane | 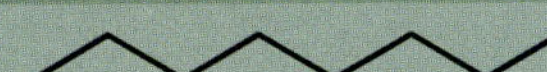 |
| 9 | Nonane |  |
| 10 | Decane |  |

**Table 1.1** Examples of Alkanes

## Alcohols

**Alcohols** are named by replacing the –e at the end of the name of the corresponding alkane with the suffix –**ol**. The chain is numbered so that the carbon attached to the hydroxyl group (–OH) gets the lowest possible number—even when there is a carbon-carbon multiple bond present. The hydroxyl group takes precedence over carbon-carbon double and triple bonds because of the higher oxidation state of the carbon when bound to an oxygen. If the alcohol is not the highest-priority functional group, then it is named as a hydroxyl substituent (**hydroxy**–). Figure 1.7 demonstrates a few alcohols and their IUPAC names.

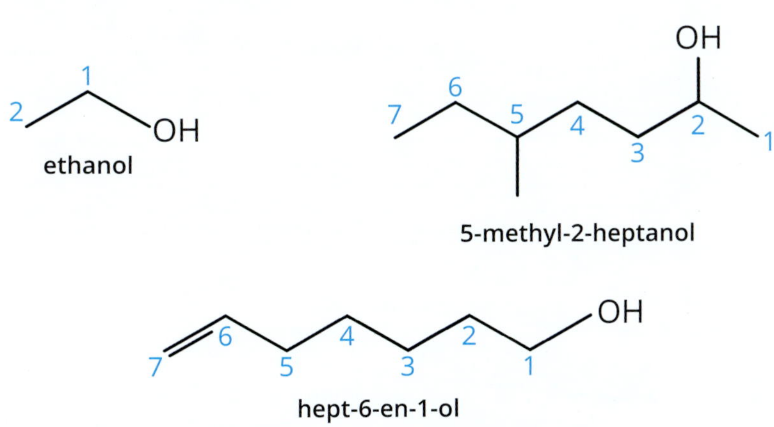


**Figure 1.7** Naming Alcohols
*When alcohols take priority, they are indicated with the suffix –ol.*

Alcohols are often referred to by their common names, rather than their IUPAC names. In this version of naming, the name of the alkyl group is followed by the word **alcohol**. Examples include ethyl alcohol (rather than ethanol) and isopropyl alcohol (rather than 2-propanol.)

Alcohols with two hydroxyl groups are called **diols** or **glycols** and are indicated with the suffix –**diol**. The entire hydrocarbon name is preserved, and –diol is added. When naming diols, one must number each hydroxyl group. For example, ethane-1,2-diol is an ethane molecule that has a hydroxyl group on each carbon. This molecule is also known by its common name, ethylene glycol. Diols with hydroxyl groups on the same carbon are called **geminal diols**; diols with hydroxyl groups on adjacent carbons are called **vicinal diols**. The difference between geminal and vicinal diols is shown in Figure 1.8. Geminal diols, or **hydrates**, are not commonly seen because they spontaneously dehydrate (lose a water molecule) to produce carbonyl compounds with the functional group C=O.

## MCAT EXPERTISE

The MCAT may use the common names for some alcohols, as well as some of the molecules we will see later. For alcohols, these include ethyl alcohol and isopropyl alcohol—know what these common names refer to!

## MNEMONIC

**Vicin**al diols are in the **vicin**ity of each other, on adjacent carbons. **Gemin**al diols—like the **Gemin**i twins—are paired on the same carbon.

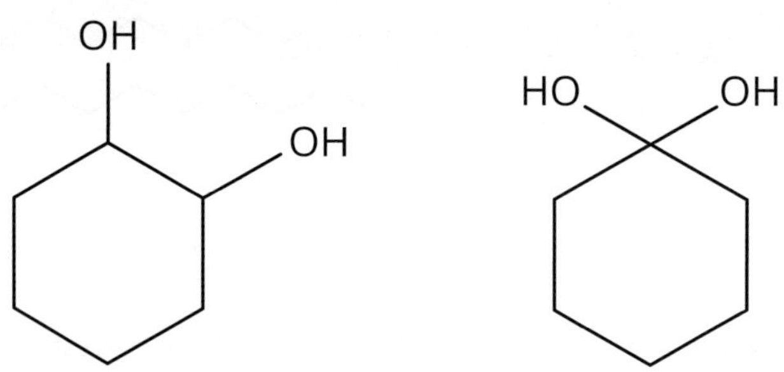


**Vicinal diol**
1, 2-cyclodihexanol

**Geminal diol**
1, 1-cyclodihexanol

**Figure 1.8** Vicinal vs. Geminal Diols
*Vicinal diols have hydroxyl groups on adjacent carbons, while geminal diols have two hydroxyl groups on the same carbon.*

## MCAT CONCEPT CHECK 1.2

Before you move on, assess your understanding of the material with these questions.

1. Fill in the correct names for the alkanes listed below. If more than one compound can be described with a given molecular formula, name the straight-chain alkane to which the formula refers and draw one alternative.

| Molecular Formula | IUPAC Name (Straight-Chain Alkane) | Alternative Structure |
|---|---|---|
| $CH_4$ | | |
| $C_2H_6$ | | |
| $C_3H_8$ | | |
| $C_4H_{10}$ | | |
| $C_5H_{12}$ | | |
| $C_6H_{14}$ | | |
| $C_7H_{16}$ | | |
| $C_8H_{18}$ | | |
| $C_9H_{20}$ | | |
| $C_{10}H_{22}$ | | |

2. In a molecule with two double bonds adjacent to each other and an alcohol, which functional group would take precedence in naming?

_______________________________________________

3. Is the following compound a geminal diol or a vicinal diol?

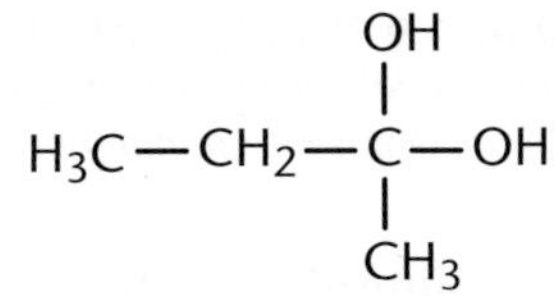


4. What are the common names for 2-propanol and ethanol?
   - 2-Propanol:

   _______________________________________________

   - Ethanol:

   _______________________________________________

## 1.3 Aldehydes and Ketones

### LEARNING OBJECTIVES

After Chapter 1.3, you will be able to:

- Distinguish aldehydes from ketones
- Recall common names for methanal, ethanal, propanal, and propanone
- Determine the highest priority functional group in a complex molecule
- Apply appropriate prefixes and suffixes when naming molecules containing aldehyde and ketone groups

Aldehydes and ketones are two classes of molecules that contain a **carbonyl group**, which is a carbon double-bonded to an oxygen. Aldehydes and ketones differ in the placement of the carbonyl group: aldehydes are **chain-terminating**, meaning that they appear at the end of a parent chain, while ketones are found in the middle of carbon chains. Aldehydes and ketones do not have any leaving groups connected to the carbonyl carbon; they are only connected to alkyl chains or, in the case of aldehydes, hydrogen atoms. As we'll examine later, carboxylic acids and their derivatives do contain leaving groups connected to the carbonyl carbon.

## Aldehydes

**Aldehydes** have a carbonyl group found at the end of the carbon chain. Because this is a terminal functional group that takes precedence over many others, it is generally attached to carbon number 1. Aldehydes are named by replacing the –e of the parent alkane with the suffix **–al**. When the aldehyde is at position 1, as is usually the case, we do not need to include this number in the chemical name. Figure 1.9 shows the IUPAC nomenclature for two aldehydes.

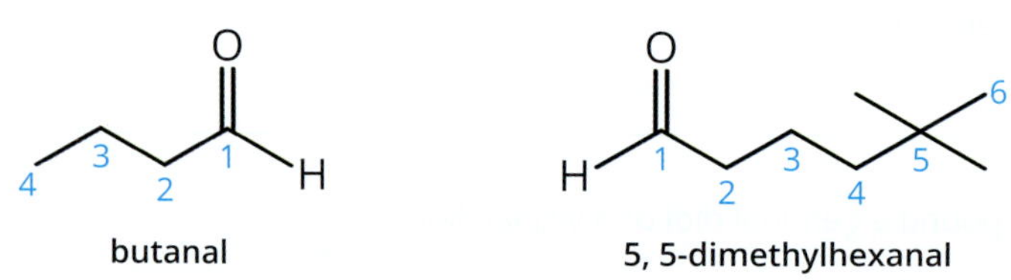


**Figure 1.9** Naming Aldehydes
*The carbonyl group of the aldehyde usually does not receive a number in the name because it is a terminal functional group.*

Methanal, ethanal, and propanal are referred to almost exclusively by their common names, *formaldehyde*, *acetaldehyde*, and *propionaldehyde*, rather than their IUPAC names. These molecules are shown in Figure 1.10.

### MCAT EXPERTISE

As is the case for alcohols, it is important to know both the common names and IUPAC names for common aldehydes and ketones. Make sure that you know what formaldehyde, acetaldehyde, and acetone are!

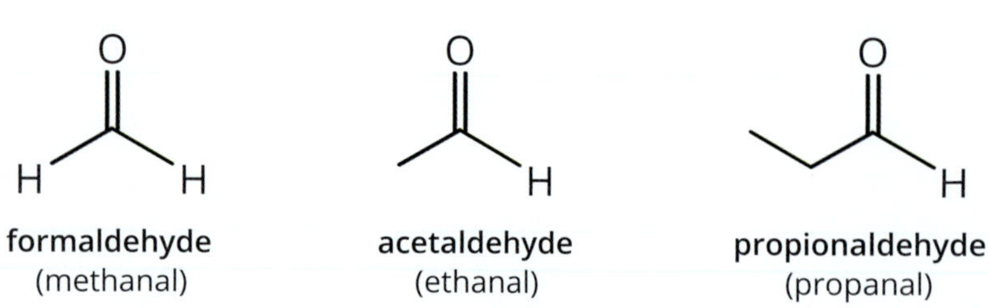


**Figure 1.10** Common Names of Aldehydes

## Ketones

**Ketones** contain a carbonyl group somewhere in the middle of the carbon chain. Because this is the case, we will always have to assign a number to the carbonyl carbon when naming ketones (except propanone, which sometimes appears without a number because it must have the ketone on carbon 2 by default). Ketones are named by replacing the –e in the name of the parent alkane with the suffix –**one**. Just as when naming other compounds, be sure to give the carbonyl the lowest possible number if it is the highest-priority group.

Ketones are commonly named by listing the alkyl groups in alphabetical order, followed by **ketone**, such as ethyl methyl ketone. *Acetone* is the smallest possible ketone molecule. Figure 1.11 includes IUPAC and common names for a number of ketones.

**BRIDGE**

Sugars are classified as either aldoses (aldehyde sugars) or ketoses (ketone sugars). Understanding nomenclature can help you to identify the structure of a sugar, as well as some of its physical properties. Carbohydrate structure is discussed in Chapter 4 of *MCAT Biochemistry Review.*

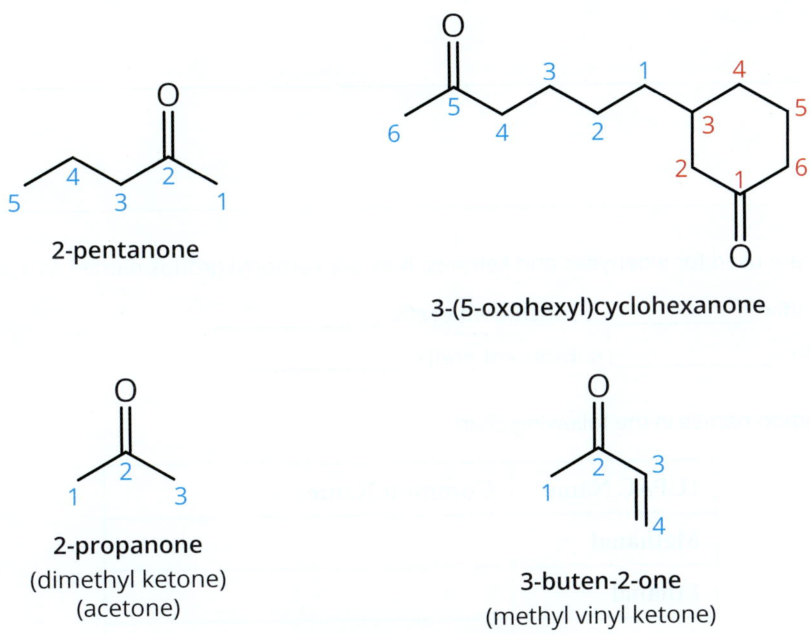


**Figure 1.11** Naming Ketones
*Common names are included in parentheses.*

In a more complex molecule with a higher-priority group that takes precedence over the carbonyl, we name aldehydes and ketones as substituents, using the prefix **oxo**–. This is in reference to the carbonyl oxygen and applies for both ketones and aldehydes. Sometimes ketones may also be indicated with the prefix **keto**–.

Another convention that you may see on the MCAT is the use of Greek letters as locants to indicate the position of a carbon relative to the carbonyl group. By this convention, the carbon *adjacent* to the carbonyl carbon is indicated by alpha ($\alpha$). Moving away from the carbonyl, the successive carbons are referred to as beta ($\beta$), gamma ($\gamma$), and delta ($\delta$) carbons, as depicted in Figure 1.12. This applies on both sides of the carbonyl in the same fashion, so the carbons on both sides of a ketone are considered alpha carbons. This will become important when we discuss $\alpha$-hydrogen acidity in Chapter 7 of *MCAT Organic Chemistry Review.*

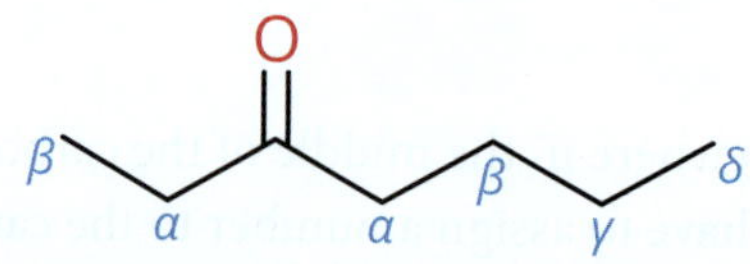


**Figure 1.12** Greek Letter Locant System
*Greek letters act as locants that identify the location of a carbon relative to a functional group, such as the ketone group in the molecule shown.*

## MCAT CONCEPT CHECK 1.3

Before you move on, assess your understanding of the material with these questions.

1. What is the difference between an aldehyde and a ketone?
   - Aldehyde:

   ______________________________

   - Ketone:

   ______________________________

2. What suffixes are used for aldehydes and ketones; how are carbonyl groups named as a substituent?
   - Aldehyde suffix: ____________; substituent prefix: ____________
   - Ketone suffix: ____________; substituent prefix: ____________

3. Fill in the common names in the following chart.

| IUPAC Name | Common Name |
|---|---|
| Methanal | |
| Ethanal | |
| Propanal | |
| Propanone | |

4. For a molecule with a double bond, an aldehyde, and an alcohol, which functional group would determine the suffix when naming?

   ______________________________

# 1.4 Carboxylic Acids and Derivatives

**LEARNING OBJECTIVES**

After Chapter 1.4, you will be able to:

- Name common carboxylic acid derivatives, including esters, amides, and anhydrides
- Differentiate between common carboxylic acid derivatives

## Carboxylic Acids

**Carboxylic acids** contain both a carbonyl group (C=O) and a hydroxyl group (−OH) on a terminal carbon. Carboxylic acids, like aldehydes, are terminal functional groups; therefore, their associated carbon is usually numbered 1. This is the most oxidized functional group that appears on the MCAT, with three bonds to oxygen; only carbon dioxide, with four bonds to oxygen, contains a more oxidized carbon. Carboxylic acids are thus the highest-priority functional group in MCAT-tested nomenclature, and all other groups are named as substituents using prefixes. Carboxylic acids are named by replacing the -e at the end of the name of the parent alkane with the suffix **-oic acid.**

Once again, the common names for carboxylic acids show up fairly often on the MCAT. *Formic acid* is the common name for methanoic acid; *acetic acid* is ethanoic acid; and *propionic acid* is propanoic acid. These compounds are shown in Figure 1.13. Be sure that you know both these common names and IUPAC names for Test Day.

**MCAT EXPERTISE**

Did you notice that some of the common names are similar between aldehydes and carboxylic acids? Remembering that formaldehyde and formic acid both refer to molecules with methane as a parent alkane—and that acetaldehyde and acetic acid contain ethane as a parent alkane—will help consolidate this information.

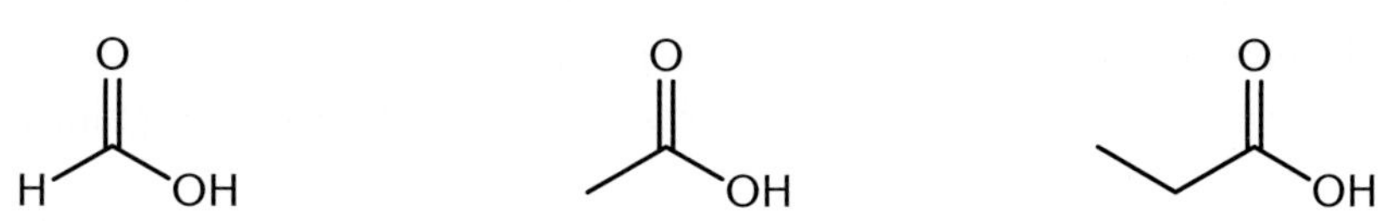


methanoic acid (formic acid) | ethanoic acid (acetic acid) | propanoic acid (propionic acid)

**Figure 1.13** Naming Carboxylic Acids
*The carboxylic acid group does not receive a number in the name because it is a terminal functional group; common names are included in parentheses.*

The carboxylic acid derivatives are the final category of functional groups. These include esters, amides, and anhydrides.

## Esters

**Esters** are common carboxylic acid derivatives. In these compounds, the hydroxyl group (−OH) is replaced with an **alkoxy group** (−OR, where R is a hydrocarbon chain). Ester nomenclature is based on the naming conventions for carboxylic acids. The first term is the alkyl name of the esterifying group. Think of this first term as an adjective describing the ester, based on the identity of the alkyl (R) group. The second term is the name of the parent acid, with **-oate** replacing the **-oic acid** suffix. For example, methanoic acid (formic acid) would form butyl methanoate with exposure to butanol under appropriate reaction conditions. Examples of ester nomenclature are shown in Figure 1.14.

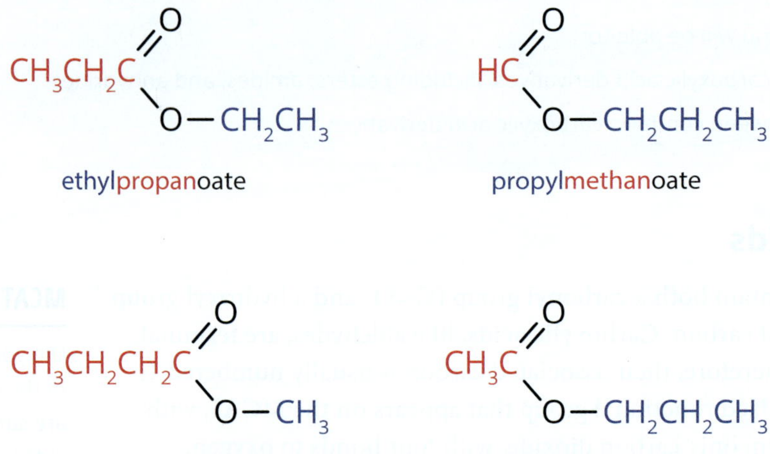

ethylpropanoate — propylmethanoate — methylbutanoate — propylethanoate

**Figure 1.14** Naming Esters
*Groups bonded directly to the ester oxygen are named as substituents and are not numbered.*

## Amides

Another group of carboxylic acid derivatives includes **amides**. In an amide, the hydroxyl group is replaced by an **amino group** (nitrogen-containing group). These compounds can be more complex—the amino nitrogen can be bonded to zero, one, or two alkyl groups. Amides are named similarly to esters, except that the suffix becomes –**amide**. Substituents attached to the nitrogen atom are labeled with a capital ***N***–, indicating that this group is bonded to the parent molecule via a nitrogen atom. These substituents are included as prefixes in the compound name and are not numbered. Several examples of amide nomenclature are included in Figure 1.15.

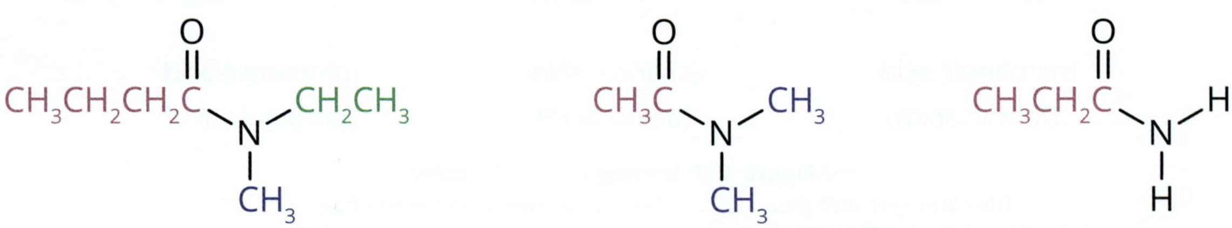

*N*-ethyl-*N*-methylbutanamide — *N*,*N*-dimethylethanamide — propanamide

**Figure 1.15** Naming Amides
*Groups bonded directly to the amide nitrogen are named as substituents with the prefix* N–, *and are not numbered.*

## Anhydrides

One final group of carboxylic acid derivatives is the **anhydrides**. In the formation of an anhydride from two carboxylic acid molecules, one water molecule is removed. Many anhydrides are cyclic, which may result from the intramolecular dehydration of a dicarboxylic acid. Anhydrides are named by replacing **acid** with **anhydride** in the name of the corresponding carboxylic acid if the anhydride is formed from only one type of carboxylic acid. If the anhydride is not symmetrical, both carboxylic acids are named (without *acid*) before *anhydride* is added to the name. Some examples of anhydrides are shown in Figure 1.16.

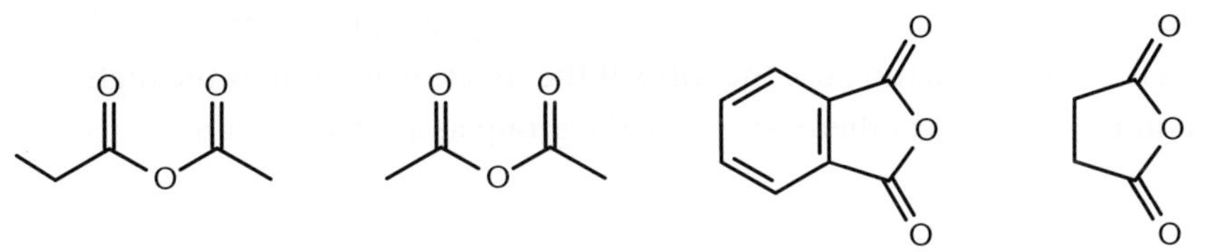

ethanoic propanoic anhydride | ethanoic anhydride (acetic anhydride) | phthalic anhydride | succinic anhydride

**Figure 1.16** Naming Anhydrides
*Phthalic anhydride and succinic anhydride are given as examples of cyclic anhydrides; their names need not be memorized.*

### MNEMONIC

Because hydro– is a prefix meaning *water*, and an– is a prefix meaning *not* or *without*, we can remember that anhydrides have had water molecules removed during formation.

### MCAT CONCEPT CHECK 1.4

Before you move on, assess your understanding of the material with these questions.

1. What would be the names of the ester, amide, and anhydride derivatives of pentanoic acid? Assume that the R group on the ester is $-CH_3$ and that the amide is unsubstituted.
   - Ester:

     ______________________________
   - Amide:

     ______________________________
   - Anhydride:

     ______________________________

2. Name the following compound:

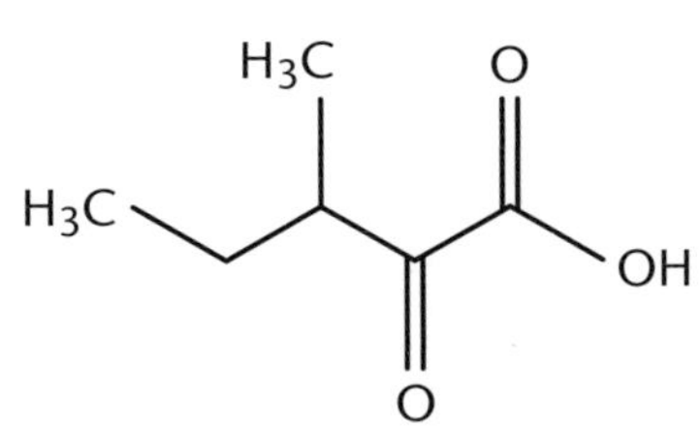

______________________________

## 1.5 Summary of Functional Groups

High Yield

### MCAT EXPERTISE

The "High-Yield" badge on this section indicates that the content is frequently tested on the MCAT.

### LEARNING OBJECTIVES

After Chapter 1.5, you will be able to:

- Apply appropriate prefixes and suffixes for common organic functional groups

Table 1.2 lists the functional groups that you will need to know for the MCAT in order of priority, with prefixes and suffixes. Carboxylic acids are the highest-priority functional group on the MCAT. In nomenclature, use the suffix if the functional group is the highest-priority group in the molecule; otherwise, name the group as a substituent using its prefix.

### KEY CONCEPT

Functional group priority is correlated with oxidation state. Carboxylic acids have the highest priority while alkanes have the lowest.

| Functional Group | Prefix | Suffix |
|---|---|---|
| Carboxylic acid | carboxy– | –oic acid |
| Anhydride | alkanoyloxycarbonyl– | anhydride |
| Ester | alkoxycarbonyl– | –oate |
| Amide | carbamoyl– or amido– | –amide |
| Aldehyde | oxo– | –al |
| Ketone | oxo– or keto– | –one |
| Alcohol | hydroxy– | –ol |
| Alkene* | alkenyl– | –ene |
| Alkyne* | alkynyl– | –yne |
| Alkane | alkyl– | –ane |

*Note: Alkenes and alkynes are considered to be tied for priority except in cyclic compounds, where alkenes have higher priority.

**Table 1.2** Major Functional Groups

## Conclusion

Now that we've worked through nomenclature, we should be able to navigate MCAT organic chemistry questions with ease and confidence. Remember that even if an MCAT question is asking about a reaction or laboratory technique, translating the name of a compound in the question stem may be a necessary step to get to the answer. We have also covered the important functional groups that will show up and have taken note of the order of priority for these groups when it comes to naming compounds. Remember, the common names can be just as important on the MCAT as the IUPAC names—so knowing both is key. Now that we know the language of organic chemistry, we will learn more about the properties of molecules in the next two chapters, and then will focus on reactions of functional groups and laboratory techniques in subsequent chapters of *MCAT Organic Chemistry Review*.

**▶ GO ONLINE**

**You've reviewed the content, now test your knowledge and critical thinking skills by completing a test-like passage set in your online resources!**

# CONCEPT SUMMARY

## IUPAC Naming Conventions

- The **International Union of Pure and Applied Chemistry** (**IUPAC**) has designated standards for naming chemical compounds. There are five steps in the process:
  - First, find the longest carbon chain in the compound that contains the highest-priority functional group. This is called the **parent chain**.
  - Second, number the chain in such a way that the highest-priority functional group receives the lowest possible number. This group will determine the **suffix** of the molecule.
  - Third, name the **substituents** with a **prefix**. Multiple substituents of a single type receive another prefix denoting how many are present (**di**–, **tri**–, **tetra**–, and so on).
  - Fourth, assign a number to each of the substituents depending on the carbon to which it is bonded.
  - Finally, complete the name by alphabetizing the substituents and separating numbers from each other by commas and from words by hyphens.

## Hydrocarbons and Alcohols

- **Alkanes** are **hydrocarbons** without any double or triple bonds. They have the general formula $C_nH_{(2n+2)}$.
- Alkanes are named according to the number of carbons present followed by the suffix –**ane**.
  - The first four alkanes are methane ($CH_4$), ethane ($C_2H_6$), propane ($C_3H_8$), and butane ($C_4H_{10}$).
  - Larger alkanes use a Greek/Latin root for the number (pentane, hexane, heptane, octane, and so on).
- **Alkenes** and **alkynes** contain double and triple bonds, respectively.
  - Alkenes are named by substituting –**ene** for the suffix and numbering the double bond by its lower-numbered carbon. Alkynes substitute –**yne** with the same numbering.
- **Alcohols** contain a hydroxyl (–OH) group, which substitutes for one or more of the hydrogens in the hydrocarbon chain.
  - Alcohols are named by substituting the suffix –**ol** or by using the prefix **hydroxy**– if a higher-priority group is present.
  - Alcohols have higher priority than double or triple bonds and alkanes.
  - Common names of alcohols include the name of the carbon chain followed by the word *alcohol*. For example, ethyl alcohol is the same compound as ethanol.
  - **Diols** contain two hydroxyl groups. They are termed **geminal** if on the same carbon or **vicinal** if on adjacent carbons.

## Aldehydes and Ketones

- Aldehydes and ketones contain a **carbonyl group**—a carbon double-bonded to an oxygen.
- **Aldehydes** have the carbonyl group on a terminal carbon that is also attached to a hydrogen atom.
  - Aldehydes are named with the suffix –**al**, or by using the prefix **oxo**– if a higher-priority group is present.
  - Common names of aldehydes include formaldehyde for methanal, acetaldehyde for ethanal, and propionaldehyde for propanal.

- **Ketones** have the carbonyl group on a nonterminal carbon.
  - Ketones are named with the suffix **–one** and share the prefix **oxo–** if a higher-priority group is present. Ketones can also be indicated by the prefix **keto–**.
  - The common names of ketones are constructed by naming the alkyl groups on either side alphabetically and adding ketone. For example, 2-butanone is called ethyl methyl ketone.
  - Acetone is significant as the smallest ketone. Its IUPAC name is propanone.
- Carbonyl-containing compounds (aldehydes, ketones, carboxylic acids, and derivatives) also create a lettering scheme for carbons. The carbon adjacent to the carbonyl carbon is the **$\alpha$-carbon**.

## Carboxylic Acids and Derivatives

- **Carboxylic acids** are the highest-priority functional group because they contain three bonds to oxygen: one from a hydroxyl group and two from a carbonyl group.
- Carboxylic acids are always terminal, although their **derivatives** may occur within a molecule.
  - Carboxylic acids are named with the suffix **–oic acid**. They are very rarely named as a prefix.
  - Common names for carboxylic acids follow the trend for aldehydes. Formic acid is methanoic acid, acetic acid is ethanoic acid, and propionic acid is propanoic acid.
- **Esters** are carboxylic acid derivatives where –OH is replaced with –OR, an **alkoxy group**.
  - Esters use the suffix **–oate** or the prefix **alkoxycarbonyl–**.
  - Common names for esters are derived from the alcohol and the carboxylic acid used during synthesis.
- **Amides** replace the hydroxyl group of a carboxylic acid with an amino group that may or may not be substituted.
  - Amides use the suffix **–amide** or the prefix **carbamoyl–** or **amido–**. Substituents attached to the amide nitrogen are designated with a capital ***N*–**.
- **Anhydrides** are formed from two carboxylic acids by dehydration. They may be symmetric (two of the same acid), asymmetric (two different acids), or cyclic (intramolecular reaction of a dicarboxylic acid).
  - Anhydrides are named using the suffix **anhydride** in place of *acid*. If the anhydride is formed from more than one carboxylic acid, both are named in alphabetical order in the name before the word **anhydride**.

## Summary of Functional Groups

- Functional groups are arranged in order of priority as follows: Carboxylic acid > anhydride > ester > amide > aldehyde > ketone > alcohol > alkene or alkyne > alkane.

## ANSWERS TO CONCEPT CHECKS

### 1.1

1. 1. Find the longest carbon chain in the compound with the highest-order functional group; 2. Number the chain; 3. Name the substituents; 4. Assign a number to each substituent; 5. Complete the name
2. 

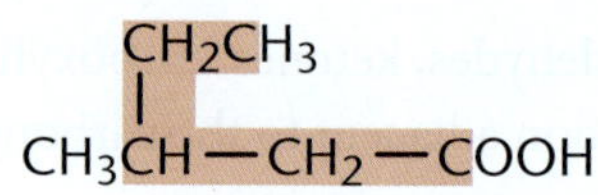


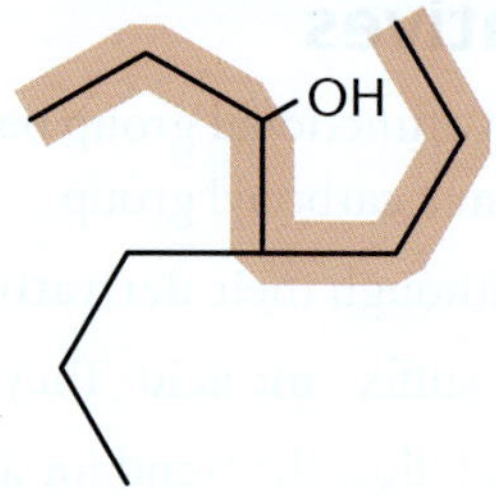


Note: There are two possible answers; however, the longest chain must include the hydroxyl group.

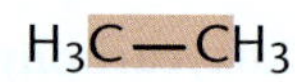


3. 

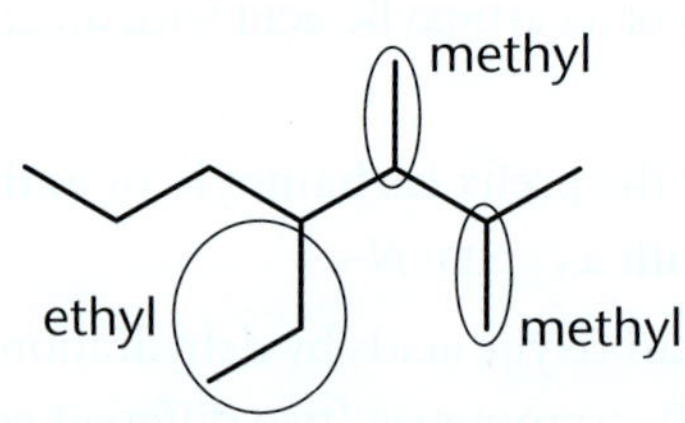


The question asks us to circle and name the substituents, but in order to determine the substituents it is necessary to identify the parent chain. So, begin by identifying the longest carbon chain that contains the highest-priority functional group. The molecule contains only alkyl functional groups, and the alkyl functional groups have the same priority, so the parent chain will be the longest continuous carbon chain (seven carbons). Once the parent chain is identified, the substituents can be circled and named as shown above.

Numbering the chain from right to left ensures that the substituents have the smallest possible locants (numbers). The substituents have already been named and numbered, so to complete the name, alphabetize the substituents (remembering that di– is ignored): 4-ethyl-2,3-dimethylheptane.

## 1.2

1.

| Molecular Formula | IUPAC Name (Straight-Chain Alkane) | Alternative Structure |
|---|---|---|
| $CH_4$ | Methane | No alternative structures |
| $C_2H_6$ | Ethane | No alternative structures |
| $C_3H_8$ | Propane | No alternative structures |
| $C_4H_{10}$ | Butane | See below |
| $C_5H_{12}$ | Pentane | See below |
| $C_6H_{14}$ | Hexane | See below |
| $C_7H_{16}$ | Heptane | See below |
| $C_8H_{18}$ | Octane | See below |
| $C_9H_{20}$ | Nonane | See below |
| $C_{10}H_{22}$ | Decane | See below |

Butane and all hydrocarbons that are larger than butane may have a branched appearance, which shortens the parent chain. An example is isobutane, properly named methylpropane, shown here. Any branched hydrocarbon with the correct number of carbons and no multiple bonds or rings is correct.

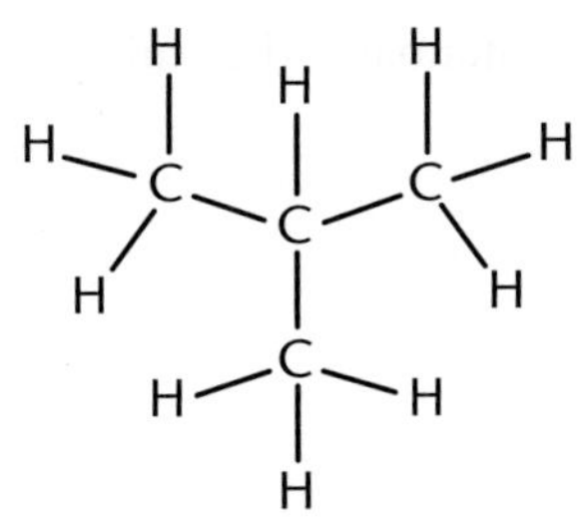

2. The alcohol would take precedence because the carbon to which it is attached has a higher oxidation state.
3. Diols are alcohols with two hydroxyl groups. In a *gemin*al diol, these hydroxyl groups are on the same carbon (*gemini* derives from the Latin for "paired" or "twins"). In a *vicin*al diol, the hydroxyls are in the *vicinity* of each other—on adjacent carbons (*vicinus* derives from the Latin for "neighbor"). Thus, the compound shown is a geminal diol.
4. Isopropyl alcohol and ethyl alcohol, respectively.

## 1.3

1. An aldehyde has a carbonyl group at the end of the chain. A ketone has a carbonyl group somewhere in the middle of the carbon chain. Another way to think of this is that the carbonyl carbon of an aldehyde has at least one bond to a hydrogen atom, whereas the carbonyl carbon of a ketone is always bonded to two other carbons.
2. Aldehydes are referred to with the suffix –al, while ketones are given the suffix –one. Carbonyl groups of both aldehydes and ketones are labeled as oxo– substituents (ketones may also be called keto– substituents).
3.

| IUPAC Name | Common Name |
|---|---|
| **Methanal** | Formaldehyde |
| **Ethanal** | Acetaldehyde |
| **Propanal** | Propionaldehyde |
| **Propanone** | Acetone |

4. Ketones and aldehydes both take precedence over both alcohols and hydrocarbon chains, and the functional group that is the highest priority determines the suffix. Because the aldehyde is chain-terminating and therefore on carbon number 1, the aldehyde would determine the suffix when naming this compound.

## 1.4

1. The ester derivative would be methyl pentanoate. The amide would be pentanamide. The anhydride would be pentanoic anhydride.
2. 3-methyl-2-oxopentanoic acid

## SCIENCE MASTERY ASSESSMENT EXPLANATIONS

1. **A**

The common name of ethanal is acetaldehyde, the common name of methanal is formaldehyde, and the common name of ethanol is ethyl alcohol. Isopropyl alcohol is the common name of 2-propanol. Propionaldehyde is the common name of propanal.

2. **C**

Aldehydes and carboxylic acids are characterized by their positions at the ends of carbon backbones and are thus considered terminal groups. As a result, the carbons to which they are attached are usually designated carbon 1. Ketones are internal by definition because there must be a carbon on either side of the carbonyl.

3. **C**

The highest-priority functional group in this molecule is the carboxyl group, so this will be a component of the backbone and provides the suffix of the molecule. This molecule is 2-methyl-3-oxopropanoic acid.

4. **A**

This molecule features an anhydride. The only other groups are hydrocarbon chains, which will provide part of the name of the parent root. Keep in mind that when a carbonyl group is present with a leaving group, the larger functional group (carboxylic acid, anhydride, ester, amide) takes priority over the carbonyl group alone. This molecule is propanoic anhydride.

5. **C**

Among the functional groups presented, carboxylic acids have the highest priority, and their compounds end with the suffix –oic acid. **(A)** denotes an alcohol, **(B)** a ketone, and **(D)** an alkyne, all of which have lower priorities than carboxylic acids. The MCAT does not test nomenclature of halides or ethers, but note that these must have lower priority than a carboxylic acid because they are less oxidized groups.

6. **A**

This molecule is 3-ethyl-4-methylhexane, not 2,3-diethylpentane. When naming alkanes, one must locate the longest carbon chain (6 carbons rather than 5 carbons), and the numbering system should give the alkyl groups the lowest possible numbers.

7. **B**

We know from the IUPAC name that we have a butanedioic acid backbone—in other words, a four-carbon backbone with carboxylic acids at either end. Adding the hydroxyl groups at carbons 2 and 3 then yields the correct structure.

8. **B**

Form– is a prefix shared by the common names of methanoic acid (formic acid) and methanal (formaldehyde).

9. **A**

The first task in naming a compound is identifying the longest carbon chain. In this case, the longest chain has seven carbons, so the parent alkane ends in –heptane. **(B)** and **(D)** can therefore be eliminated. Then, we must make sure that the carbons are numbered so that the substituents' position numbers are as small as possible. This compound has two methyl groups; minimizing their position numbers requires us to number the chain from right to left. These methyl groups are attached to carbons 2 and 5, so the correct IUPAC name is 2,5-dimethylheptane. **(C)** is incorrect because the position numbers of the substituents are not minimized.

10. **D**

We begin by finding the longest carbon chain; because there are no non-alkyl groups, we don't need to worry about any other groups' priorities. We then number our carbons such that the lowest possible combination of numbers is given to the various substituents. Then substituents are organized alphabetically, not numerically—eliminating **(C)**.

11. **B**

We know right away that **(C)** and **(D)** will be incorrect because a hydroxyl group is of higher priority than a methyl group. We also know that we will number the carbon chain so that the hydroxyl group receives the lowest possible position. Therefore, this molecule is 2-methyl-2-butanol, which starts with the prefix 2-methyl.

12. **C**

The suffix –amide in nicotinamide indicates that this compound contains an amide functional group. The prefix diphospho– indicates that there are two phosphate groups as well. Even if we did not know the prefix phospho– from this chapter, we should recognize that nucleotides, mentioned in the name of the compound, contain a sugar, a phosphate group, and a nitrogenous base. The structure of $NAD^+$, the oxidized form of NADH, is shown below.

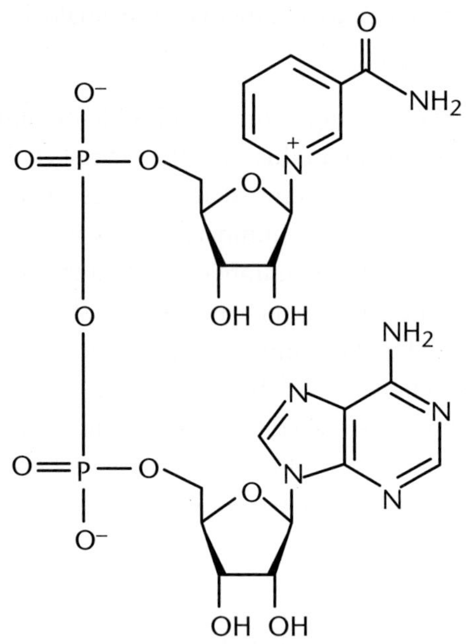

13. **A**

We can use the name acetylformic acid to figure out what our functional groups are. The prefix acet– refers to a two-carbon unit with one carbon in a carbonyl group—think of acetic acid, acetic anhydride, or acetaldehyde. The carbonyl carbon is the point of attachment to another functional group. Formic acid is a single-carbon carboxylic acid. Therefore, acetylformic acid is an acetyl group directly attached to formic acid, as shown in **(A)**. **(B)** shows acetic acid, or vinegar; **(C)** shows glucose; and **(D)** shows formic acid.

14. **B**

Acetic anhydride is the common name for ethanoic anhydride. Methyl formate is the common name for methyl methanoate; we can infer this from the common root form– and the ester suffix –oate (which is sometimes shortened to –ate for pronunciation purposes). Formic acid is the common name for methanoic acid, but this is a carboxylic acid—not a derivative.

15. **C**

Draw out the molecule, and you will see that the longest carbon chain with the substituents at the lowest possible carbon numbers is actually different from the one chosen in the original name. The correct IUPAC name for this molecule is 3-ethyl-4-methylhexane.

**GO ONLINE**

**Consult your online resources for additional practice.**

## SHARED CONCEPTS

**Organic Chemistry Chapter 4**
Analyzing Organic Reactions

**Organic Chemistry Chapter 5**
Alcohols

**Organic Chemistry Chapter 6**
Aldehydes and Ketones I

**Organic Chemistry Chapter 8**
Carboxylic Acids

**Organic Chemistry Chapter 9**
Carboxylic Acid Derivatives

**Organic Chemistry Chapter 10**
Nitrogen- and Phosphorus-Containing Compounds

CHAPTER 2

# ISOMERS

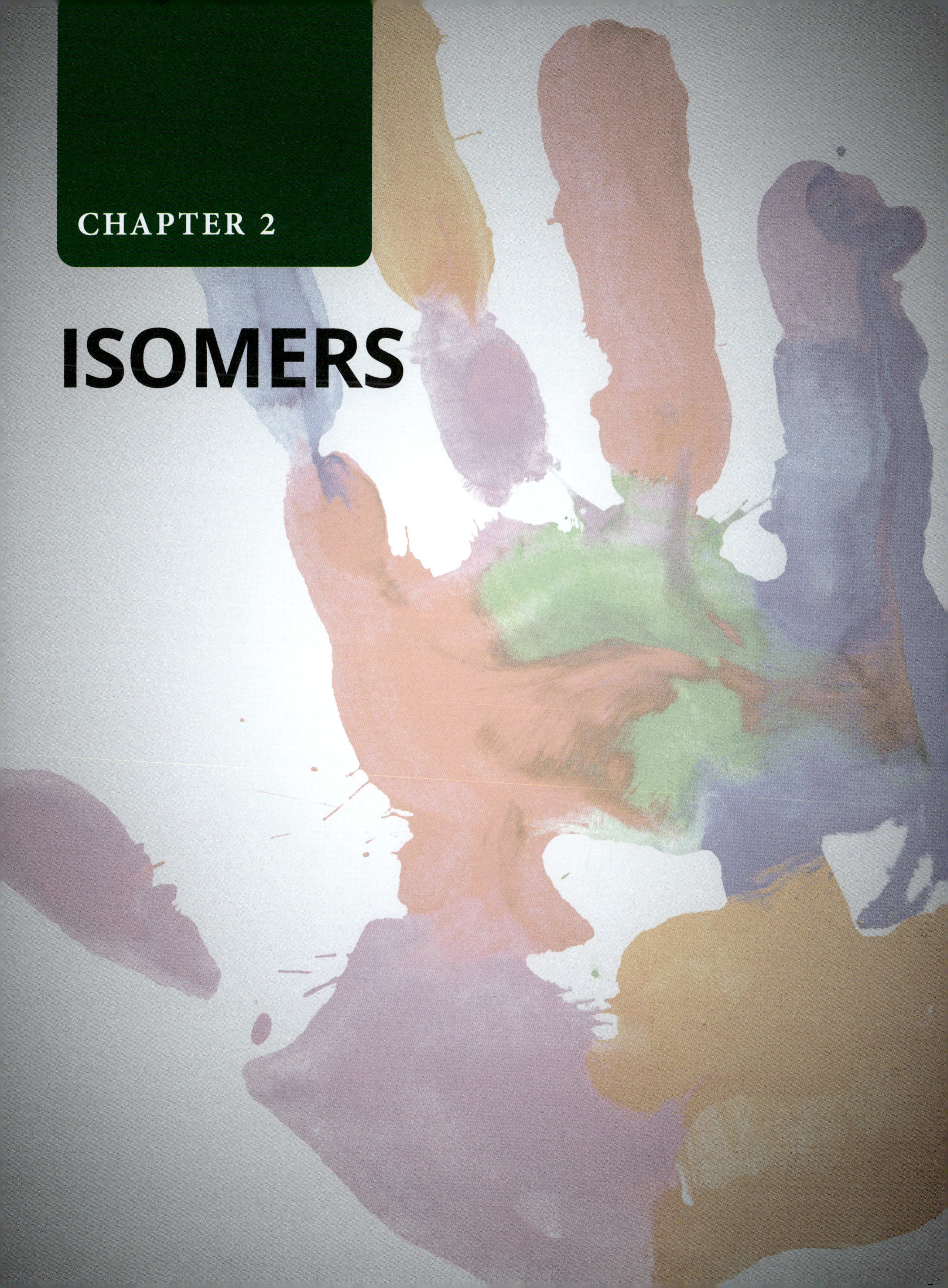

# SCIENCE MASTERY ASSESSMENT

Every pre-med knows this feeling: there is so much content I have to know for the MCAT! How do I know what to do first or what's important?

While the high-yield badges throughout this book will help you identify the most important topics, this Science Mastery Assessment is another tool in your MCAT prep arsenal. This quiz (which can also be taken in your online resources) and the guidance below will help ensure that you are spending the appropriate amount of time on this chapter based on your personal strengths and weaknesses. Don't worry though—skipping something now does not mean you'll never study it. Later on in your prep, as you complete full-length tests, you'll uncover specific pieces of content that you need to review and can come back to these chapters as appropriate.

## How to Use This Assessment

### If you answer 0–7 questions correctly:

Spend about 1 hour to read this chapter in full and take limited notes throughout. Follow up by reviewing **all** quiz questions to ensure that you now understand how to solve each one.

### If you answer 8–11 questions correctly:

Spend 20–40 minutes reviewing the quiz questions. Beginning with the questions you missed, read and take notes on the corresponding subchapters. For questions you answered correctly, ensure your thinking matches that of the explanation and you understand why each choice was correct or incorrect.

### If you answer 12–15 questions correctly:

Spend less than 20 minutes reviewing all questions from the quiz. If you missed any, then include a quick read-through of the corresponding subchapters, or even just the relevant content within a subchapter, as part of your question review. For questions you got correct, ensure your thinking matches that of the explanation and review the Concept Summary at the end of the chapter.

1. Which of the following does NOT show optical activity?
   - **A.** (*R*)-2-butanol
   - **B.** (*S*)-2-butanol
   - **C.** A solution containing 1 M (*R*)-2-butanol and 2 M (*S*)-2-butanol
   - **D.** A solution containing 2 M (*R*)-2-butanol and 2 M (*S*)-2-butanol

2. How many stereoisomers exist for the following aldehyde?

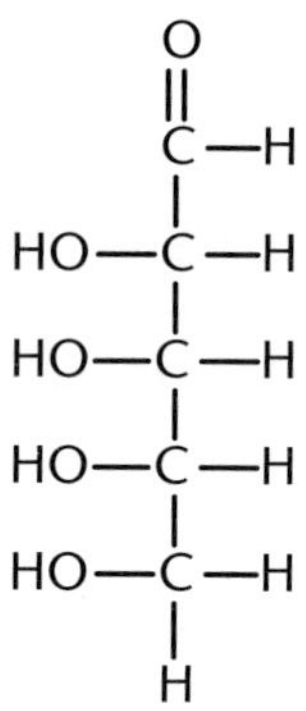

   - **A.** 2
   - **B.** 8
   - **C.** 9
   - **D.** 16

3. Which of the following compounds is optically inactive?

**A.**

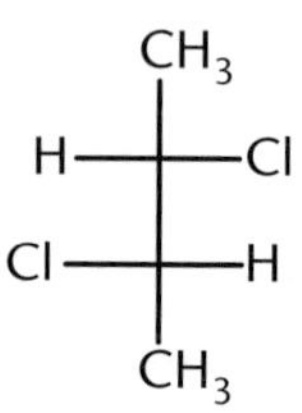

**B.**

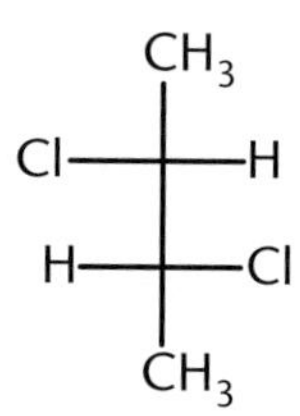

**C.**

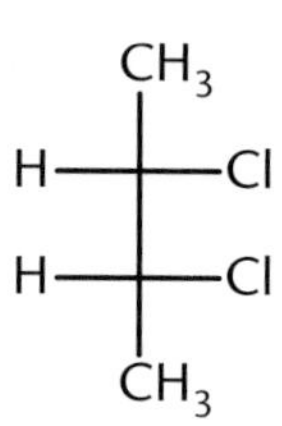

**D.**

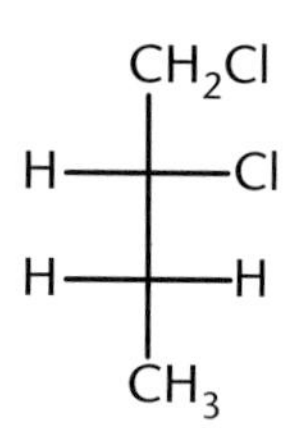

4. Cholesterol, shown below, contains how many chiral centers?

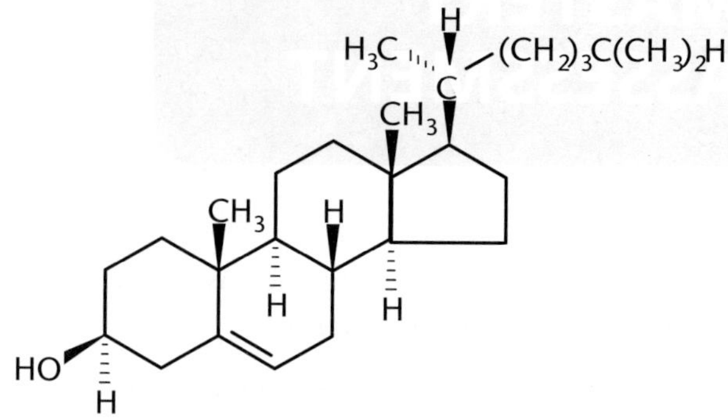

cholesterol

   - **A.** 5
   - **B.** 7
   - **C.** 8
   - **D.** 9

5. Which isomer of the following compound is the most stable?

**A.**

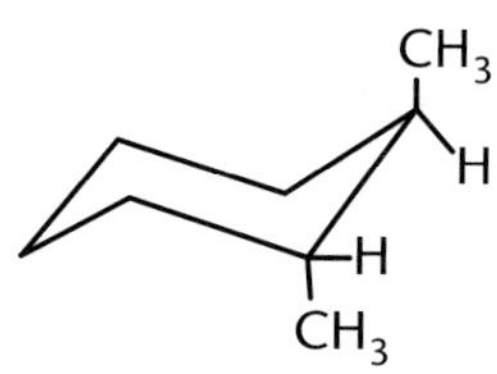

**B.**

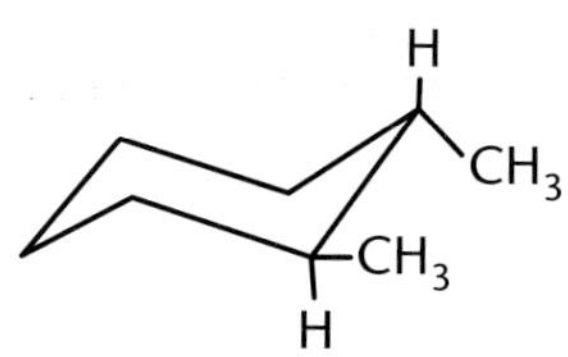

**C.**

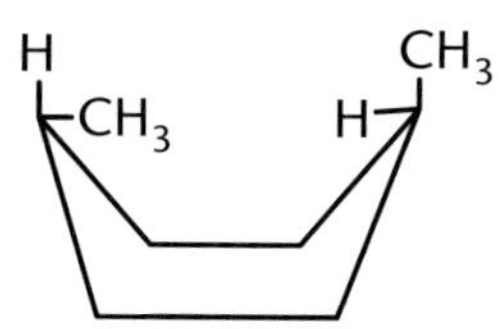

**D.** They are all equally stable.

6. The following reaction results in:

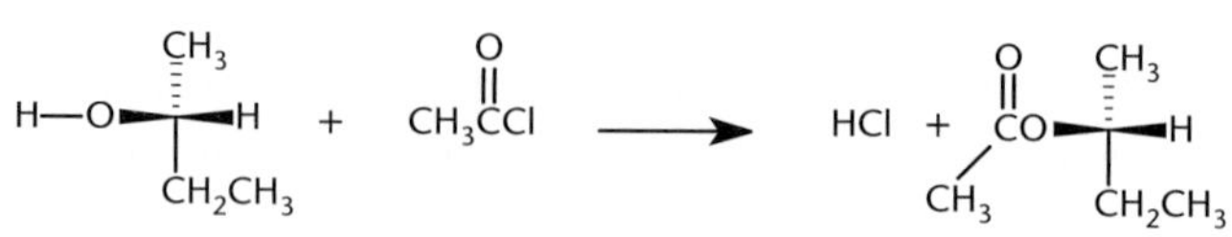

   - **A.** retention of relative configuration and a change in the absolute configuration.
   - **B.** a change in the relative and absolute configurations.
   - **C.** retention of the relative and absolute configurations.
   - **D.** retention of the absolute configuration and a change in the relative configuration.

7. The following molecules are considered to be:

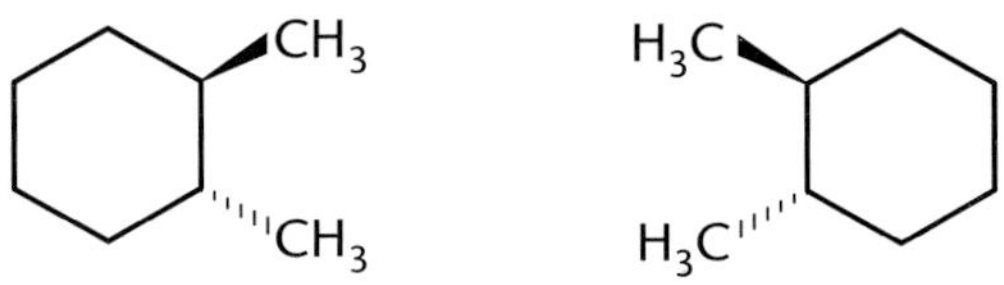


   A. enantiomers.
   B. diastereomers.
   C. *meso* compounds.
   D. structural isomers.

8. (+)-Glyceraldehyde and (−)-glyceraldehyde refer to the (*R*) and (*S*) forms of 2,3-dihydroxypropanal, respectively. These molecules are considered:
   A. enantiomers.
   B. diastereomers.
   C. *meso* compounds.
   D. structural isomers.

9. Consider (*E*)-2-butene and (*Z*)-2-butene. This is a pair of what type(s) of isomers?
   I. *Cis–trans* isomers
   II. Diastereomers
   III. Enantiomers
   A. I only
   B. II only
   C. I and II only
   D. I and III only

10. 3-methylpentane and hexane are related in that they are:
   A. enantiomers.
   B. diastereomers.
   C. constitutional isomers.
   D. conformational isomers.

11. (*R*)-2-chloro-(*S*)-3-bromobutane and (*S*)-2-chloro-(*S*)-3-bromobutane are:
   A. enantiomers.
   B. diastereomers.
   C. *meso* compounds.
   D. the same molecule.

12. A scientist takes a 0.5 $\frac{\text{g}}{\text{ml}}$ solution of an unknown pure dextrorotatory organic molecule and places it in a test tube with a diameter of 1 cm. He observes that a plane of polarized light is rotated 12° under these conditions. What is the specific rotation of this molecule?
   A. −240°
   B. −24°
   C. +24°
   D. +240°

13. Omeprazole is a proton pump inhibitor commonly used in gastroesophageal reflux disease. When omeprazole, a racemic mixture, went off-patent, pharmaceutical companies began to manufacture esomeprazole, the (*S*)-enantiomer of omeprazole, by itself. Given 1 M solutions of omeprazole and esomeprazole, which solution(s) would likely exhibit optical activity?
   A. Omeprazole only
   B. Esomeprazole only
   C. Both omeprazole and esomeprazole
   D. Neither omeprazole nor esomeprazole

14. (2*R*,3*S*)-2,3-dihydroxybutanedioic acid and (2*S*,3*R*)-2,3-dihydroxybutanedioic acid are:
   I. *meso* compounds.
   II. the same molecule.
   III. enantiomers.
   A. I only
   B. III only
   C. I and II only
   D. I and III only

15. If the methyl groups of butane are 120° apart, as seen in a Newman projection, this molecule is in its:
   A. highest-energy *gauche* form.
   B. lowest-energy staggered form.
   C. middle-energy eclipsed form.
   D. highest-energy eclipsed form.

## Answer Key

1. **D** (See section 2.3)
2. **B** (See section 2.2)
3. **C** (See section 2.3)
4. **C** (See section 2.3)
5. **B** (See section 2.1)
6. **C** (See section 2.3)
7. **A** (See section 2.3)
8. **A** (See section 2.3)
9. **C** (See section 2.2)
10. **C** (See section 2.1)
11. **B** (See section 2.2)
12. **D** (See section 2.3)
13. **B** (See section 2.3)
14. **C** (See section 2.2)
15. **C** (See section 2.1)

*The relevant section of the chapter to review for each question is given in parentheses after the correct answer. Detailed explanations can be found at the end of the chapter.*

CHAPTER 2

# ISOMERS

## In This Chapter



## Introduction

An important way that we distinguish between molecules is by identifying **isomers** of the same compound—those that have the same molecular formula but different structures. Keep in mind that isomerism describes a relationship; just as there must be at least two children to have siblings, two molecules can be isomers to each other, but no molecule can be an isomer by itself. Throughout this chapter, we will learn how to identify these relationships and describe the similarities and differences between isomers. Figure 2.1 shows the isomer classes that we will learn more about and how they are related—feel free to come back to this figure as a reference after you have read through the more detailed explanations.

### CHAPTER PROFILE

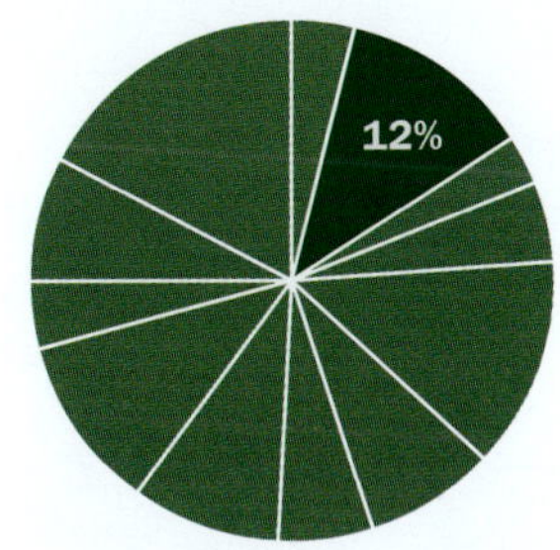


The content in this chapter should be relevant to about 12% of all questions about organic chemistry on the MCAT.

This chapter covers material from the following AAMC content categories:

**1D:** Principles of bioenergetics and fuel molecule metabolism

**5B:** Nature of molecules and intermolecular interactions

**5C:** Separation and purification methods

**5D:** Structure, function, and reactivity of biologically-relevant molecules

### KEY CONCEPT

Isomers have the same molecular formula, but different structures.

## 2.1 Structural Isomers

### LEARNING OBJECTIVES

After Chapter 2.1, you will be able to:

- Describe the shared and unique properties of structural isomers
- Explain what physical and chemical properties are
- Identify structural isomers

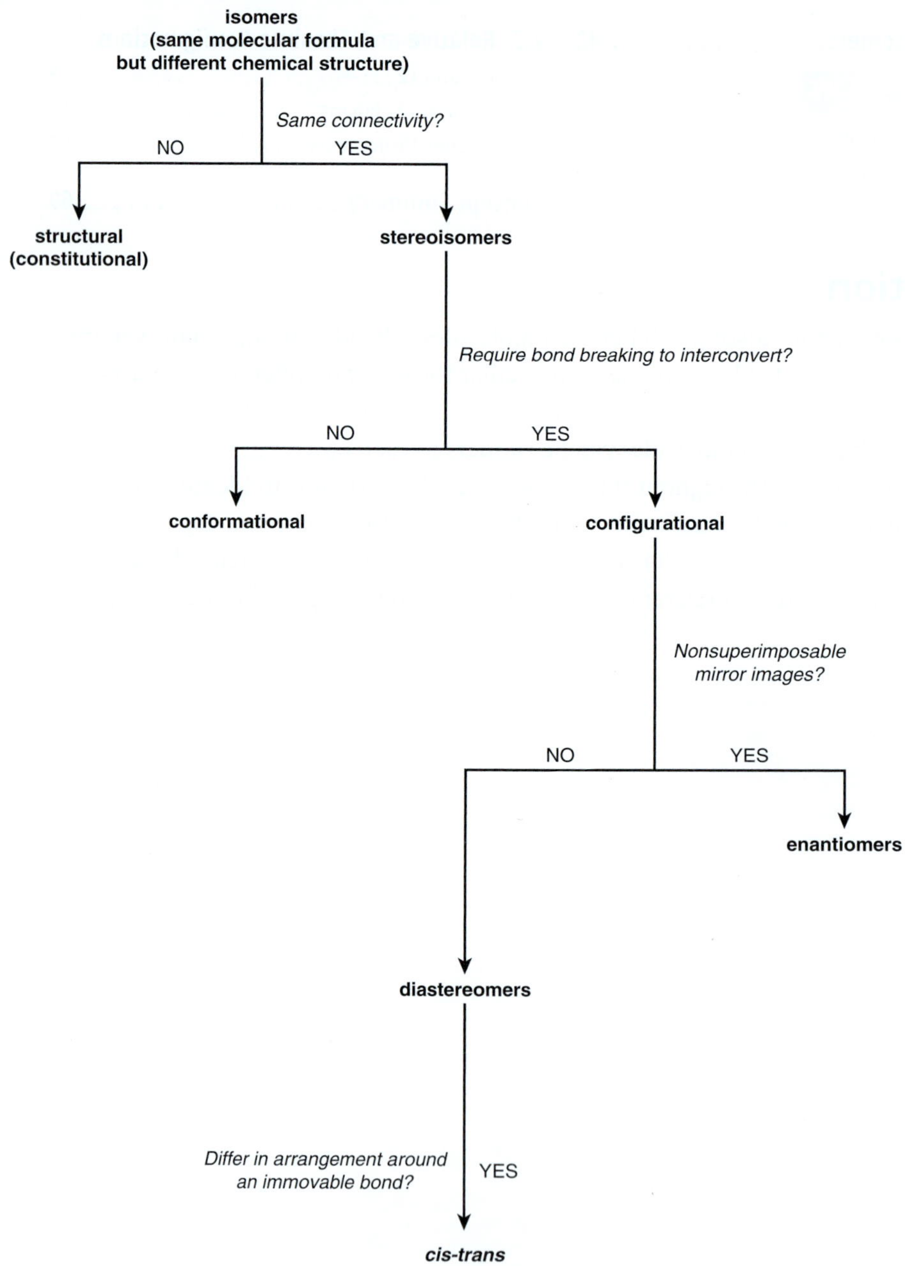


**Figure 2.1** Flowchart of Isomer Relationships

As suggested by the flowchart in Figure 2.1, structural isomers are the least similar of all isomers. In fact, the only thing that **structural isomers** (also called **constitutional isomers**) share is their molecular formula, meaning that their molecular weights must be the same. Aside from this similarity, structural isomers are widely varied, with different chemical and physical properties. For example, five different structural isomers of $C_6H_{14}$ are shown in Figure 2.2. Each of these molecules looks completely different but has the same number of carbon and hydrogen atoms.

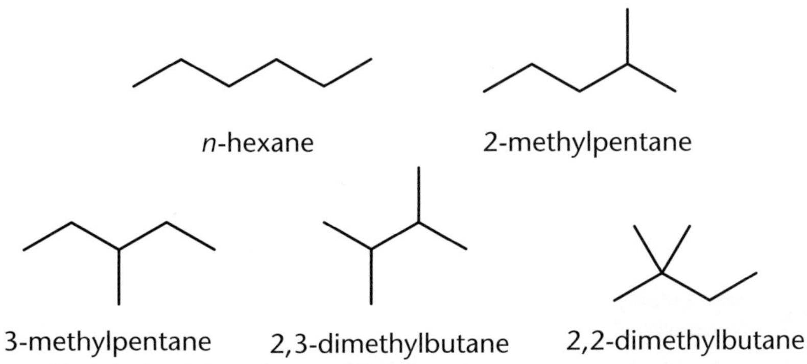


**Figure 2.2** Structural (Constitutional) Isomers of $C_6H_{14}$

Physical and chemical properties are prime MCAT material and are often tested in the context of isomerism. **Physical properties** are characteristics of processes that don't change the composition of matter, such as melting point, boiling point, solubility, odor, color, and density. **Chemical properties** have to do with the reactivity of the molecule with other molecules and result in changes in chemical composition. In organic chemistry, the chemical properties of a compound are generally dictated by the functional groups in the molecule.

## KEY CONCEPT

Physical properties: no change in composition of matter; examples include melting point, boiling point, solubility, odor, color, density.

Chemical properties: reactivity of molecule, resulting in change in composition; generally attributable to functional groups in the molecule.

## MCAT CONCEPT CHECK 2.1

Before you move on, assess your understanding of the material with these questions.

1. What property or properties do structural isomers have in common?

______________________________

2. Of the compounds cyclopropanol, 2-propanol, acetone, and prop-2-ene-1-ol, which are structural isomers of each other?

______________________________

3. What are physical properties? Give three examples of physical properties.

   •

   •

   •

4. What are chemical properties?

## 2.2 Stereoisomers High Yield

### LEARNING OBJECTIVES

After Chapter 2.2, you will be able to:

- Differentiate between conformational and configurational isomers
- Distinguish enantiomers from diastereomers
- Identify enantiomers, diastereomers, and *meso* compounds
- Convert between Newman and 3D molecular projections

Like structural isomers—and all isomers, for that matter—stereoisomers have the same chemical formula. Unlike structural isomers, however, **stereoisomers** also share the same atomic connectivity. In other words, they have the same structural backbone. Stereoisomers differ in how these atoms are arranged in space (their wedge-and-dash pattern), and all isomers that are not structural isomers fall under this category. The largest distinction within this class is between conformational and configurational isomers. **Conformational isomers** or **conformers** differ in rotation around single ($\sigma$) bonds; **configurational isomers** can be interconverted only by breaking bonds.

## Conformational Isomers

Of all of the isomers, conformational isomers are the most similar. Conformational isomers are, in fact, the same molecule, only at different points in their natural rotation around single ($\sigma$) bonds.

While double bonds hold molecules in a specific position (as explained with *cis–trans* isomers later), single bonds are free to rotate. Conformational isomers arise from the fact that varying degrees of rotation around single bonds can create different levels of strain. These conformations are easy to see when the molecule is depicted in a **Newman projection**, in which the molecule is visualized along a line extending through a carbon–carbon bond axis. The classic example for demonstrating conformational isomerism in a straight chain is butane, which is shown in Figure 2.3.

### MNEMONIC

Con**FORM**ational = free-**FORM** dance (free rotation around single bonds without bond breaking)

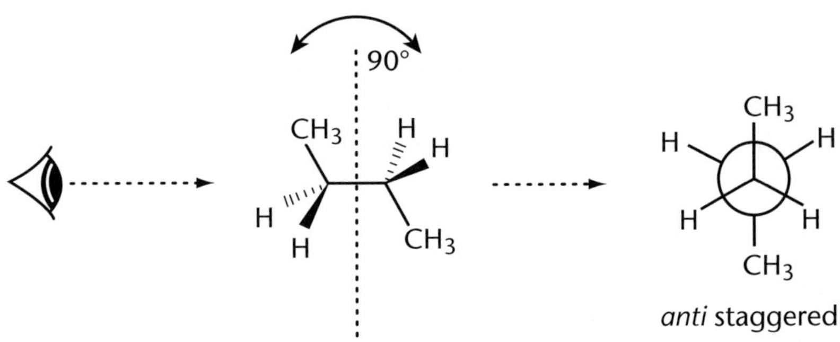


**Figure 2.3** Newman Projection of Butane
*Depiction of different atoms' positions from the point of view of the C-2 to C-3 bond axis.*

## Straight-Chain Conformations

For butane, the most stable conformation occurs when the two methyl groups (containing C-1 and C-4) are oriented 180° away from each other. In this position, there is minimal steric repulsion between the atoms' electron clouds because they are as far apart as they can possibly be. Thus, the atoms are "happiest" and in their lowest-energy state. Because there is no overlap of atoms along the line of sight (besides C-2 and C-3), the molecule is said to be in a **staggered** conformation. Specifically, it is called the ***anti*** conformation because the two largest groups are antiperiplanar (in the same plane, but on opposite sides) to each other. This is the most energetically favorable type of staggered conformation. The other type of staggered conformation, called ***gauche***, occurs when the two largest groups are 60° apart.

### MNEMONIC

It's ***gauche*** (unsophisticated or awkward) for one methyl group to stand too close to another group. Groups are **eclipsed** when they are completely in line with one another—just like a solar or lunar eclipse.

To convert from the *anti* to the *gauche* conformation, the molecule must pass through an **eclipsed** conformation in which the two methyl groups are 120° apart and overlap with the hydrogen atoms on the adjacent carbon. When the two methyl groups directly overlap each other with 0° separation, the molecule is said to be **totally eclipsed** and is in its highest-energy state. Totally eclipsed conformations are the least favorable energetically because the two largest groups are synperiplanar (in the same plane, on the same side). The different staggered and eclipsed conformations are demonstrated in Figures 2.3 and 2.4. For compounds larger than butane, the name of the conformation is decided by the relative positions of the two largest substituents about a given carbon–carbon bond.

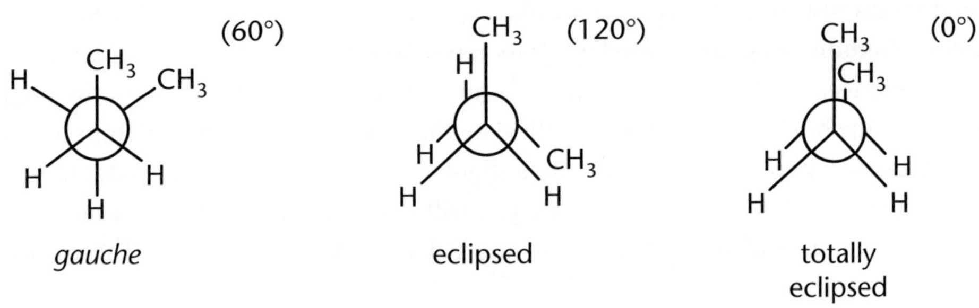


**Figure 2.4** Stability of Straight-Chain Conformational Isomers
*Degree measurements indicate the angle between the two largest substituents about the carbon–carbon bond.*

Figure 2.5 shows the plot of potential energy vs. degree of rotation about the bond between C-2 and C-3 in butane. It shows the relative minima and maxima of potential energy of the molecule throughout its various conformations. Remember that every molecule wants to be in the lowest energy state possible, so the higher the energy, the less time the molecule will spend in that energetically unfavorable state.

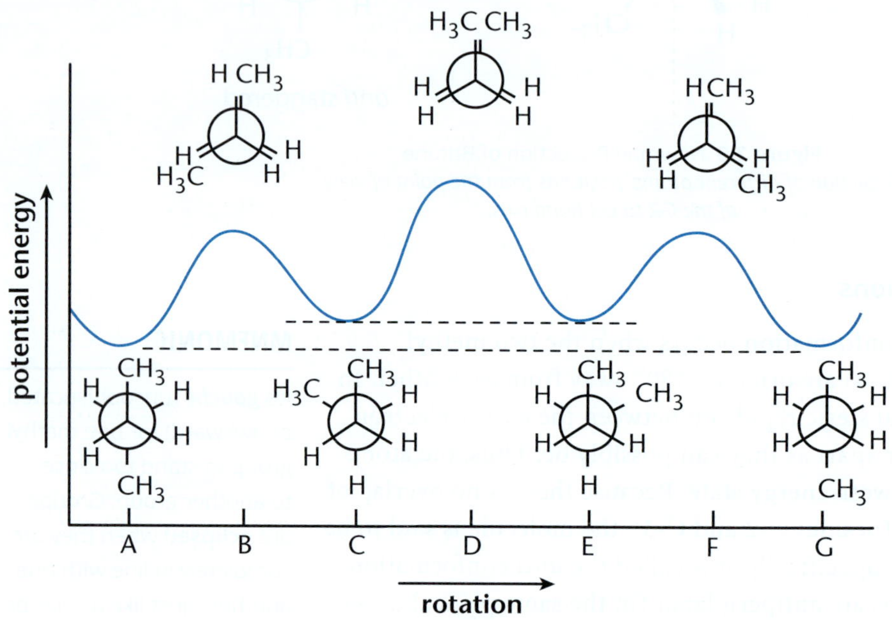


**Figure 2.5** Potential Energy vs. Degree of Rotation about the C-2 to C-3 Bond in Butane

### KEY CONCEPT

Notice that the *anti* staggered isomer (A and G) has the lowest energy, whereas the totally eclipsed isomer (D) has the highest energy.

These conformational interconversion barriers are small ($19 \frac{\text{kJ}}{\text{mol}}$ between *anti* staggered butane and totally eclipsed butane) and are easily overcome at room temperature. Nevertheless, at very low temperatures, conformational interconversions are dramatically slow. If the molecules do not possess sufficient energy to cross the energy barrier, they may not rotate at all (as happens to all molecules at absolute zero).

## Cyclic Conformations

Cycloalkanes can be either fairly stable compounds or fairly unstable—depending on **ring strain**. Ring strain arises from three factors: angle strain, torsional strain, and nonbonded strain (sometimes referred to as steric strain). **Angle strain** results when bond angles deviate from their ideal values by being stretched or compressed. **Torsional strain** results when cyclic molecules must assume conformations that have eclipsed or *gauche* interactions. **Nonbonded strain (van der Waals repulsion)** results when *nonadjacent* atoms or groups compete for the same space. Nonbonded strain is the dominant source of steric strain in the **flagpole interactions** of the cyclohexane boat conformation. To alleviate the strain, cycloalkanes attempt to adopt various nonplanar conformations. Cyclobutane puckers into a slight "V" shape; cyclopentane adopts what is called an envelope conformation; and cyclohexane (the one you will undoubtedly see the most on the MCAT) exists mainly in three conformations called the **chair**, **boat**, and **twist**- or **skew-boat** forms. These cycloalkanes are shown in Figure 2.6.

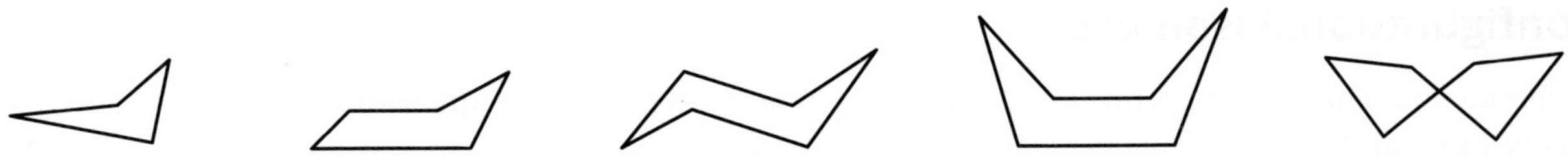

puckered cyclobutane | envelope cyclopentane | chair cyclohexane | boat cyclohexane | twist-boat cyclohexane

**Figure 2.6** Conformations of Cycloalkanes

The most stable conformation of cyclohexane is the chair conformation, which minimizes all three types of strain. The hydrogen atoms that are perpendicular to the plane of the ring (sticking up or down) are called **axial**, and those parallel (sticking out) are called **equatorial**. The axial–equatorial orientations alternate around the ring; that is, if the wedge on C-1 is an axial group, the dash on C-2 will also be axial, the wedge on C-3 will be axial, and so on.

Cyclohexane can undergo a **chair flip** in which one chair form is converted to the other. In this process, the cyclohexane molecule briefly passes through a fourth conformation called the **half-chair** conformation. After the chair flip, all axial groups become equatorial and all equatorial groups become axial. All dashes remain dashes, and all wedges remain wedges. This interconversion can be slowed if a bulky group is attached to the ring; *tert*-butyl groups are classic examples of bulky groups on the MCAT. For substituted rings, the bulkiest group will favor the equatorial position to reduce nonbonded strain (flagpole interactions) with axial groups in the molecule, as shown in Figure 2.7.

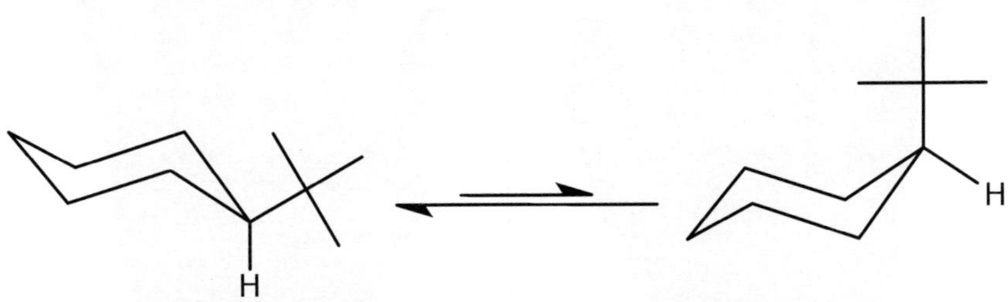


**Figure 2.7** Axial and Equatorial Positions in Cyclohexane
*During a chair flip, axial components become equatorial and vice versa. However, components pointing "up" (wedge) remain up and components pointing "down" (dash) remain down.*

In rings with more than one substituent, the preferred chair form is determined by the larger group, which will prefer the equatorial position. These rings also have associated nomenclature. If both groups are located on the same side of the ring, the molecule is called ***cis***; if they are on opposite sides of the ring, it is called ***trans***, as shown in Figure 2.8. These same terms are used for molecules with double bonds, as explained later in this chapter.

*cis*-1,2-dimethylcyclohexane | *trans*-1,2-dimethylcyclohexane

**Figure 2.8** Nomenclature of Rings with Multiple Substituents

## Configurational Isomers

Unlike conformational isomers that interconvert by simple bond rotation, **configurational isomers** can only change from one form to another by breaking and reforming covalent bonds. The two categories of configurational isomers are enantiomers and diastereomers. Both enantiomers and diastereomers can also be considered **optical isomers** because the different spatial arrangement of groups in these molecules affects the rotation of plane-polarized light.

### Chirality

An object is considered **chiral** if its mirror image cannot be superimposed on the original object; this implies that the molecule lacks an internal plane of symmetry. Chirality can also be thought of as handedness. In fact, one of the easiest visualizations of chirality is to think of a pair of hands, as shown in Figure 2.9. Although essentially identical, the left hand will not be able to fit into a right-handed glove. **Achiral** objects have mirror images that *can* be superimposed; for example, a fork is identical to its mirror image and is therefore achiral.

**KEY CONCEPT**

Chirality = handedness

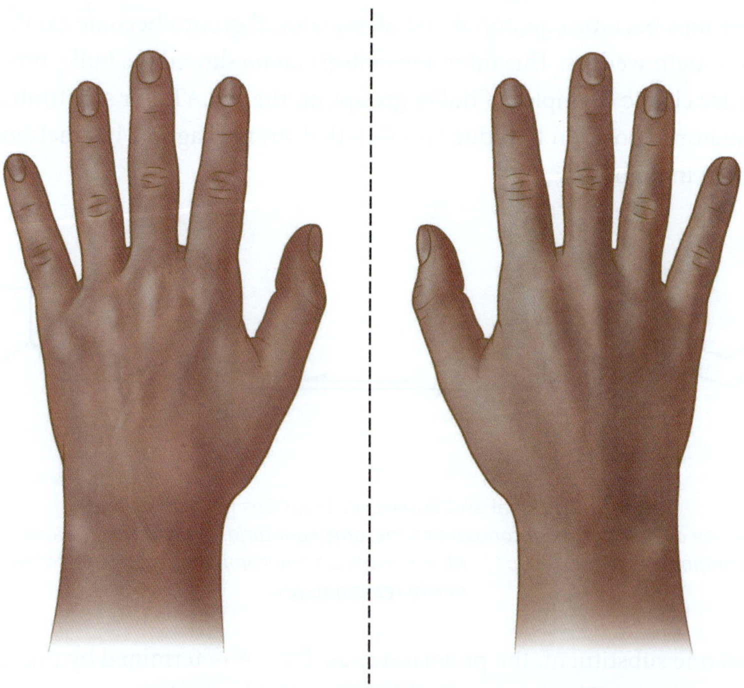

**Figure 2.9** Hands as Examples of Chiral Structures
*Each hand has a nonsuperimposable mirror image.*

On the MCAT, you will often see this concept tested when there is a carbon atom with four different substituents. This carbon will be an asymmetrical core of optical activity and is known as a **chiral center**. As mentioned earlier, chiral centers lack a plane of symmetry. For example, the C-1 carbon atom in 1-bromo-1-chloroethane has four different substituents. As shown in Figure 2.10, this molecule is chiral because it is not superimposable on its mirror image.

**MCAT EXPERTISE**

Whenever you see a carbon with four different substituents, think chirality.

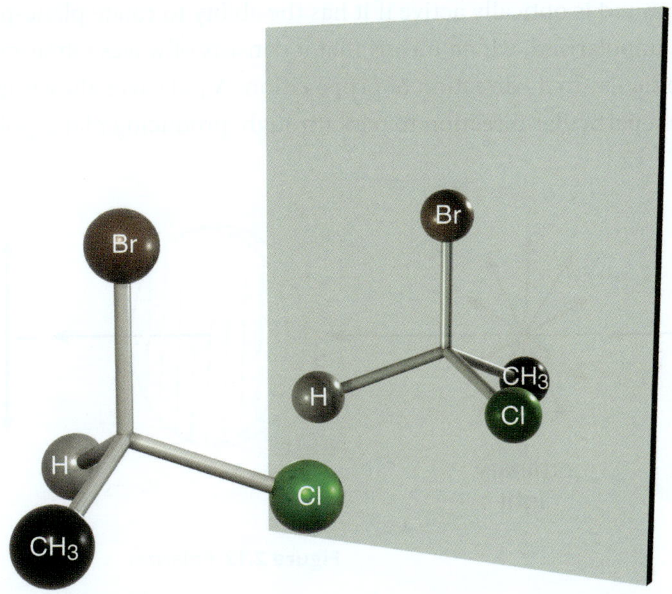


**Figure 2.10** Enantiomers of 1-Bromo-1-Chloroethane

Two molecules that are nonsuperimposable mirror images of each other are called **enantiomers**. Molecules may also be related as **diastereomers**. These molecules are chiral and share the same connectivity but are not mirror images of each other. This is because they differ at some (but not all) of their multiple chiral centers.

Alternatively, a carbon atom with only *three different* substituents, such as 1,1-dibromoethane, has a plane of symmetry and is therefore **achiral**. A simple 180° rotation around a vertical axis, as shown in Figure 2.11, allows the compound to be superimposed upon its mirror image.

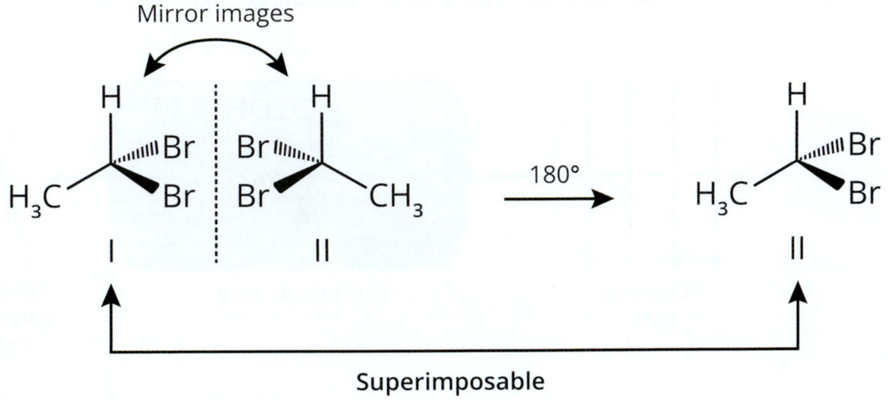


**Figure 2.11** Rotation of an Achiral Molecule

## Enantiomers

**Enantiomers** (nonsuperimposable mirror images) have the same connectivity but opposite configurations at every chiral center in the molecule. Enantiomers have identical physical and chemical properties with two notable exceptions: optical activity and reactions in chiral environments. A real-world example of this is the difference in smell between some enantiomers; for instance, (+)-carvone smells like caraway, while its enantiomer, (−)-carvone, smells like spearmint.

### KEY CONCEPT

Enantiomers have nearly identical physical properties and chemical properties, but they rotate plane-polarized light in opposite directions and react differently in chiral environments.

A compound is optically active if it has the ability to rotate plane-polarized light. Ordinary light is unpolarized, which means that it consists of waves vibrating in all possible planes perpendicular to its direction of propagation. A polarizer allows light waves oscillating only in a particular direction to pass through, producing plane-polarized light, as shown in Figure 2.12.

## BRIDGE

While rotation of plane-polarized light can be tested in organic chemistry questions, the polarization of light *itself* is fair game as a physics question. Be sure to review light polarization, discussed in Chapter 8 of *MCAT Physics and Math Review.*

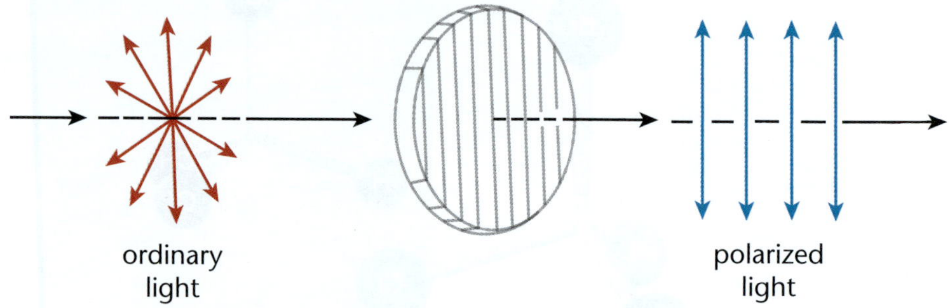


**Figure 2.12** Polarizer

**Optical activity** refers to the rotation of this plane-polarized light by a chiral molecule. At the molecular level, one enantiomer will rotate plane-polarized light to the same magnitude but in the opposite direction of its mirror image (assuming concentration and path lengths are equal). For example, as shown in Figure 2.13, (+)-lactic acid will take polarized light and rotate it clockwise (+2.6°), while (−)-lactic acid will take polarized light and rotate it in the opposite counter-clockwise direction (−2.6°). A compound that rotates the plane of polarized light to the right, or clockwise, is dextrorotatory (d-) and is labeled (+). A compound that rotates light toward the left, or counterclockwise, is levorotatory (l-) and is labeled (−). The direction of rotation cannot be determined from the structure of a molecule and must be determined experimentally. That is, it is not related to the absolute configuration of the molecule.

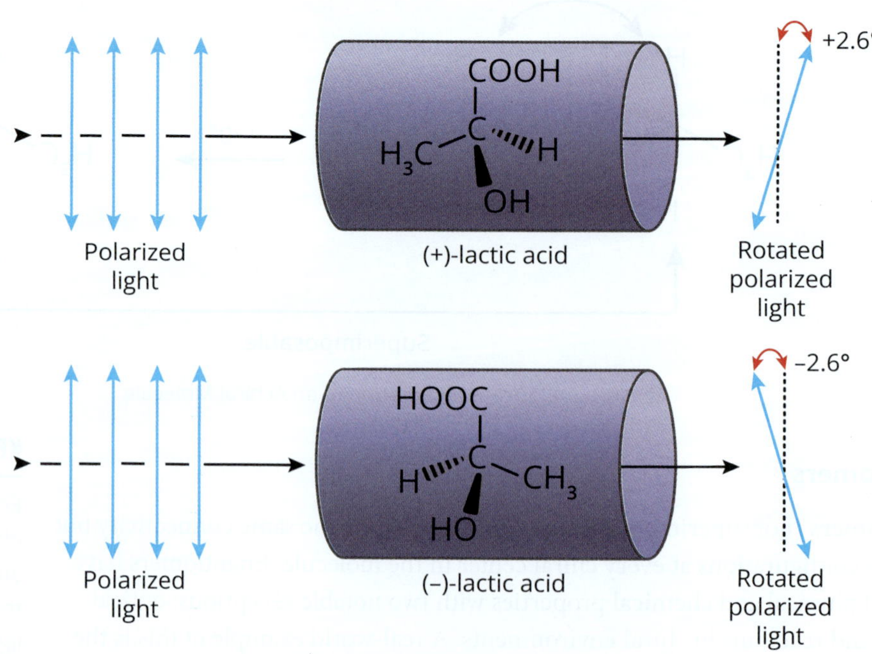


**Figure 2.13** Rotation of Light by Enantiomers

The amount of rotation depends on the number of molecules that a light wave encounters. This depends on two factors: the concentration of the optically active compound and the length of the tube through which the light passes. Chemists have set standard conditions of 1 $\frac{\text{g}}{\text{mL}}$ for concentration and 1 dm (10 cm) for length to compare the optical activities of different compounds. Rotations measured at different concentrations and tube lengths can be converted to a standardized **specific rotation** using the following equation:

$$[\alpha] = \frac{\alpha_{\text{obs}}}{c \times l}$$

**Equation 2.1**

where $[\alpha]$ is specific rotation in degrees, $\alpha_{\text{obs}}$ is the observed rotation in degrees, $c$ is the concentration in $\frac{\text{g}}{\text{mL}}$, and $l$ is the path length in dm.

When both (+) and (−) enantiomers are present in equal concentrations, they form a **racemic mixture**. In these solutions, the rotations cancel each other out, and no optical activity is observed. If enantiomerism is analogous to handedness, racemic mixtures are the equivalent of ambidexterity. These solutions possess no handedness overall and will not rotate plane-polarized light.

The fact that enantiomers have identical physical and chemical properties prompts a question about racemic mixtures: How can one separate the mixture into its two constituent isomers? The answer lies in the relationship between enantiomers and diastereomers. Reacting two enantiomers with a single enantiomer of another compound will, by definition, lead to two diastereomers. Imagine, for example, two enantiomers that contain only one chiral carbon; these compounds could be labeled (+) and (−). If each is reacted with only the (+) enantiomer of another compound, two products would result: (+,+) and (−,+). Because these two products differ at some—but not all—chiral centers, they are necessarily diastereomers. Diastereomers have different physical properties, as we will explore momentarily. These differences enable one to separate these products by common laboratory techniques such as crystallization, filtration, distillation, and others. Once separated, these diastereomers can be reacted to regenerate the original enantiomers.

**KEY CONCEPT**

The system for labeling optical activity always uses d- or (+) to refer to clockwise rotation of plane-polarized light, while l- and (−) always go together and refer to counterclockwise rotation of plane-polarized light. Do not confuse this with D- or L- labels on carbohydrates or amino acids, which are based on the absolute configuration of glyceraldehyde. (*R*) and (*S*) also refer to absolute configuration, which is determined by structure. Optical activity does not consistently align with the other systems.

**KEY CONCEPT**

A racemic mixture displays no optical activity.

### Diastereomers

**Diastereomers** are non-mirror-image configurational isomers. Diastereomers occur when a molecule has two or more stereogenic centers and differs at some, but not all, of these centers. The term diastereomer encompasses any stereoisomer that is not an enantiomer. For any molecule with *n* chiral centers, there are $2^n$ possible stereoisomers. Thus, if a compound has two chiral carbon atoms, it has a maximum of four possible stereoisomers, as shown in Figure 2.14.

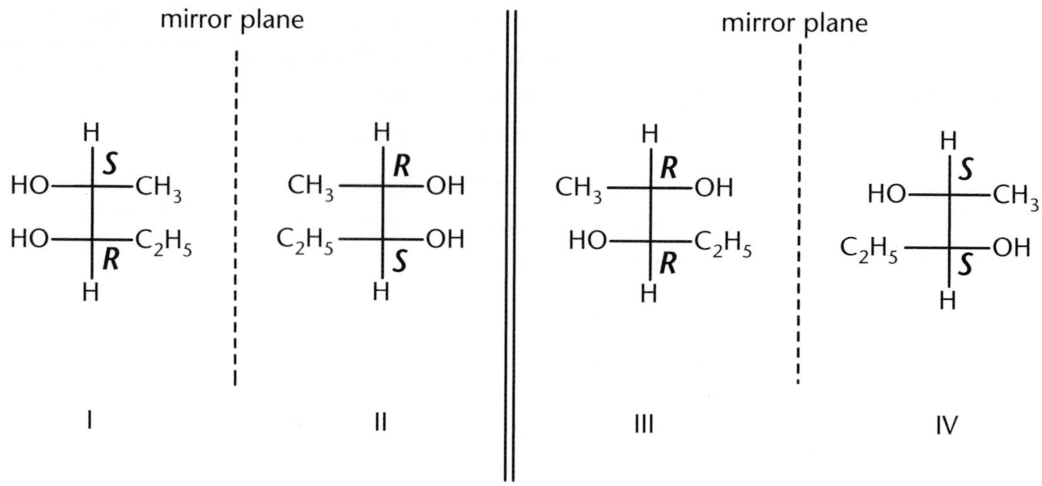


**Figure 2.14** $2^n$ Possible Stereoisomers ($n$ = chiral centers)
*Four stereoisomers with two chiral centers; enantiomers = I/II and III/IV pairs, and all other combinations are diastereomers.*

In this image, one can see that I and II are mirror images of each other and are therefore enantiomers of each other. Similarly, III and IV are enantiomers. However, I and III are not. These are stereoisomers that are not mirror images and are thus diastereomers. Notice that other combinations of non-mirror-image stereoisomers are also diastereomers: I and IV, II and III, and II and IV.

Diastereomers have different chemical properties. However, they might behave similarly in particular reactions because they have the same functional groups. Because they have different arrangements in space, they will consistently have different physical properties. Diastereomers will also rotate plane-polarized light; however, knowing the specific rotation of one diastereomer gives no indication of the specific rotation of another diastereomer. This is a stark contrast from enantiomers, which will always have equal-magnitude rotations in opposite directions.

### *Cis–Trans* Isomers

***Cis–trans* isomers** (formerly called **geometric isomers**) are a specific subtype of diastereomers in which substituents differ in their position around an immovable bond, such as a double bond, or around a ring structure, such as a cycloalkane in which the rotation of bonds is greatly restricted. In simple compounds with only one substituent on either side of the immovable bond, we use the terms ***cis*** and ***trans***. If two substituents are on the same side of the immovable bond, the molecule is considered *cis*. If they are on opposite sides, it is considered *trans*. Figure 2.15 shows *cis*- and *trans*-2-butene, where the notation *cis* is used when the two methyl groups are on the same side of the double bond, while the notation *trans* is used when they are on different sides of the double bond. For more complicated compounds with polysubstituted double bonds, the more systematic (*E*)/(*Z*) nomenclature is used instead, where (*Z*) indicates the higher-priority groups are on the same side and (*E*) indicates they are on opposite side, as described in the next section.

#### MCAT EXPERTISE

While the MCAT is up-to-date with science, it is still possible to see older terms for some concepts on Test Day. Thus, it's important to know not only the current name, *cis–trans* isomers, but also the older name, geometric isomers.

*cis*-2-butene *trans*-2-butene

**Figure 2.15** *Cis* and *Trans* Isomers of Butene

### *Meso* Compounds

For a molecule to have optical activity, it must not only have chiral centers within it, but must also lack a plane of symmetry. Thus, if a plane of symmetry exists, the molecule is not optically active even if it possesses chiral centers. This plane of symmetry can occur either through the chiral center or between chiral centers. A molecule with chiral centers that has an internal plane of symmetry is called a ***meso* compound**, an example of which is shown in Figure 2.16.

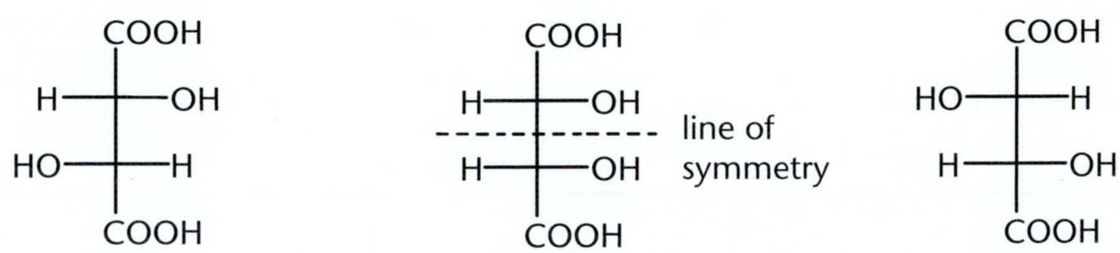


L-tartaric acid *meso*-tartaric acid D-tartaric acid

**Figure 2.16** Example of a *Meso* Compound

As shown in this image, D- and L-tartaric acid are both optically active, but *meso*-tartaric acid has a plane of symmetry and is not optically active. This means that even though *meso*-tartaric acid has two chiral carbon atoms, the molecule as a whole does not display optical activity. *Meso* compounds are essentially the molecular equivalent of a racemic mixture.

**KEY CONCEPT**

*Meso* compounds are made up of two halves that are mirror images. Thus, as a whole they are not optically active.

**MCAT CONCEPT CHECK 2.2**

Before you move on, assess your understanding of the material with these questions.

1. What is the difference between a conformational and a configurational isomer?
   - Conformational:

   ______________________________

   - Configurational:

   ______________________________

2. Consider the six pairs that the following four molecules can make. Which pairs are enantiomers? Diastereomers?

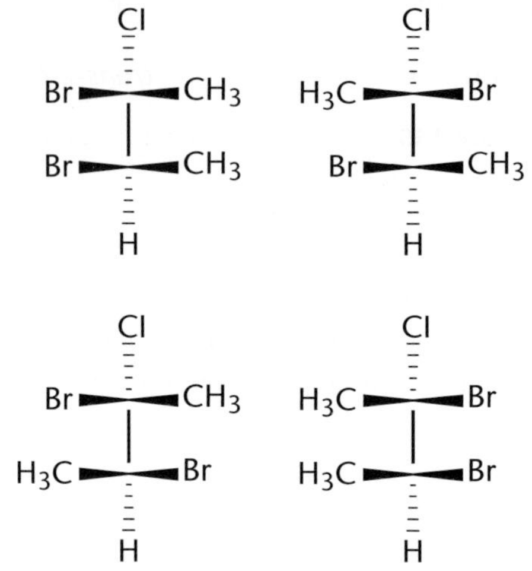


3. What is a *meso* compound?

---

4. Complete the Newman projection for the following compound:

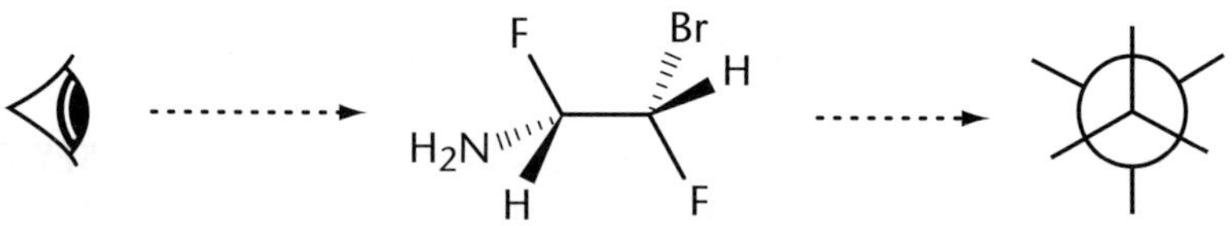


## 2.3 Relative and Absolute Configurations

**LEARNING OBJECTIVES**

After Chapter 2.3, you will be able to:

- Name *cis*, *trans*, *E*, and *Z* molecules using appropriate nomenclature
- Apply Cahn–Ingold–Prelog priority rules to molecules with up to four substituents

The **configuration** of a stereoisomer refers to the spatial arrangement of the atoms or groups in the molecule. The **relative configuration** of a chiral molecule is its configuration in relation to another chiral molecule (often through chemical interconversion). We can use the relative configuration to determine whether molecules are enantiomers, diastereomers, or the same molecule. On the other hand, the **absolute conformation** of a chiral molecule describes the exact spatial arrangement of these atoms or groups, independent of other molecules.

## (*E*) and (*Z*) Forms

(*E*) and (*Z*) nomenclature is used for compounds with polysubstituted double bonds. Recall that simpler double-bond-containing compounds can use the *cis–trans* system. To determine the (*E*)/(*Z*) designation, one starts by identifying the highest-priority substituent attached to each double-bonded carbon. Using the **Cahn–Ingold–Prelog priority rules**, priority is assigned based on the atom bonded to the double-bonded carbons: the higher the atomic number, the higher the priority. If the atomic numbers are equal, priority is determined by the next atoms outward; again, whichever group contains the atom with the highest atomic number is given top priority. If a tie remains, the atoms in this group are compared one-by-one in descending atomic number order until the tie is broken. The alkene is named (*Z*) (German: *zusammen*, "together") if the two highest-priority substituents on each carbon are on the same side of the double bond and (*E*) (*entgegen*, "opposite") if they are on opposite sides, as shown in Figure 2.17.

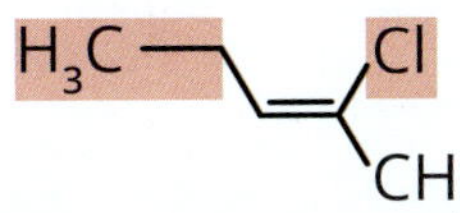


(*Z*)-2-chloro-2-pentene

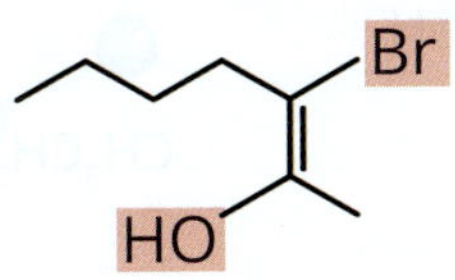


(*E*)-3-bromohept-2-ene-2-ol

**Figure 2.17** (*E*) and (*Z*) Designations of Alkenes

**MNEMONIC**

***Z*** = "**z**"ame side;
***E*** = "**e**"pposite side

## (*R*) and (*S*) Forms

(*R*) and (*S*) nomenclature is used for chiral (stereogenic) centers in molecules. We go through a set sequence to determine this absolute configuration:

### Step 1: Assign Priority

Using the Cahn–Ingold–Prelog priority rules described earlier, assign priority to the four substituents, looking only at the atoms directly attached to the chiral center. Once again, higher atomic number takes priority over lower atomic number. If the atomic numbers are equal, priority is determined by the combination of the atoms attached to these atoms; if there is a double bond, it is counted as two individual bonds to that atom. If a tie is encountered, work outward from the stereocenter until the tie is broken. An example is shown in Figure 2.18.

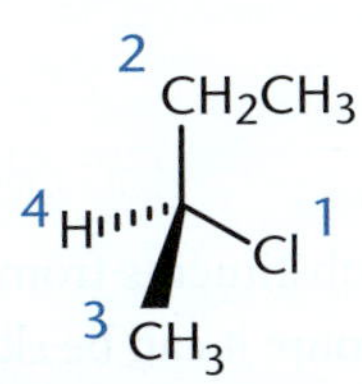


**Figure 2.18** Applying the Cahn–Ingold–Prelog Priority Rules to Determine Absolute Configuration
*Assign priority by the highest atomic number.*

### Step 2 (Classic Version): Arrange in Space

Orient the molecule in three-dimensional space so that the atom with the lowest priority (usually a hydrogen atom) is at the back of the molecule. Another way to think of this is to arrange the point of view so that the line of sight proceeds down the bond from the asymmetrical carbon atom (the chiral center) to the substituent with lowest priority. The three substituents with higher priority should then radiate out from the central carbon, coming out of the page, as shown in Figure 2.19.

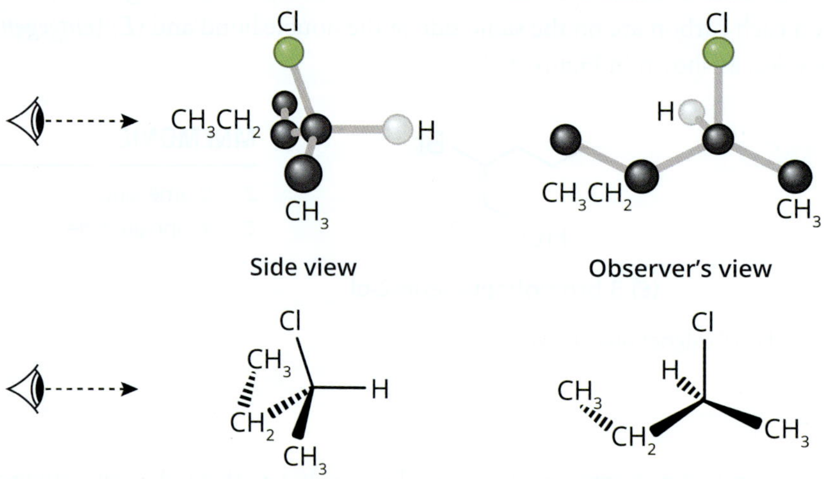


**Figure 2.19** Placing the Lowest-Priority Group in the Back

### Step 2 (Modified Version): Invert the Stereochemistry

If it is difficult to visualize rotating three-dimensional structures, one can simplify this process by remembering one simple rule: *any time two groups are switched on a chiral carbon, the stereochemistry is inverted.* By this logic, we can simply switch the lowest-priority group with the group at the back of the molecule (the substituent projecting into the page). We can then proceed to Step 3, keeping in mind that we have now changed the molecule to the opposite configuration. Therefore, if we use this modified step, we need to remember to switch our final answer (either (*R*) to (*S*), or (*S*) to (*R*)). This is a strategy we'll commonly use on Fischer diagrams, as described below.

### Step 3: Draw a Circle

Now, imagine drawing a circle connecting the substituents from number 1 to 2 to 3. Pay no attention to the lowest-priority group; it can be skipped because it projects directly into the page. If the circle is drawn counterclockwise, the asymmetric atom is called (**S**) (Latin: *sinister*, "left"). If it is clockwise, it is called (***R***) (*rectus*, "right"), as shown in Figure 2.20. Remember to correct the stereochemistry if the modified version of Step 2 was used.

**KEY CONCEPT**

When assigning priority, look only at the first atom attached to the chiral carbon, not at the group as a whole. The higher the atomic number of this first atom, the higher the priority—this same system is used to determine priority for both (*E*) and (*Z*) forms, as well as (*R*) and (*S*) forms.

**MNEMONIC**

A clockwise arrangement is like turning a steering wheel clockwise, which makes a car turn **R**ight—so the chirality at that center is (***R***).

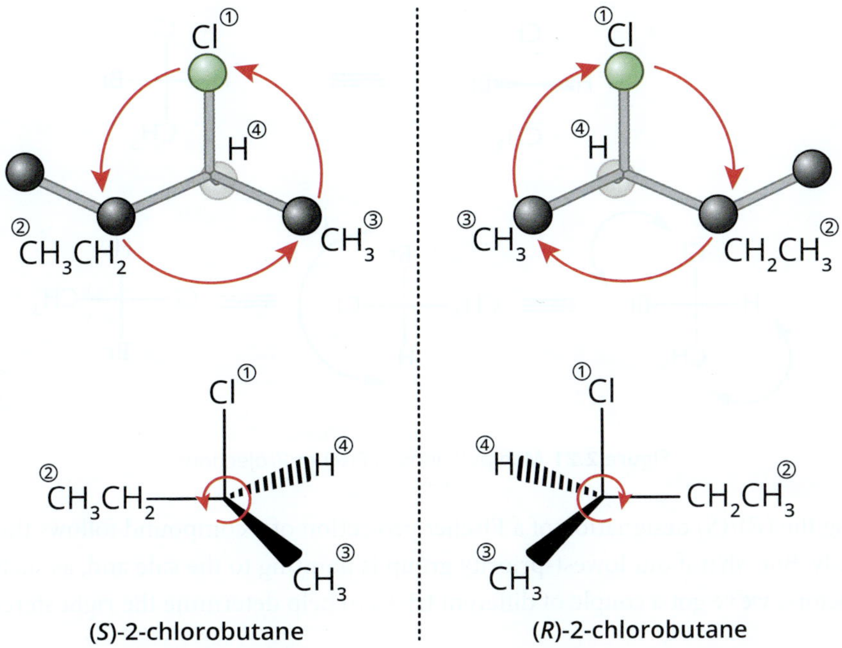


**Figure 2.20** Drawing a Circle to Determine Absolute Configuration
*Counterclockwise = (S); clockwise = (R)*

### Step 4: Write the Name

Once the (*R*)/(*S*) designation has been determined, the name can be written out. (*R*) and (*S*) are put in parentheses and separated from the rest of the name by a hyphen. If we have a compound with more than one chiral center, location is specified by a number preceding the *R* or *S* within the parentheses and without a hyphen.

## Fischer Projections

On the MCAT, one way to represent three-dimensional molecules is by a **Fischer projection**. In this system, horizontal lines indicate bonds that project out from the plane of the page (wedges), whereas vertical lines indicate bonds going into the plane of the page (dashes). The point of intersection of the lines represents a carbon atom.

**KEY CONCEPT**

To determine the absolute configuration at a chiral center:

1. Assign priority by atomic number
2. Arrange the molecule with the lowest-priority substituent in the back (or invert the stereochemistry by switching two substituents)
3. Draw a circle around the molecule from highest to lowest priority (1 to 2 to 3)
4. Clockwise = (*R*); counterclockwise = (*S*)

To determine configurations using Fischer projections, we follow the same rules listed above. Once again, we have to make sure that the lowest-priority group projects into the page. A benefit of Fischer projections is that the lowest-priority group can be on the top or bottom of the molecule and still project into the page.

Another advantage is that we can manipulate Fischer projections without changing the compound. As mentioned before, switching two substituents around a chiral carbon will invert the stereochemistry ((*R*) to (*S*), or (*S*) to (*R*)). Rotating a Fischer projection in the plane of the page by 90° will also invert the stereochemistry of the molecule. By extension, interchanging any *two* pairs of substituents will revert the compound back to its original stereochemistry, and rotating a Fischer projection in the plane of the page by 180° will also retain the stereochemistry of the molecule. These manipulations are shown in Figure 2.21.

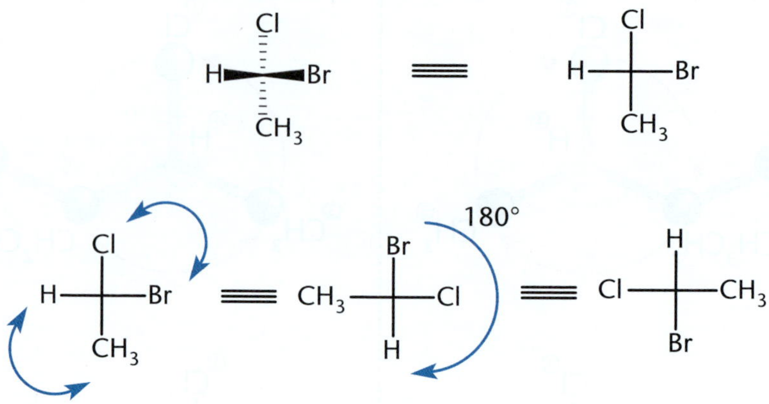


**Figure 2.21** Manipulations of Fischer Projections

Again, determining the (*R*)/(*S*) designation of a Fischer projection of a compound follows the same rules as described previously. But what if our lowest-priority group is pointing to the side and, as such, pointing out of the page? Just as before, we've got a couple of different tricks to help determine the right stereochemistry.

### Option 1: Make 0 Switches

Go ahead and determine the order of substituents as normal, drawing a circle from 1 to 2 to 3. Remember, number 4 doesn't count, so just skip right over it when determining the order. Then, obtain the (*R*)/(*S*) designation. The *true* designation will be the opposite of what you just obtained.

### Option 2: Make 1 Switch

Swap the lowest-priority group with one of the groups on the vertical axis. Obtain the (*R*)/(*S*) designation and, once again, the *true* designation will be the opposite of what you just found.

### Option 3: Make 2 Switches

In this method, start with option 2, moving the lowest-priority group into the correct position. Then, switch the other two groups as well. Because we made two switches, this molecule will have the *same* designation as the initial molecule. This is the same as holding one substituent in place and rotating the other three in order.

**MCAT EXPERTISE**

Determine which option you prefer for Fischer projection (*R*)/(*S*) designation and stick with it. It's more efficient to have a consistent method than to use all three interchangeably.

## MCAT CONCEPT CHECK 2.3

Before you move on, assess your understanding of the material with these questions.

1. How is priority assigned under the Cahn–Ingold–Prelog priority rules?

   ______________________________________________

2. Name the following compound using *E*/*Z* nomenclature:

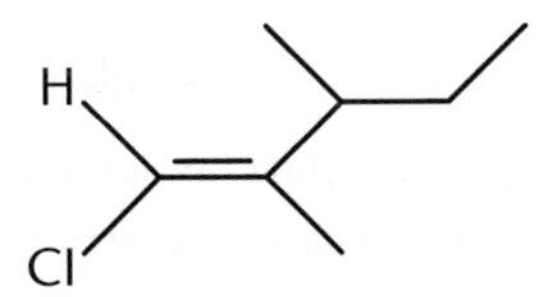


   ______________________________________________

3. For each of the Fischer projection manipulations listed below, is stereochemistry retained or inverted?
   - Switching a pair of substituents: ____________________
   - Switching two pairs of substituents: ____________________
   - Rotating the molecule 90°: ____________________
   - Rotating the molecule 180°: ____________________

## Conclusion

Throughout this chapter, we've seen just how many different molecules can be derived from the same molecular formula. This information is going to be essential on the MCAT—not only for questions on isomerism itself but on every single organic chemistry question you encounter. Most of the compounds we come across will have different possible isomers, and you need to be prepared to differentiate among them to find the one and only correct answer. In the next chapter, we'll explore how organic molecules are held together through discussions of hybridized orbitals and resonance.

### ▶ GO ONLINE

**You've reviewed the content, now test your knowledge and critical thinking skills by completing a test-like passage set in your online resources!**

# CONCEPT SUMMARY

## Structural Isomers

- **Structural isomers** share only a molecular formula.
- They have different physical and chemical properties.

## Stereoisomers

- **Conformational isomers** differ by rotation around a single ($\sigma$) bond.
  - **Staggered conformations** have groups 60° apart, as seen in a **Newman projection**. In ***anti*** **staggered** molecules, the two largest groups are 180° apart, and strain is minimized. In ***gauche*** **staggered** molecules, the two largest groups are 60° apart.
  - **Eclipsed conformations** have groups directly in front of each other as seen in a Newman projection. In **totally eclipsed conformations**, the two largest groups are directly in front of each other and strain is maximized.
  - The strain in cyclic molecules comes from **angle strain** (created by stretching or compressing angles from their normal size), **torsional strain** (from eclipsing conformations), and **nonbonded strain** (from interactions between substituents attached to nonadjacent carbons). Cyclic molecules will usually adopt nonplanar shapes to minimize this strain.
  - Substituents attached to cyclohexane can be classified as **axial** (sticking up or down from the plane of the molecule) or **equatorial** (in the plane of the molecule). Axial substituents create more nonbonded strain.
  - In cyclohexane molecules with multiple substituents, the largest substituent will usually take the equatorial position to minimize strain.
- **Configurational isomers** can only be interchanged by breaking and reforming bonds.
  - **Enantiomers** are nonsuperimposable mirror images and thus have opposite stereochemistry at every chiral carbon. They have the same chemical and physical properties except for rotation of plane-polarized light and reactions in a chiral environment.
  - **Optical activity** refers to the ability of a molecule to rotate plane-polarized light: d- or (+) molecules rotate light to the right; l- or (−) molecules rotate light to the left.
  - **Racemic mixtures**, with equal concentrations of two enantiomers, will not be optically active because the two enantiomers' rotations cancel each other out.
  - ***Meso*** **compounds**, with an internal plane of symmetry, will also be optically inactive because the two sides of the molecule cancel each other out.
  - **Diastereomers** are non-mirror-image stereoisomers. They differ at some, but not all, chiral centers. They have different chemical and physical properties.
  - ***Cis–trans*** isomers are a subtype of diastereomers in which groups differ in position about an immovable bond (such as a double bond or in a cycloalkane).
- **Chiral centers** have four different groups attached to the central carbon.

## Relative and Absolute Configurations

- **Relative configuration** gives the stereochemistry of a compound in comparison to another molecule.
- **Absolute configuration** gives the stereochemistry of a compound without having to compare to other molecules.
  - Absolute configuration uses the **Cahn–Ingold–Prelog priority rules**, in which priority is given by looking at the atoms connected to the chiral carbon or double-bonded carbons; whichever has the highest atomic number gets highest priority. If there is a tie, one moves outward from the chiral carbon or double-bonded carbon until the tie is broken.
- An alkene is (***Z***) if the highest-priority substituents are on the same side of the double bond and (***E***) if on opposite sides.
- A stereocenter's configuration is determined by putting the lowest priority group in the back and drawing a circle from group 1 to 2 to 3 in descending priority. If this circle is clockwise, the stereocenter is (***R***); if it is counterclockwise, the stereocenter is (***S***).
- Vertical lines in **Fischer diagrams** go into the plane of the page (dashes); horizontal lines come out of the plane of the page (wedges).
  - Switching one pair of substituents in a Fischer diagram inverts the stereochemistry of the chiral center. Switching two pairs retains the stereochemistry.
  - Rotating a Fischer diagram 90° inverts the stereochemistry of the chiral center. Rotating 180° retains the stereochemistry.

## ANSWERS TO CONCEPT CHECKS

### 2.1

1. Structural isomers share a molecular formula, and not necessarily anything else.
2. Cyclopropanol, acetone, and prop-2-ene-1-ol are all structural isomers of each other with the chemical formula $C_3H_6O$. 2-Propanol has the chemical formula $C_3H_8O$.
3. Physical properties are aspects of a compound that do not play a role in changing chemical composition. Examples include melting point, boiling point, solubility, odor, color, and density.
4. Chemical properties are aspects of a compound that change chemical composition; in organic chemistry, chemical properties are usually dictated by the reactivity of various functional groups.

### 2.2

1. Conformational isomers are stereoisomers with the same molecular connectivity at different points of rotation around a single bond. Configurational isomers are stereoisomers with differing molecular connectivity.
2. Enantiomers are nonsuperimposable mirror images. That means the molecules must be mirror images that are different from one another (superimposable mirror images represent the same object). The molecules on the top-left and bottom-right are nonsuperimposable mirror images and therefore enantiomers. The same is true for the top-right and bottom-left. All other combinations are diastereomeric because the pairs differ at some, but not all, stereocenters.
3. A *meso* compound contains chiral centers but also has an internal plane of symmetry. This means that the molecule is overall achiral and will not rotate plane-polarized light.
4. 

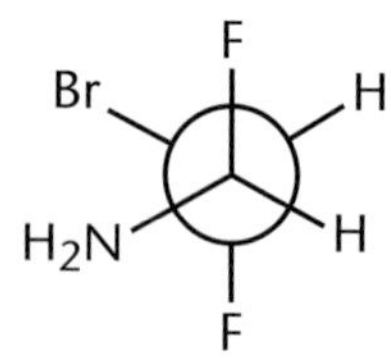


### 2.3

1. Priority is assigned by atomic number: the atom connected to the stereocenter or double-bonded carbon with the highest atomic number gets highest priority. If there is a tie, one works outward from the stereocenter or double-bonded carbon until the tie is broken.
2. The highest-priority functional group is an alkene, and the longest carbon chain that contains the double bond is five carbons long. So, the root will be *pent–* and the suffix will be *–ene*. There are three substituents: a chlorine and two methyls. Number the chain to give the double bond the lowest possible number, in this case from left to right. Bringing it all together gives 1-chloro-2,3-dimethyl-1-pentene. However, there are two possible configurations around the double bond. To determine (*E*)/(*Z*) designation, start by identifying the highest-priority substituents attached to each double-bonded carbon. The chlorine and butyl groups are the highest-priority substituents and are on opposite sides of the double bond (in addition to being on opposite ends of the double bond), so this molecule is (*E*)-1-chloro-2,3-dimethyl-1-pentene.
3. Switching a pair of substituents inverts stereochemistry; switching two pairs retains it. Rotating the molecule 90° inverts stereochemistry; rotating 180° retains it.

# SCIENCE MASTERY ASSESSMENT EXPLANATIONS

1. **D**

This is a racemic mixture of 2-butanol because it consists of equimolar amounts of (*R*)-2-butanol and (*S*)-2-butanol. The (*R*)-2-butanol molecule rotates the plane of polarized light in one direction, and the (*S*)-2-butanol rotates it by the same angle but in the opposite direction; as a result, no net rotation of polarized light is observed.

2. **B**

The maximum number of stereoisomers of a compound equals $2^n$, where *n* is the number of chiral carbons in the compound. In this molecule, C-1 (the aldehydic carbon) is not chiral, nor is C-5 (because it is attached to two hydrogen atoms). Therefore, with three chiral centers, there are $2^3 = 8$ stereoisomers.

3. **C**

This answer choice is an example of a *meso* compound—a compound that contains chiral centers but has an internal plane of symmetry:

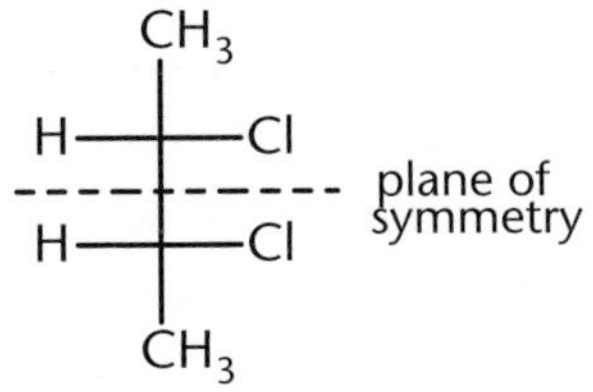


Owing to this internal plane of symmetry, the molecule is achiral and, hence, optically inactive. **(A)** and **(B)** are enantiomers of each other and will certainly show optical activity on their own. **(D)**, because it contains a chiral carbon and no internal plane of symmetry, is optically active as well.

4. **C**

To be considered a chiral center, a carbon must have four different substituents. There are eight stereocenters in this molecule, which are marked below with asterisks.

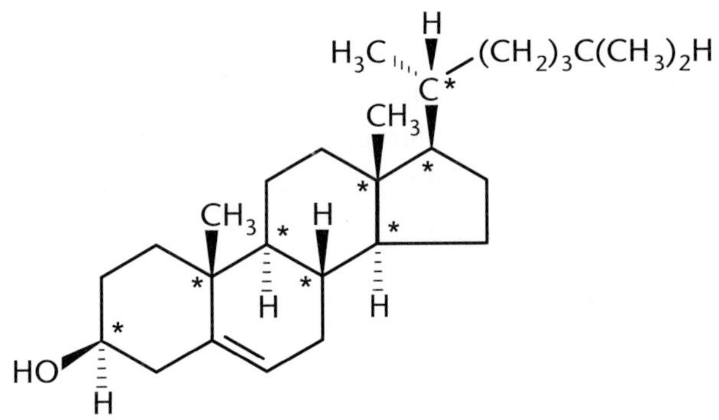


cholesterol

The other carbons are not chiral for various reasons. Many are bonded to two hydrogens; others participate in double bonds, which count as two bonds to the same atom.

5. **B**

This molecule is a chair conformation in which the two equatorial methyl groups are *trans* to each other. Because the axial methyl hydrogens do not compete for the same space as the hydrogens attached to the ring, this conformation ensures the least amount of steric strain. **(A)** would be less stable because the diaxial methyl group hydrogens are closer to the hydrogens on the ring, causing greater steric strain. **(C)** is incorrect because it is in the more unstable boat conformation.

6. **C**

The relative configuration is retained because the bonds of the stereocenter are not broken; thus, the positions of groups around the chiral carbon are maintained. The absolute configuration is also retained because both the reactant and product are (*R*).

7. **A**

These compounds are nonsuperimposable mirror images. To make analysis a bit easier, we can rotate structure II 180° to look like structure III. Structures I and III more clearly have opposite stereochemistry at every chiral center, meaning that they are enantiomers.

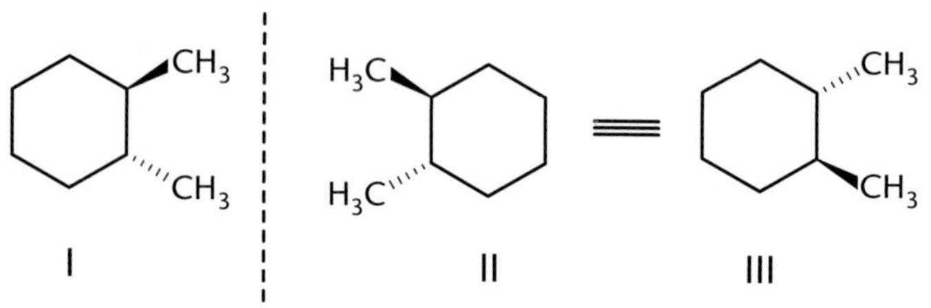


**(B)** is incorrect because diastereomers are stereoisomers that are not mirror images of each other. **(C)** is incorrect because *meso* compounds must contain a plane of symmetry, which neither of these molecules has. **(D)** is incorrect because structural isomers are compounds with the same molecular formula but different atomic connections. The connectivity in these two molecules is the same, which means that they are stereoisomers, not structural isomers.

8. **A**

(+)-Glyceraldehyde and (−)-glyceraldehyde, or (*R*)- and (*S*)-2,3-dihydroxypropanal, are enantiomers. Enantiomers are nonsuperimposable mirror images. Each has only one chiral center (C-2), which has opposite absolute configuration in these two molecules.

9. **C**

(*E*)-2-butene can also be called *trans*-2-butene; (*Z*)-2-butene can also be called *cis*-2-butene. As such, they are *cis–trans* isomers. Remember that *cis–trans* isomers are a subtype of diastereomers in which the position of substituents differs about an immovable bond. Diastereomers are molecules that are non-mirror-image stereoisomers (molecules with the same atomic connectivity). These are not enantiomers because they are not mirror images of each other.

10. **C**

Because they have the same molecular formula but different atomic connectivity, 3-methylpentane and hexane are constitutional isomers.

11. **B**

These two molecules are stereoisomers of one another, but are *not* nonsuperimposable mirror images. Therefore, they are diastereomers. Note that these molecules differ by at least one, but not all, chiral carbons.

12. **D**

Remember that the equation for specific rotation is $[\alpha] = \frac{\alpha_{obs}}{c \times l}$. In this example, $\alpha_{obs}$ is +12° (remember that dextrorotatory, or clockwise, rotation is considered positive), $c = 0.5\,\frac{g}{mL}$, $l = 1\text{ cm} = 0.1\text{ dm}$. Remember that path length is always measured in decimeters when calculating specific rotation. Therefore, the specific rotation can be calculated as:

$$[\alpha] = \frac{\alpha_{obs}}{c \times l} = \frac{+12}{\left(0.5\,\frac{g}{mL}\right) \times (0.1\text{ dm})} = +240°$$

13. **B**

Racemic mixtures like omeprazole contain equimolar amounts of two enantiomers and thus have no observed optical activity. Each of the two enantiomers causes rotation in opposite directions, so their effects cancel out. Esomeprazole only contains one of the two enantiomers and thus should cause rotation of plane-polarized light.

14. **C**

Draw out these structures. The two names describe the same molecule, which also happens to be a *meso* compound because it contains a plane of symmetry. These compounds are not enantiomers because they are superimposable mirror images of one another, *not* nonsuperimposable mirror images. These compounds are better termed *meso*-2,3-dihydroxybutanedioic acid:

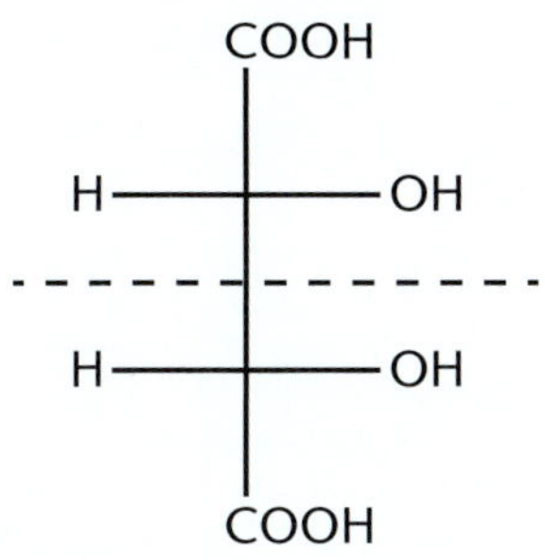


15. **C**

In butane, the position at which the two methyl groups are 120° apart is an eclipsed conformation. This has a moderate amount of energy, although not as high as a totally eclipsed conformation in which the two methyl groups are 0° apart.

**GO ONLINE**

**Consult your online resources for additional practice.**

## EQUATIONS TO REMEMBER

(2.1) **Specific rotation:** $[\alpha] = \frac{\alpha_{\text{obs}}}{c \times l}$

## SHARED CONCEPTS

**Biochemistry Chapter 1**
Amino Acids, Peptides, and Proteins

**Biochemistry Chapter 4**
Carbohydrate Structure and Function

**General Chemistry Chapter 3**
Bonding and Chemical Interactions

**Organic Chemistry Chapter 3**
Bonding

**Organic Chemistry Chapter 4**
Analyzing Organic Reactions

**Physics and Math Chapter 8**
Light and Optics

CHAPTER 3

# BONDING

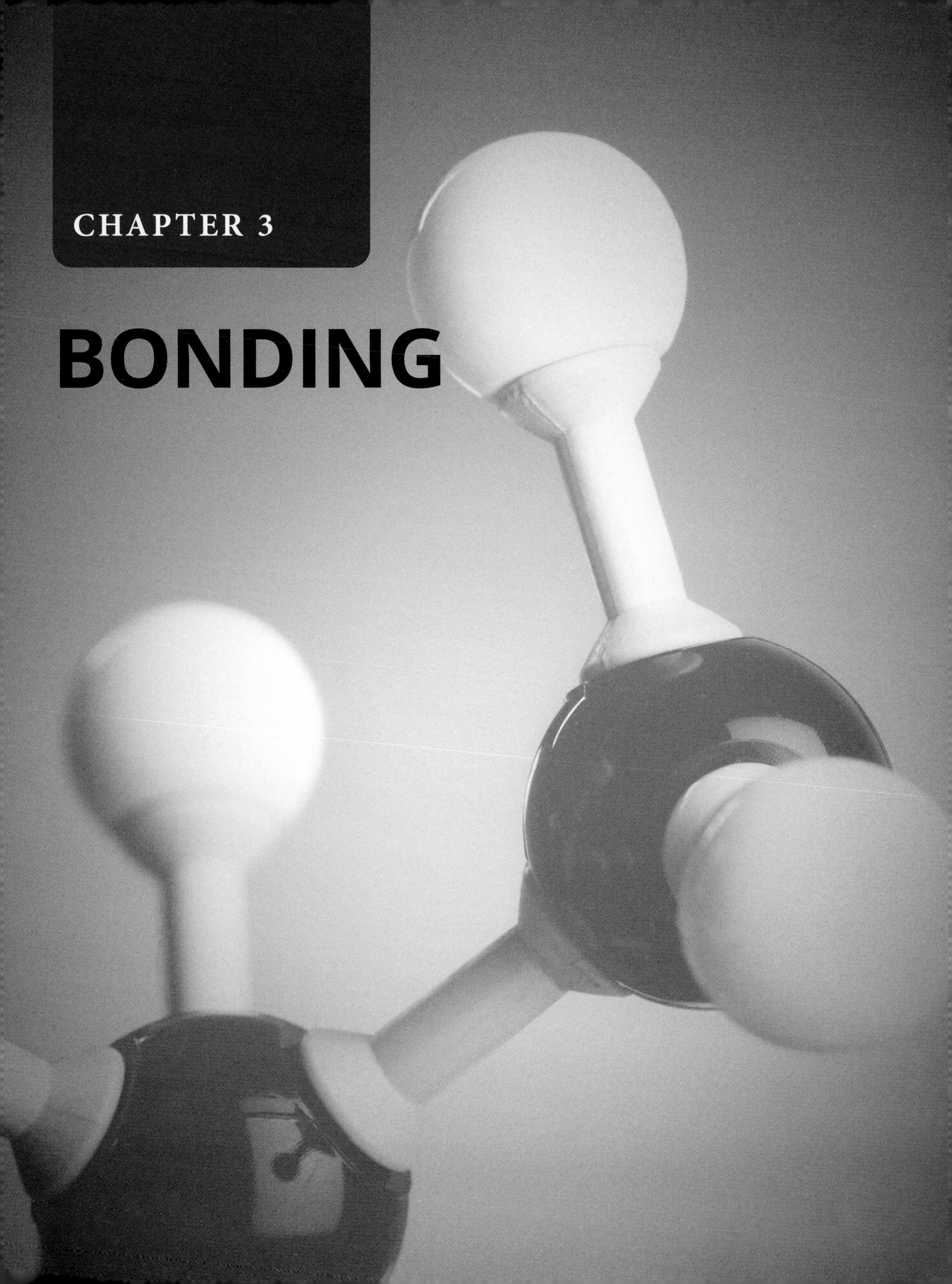

# SCIENCE MASTERY ASSESSMENT

Every pre-med knows this feeling: there is so much content I have to know for the MCAT! How do I know what to do first or what's important?

While the high-yield badges throughout this book will help you identify the most important topics, this Science Mastery Assessment is another tool in your MCAT prep arsenal. This quiz (which can also be taken in your online resources) and the guidance below will help ensure that you are spending the appropriate amount of time on this chapter based on your personal strengths and weaknesses. Don't worry though—skipping something now does not mean you'll never study it. Later on in your prep, as you complete full-length tests, you'll uncover specific pieces of content that you need to review and can come back to these chapters as appropriate.

## How to Use This Assessment

### If you answer 0–7 questions correctly:

Spend about 1 hour to read this chapter in full and take limited notes throughout. Follow up by reviewing **all** quiz questions to ensure that you now understand how to solve each one.

### If you answer 8–11 questions correctly:

Spend 20–40 minutes reviewing the quiz questions. Beginning with the questions you missed, read and take notes on the corresponding subchapters. For questions you answered correctly, ensure your thinking matches that of the explanation and you understand why each choice was correct or incorrect.

### If you answer 12–15 questions correctly:

Spend less than 20 minutes reviewing all questions from the quiz. If you missed any, then include a quick read-through of the corresponding subchapters, or even just the relevant content within a subchapter, as part of your question review. For questions you got correct, ensure your thinking matches that of the explanation and review the Concept Summary at the end of the chapter.

1. Within one principal energy level, which subshell has the least energy?
   - **A.** *s*
   - **B.** *p*
   - **C.** *d*
   - **D.** *f*

2. Which of the following compounds possesses at least one $\sigma$ bond?
   - **A.** $CH_4$
   - **B.** $C_2H_2$
   - **C.** $C_2H_4$
   - **D.** All of the above contain at least one $\sigma$ bond.

3. A carbon atom participates in one double bond. As such, this carbon contains orbitals with:
   - **A.** hybridization between the *s*-orbital and one *p*-orbital.
   - **B.** hybridization between the *s*-orbital and two *p*-orbitals.
   - **C.** hybridization between the *s*-orbital and three *p*-orbitals.
   - **D.** unhybridized *s* character.

4. The hybridizations of the carbon and nitrogen atoms in $CN^-$ are:
   - **A.** $sp^3$ and $sp^3$, respectively.
   - **B.** $sp^3$ and $sp$, respectively.
   - **C.** $sp$ and $sp^3$, respectively.
   - **D.** $sp$ and $sp$, respectively.

5. Which of the following hybridizations does the Be atom in $BeH_2$ assume?
   - **A.** $sp$
   - **B.** $sp^2$
   - **C.** $sp^3$
   - **D.** $sp^3d$

6. Two atomic orbitals may combine to form:
   - **I.** a bonding molecular orbital.
   - **II.** an antibonding molecular orbital.
   - **III.** hybridized orbitals.
   - **A.** I only
   - **B.** III only
   - **C.** I and II only
   - **D.** I, II, and III

7. Molecular orbitals can contain a maximum of:
   - **A.** one electron.
   - **B.** two electrons.
   - **C.** four electrons.
   - **D.** $2n^2$ electrons, where *n* is the principal quantum number of the combining atomic orbitals.

8. $\pi$ bonds are formed by which of the following orbitals?
   - **A.** Two *s*-orbitals
   - **B.** Two *p*-orbitals
   - **C.** One *s*- and one *p*-orbital
   - **D.** Two $sp^2$-hybridized orbitals

9. How many $\sigma$ bonds and $\pi$ bonds are present in the following compound?

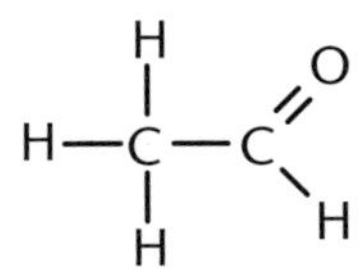


A. Six $\sigma$ bonds and one $\pi$ bond
B. Six $\sigma$ bonds and two $\pi$ bonds
C. Five $\sigma$ bonds and one $\pi$ bond
D. Five $\sigma$ bonds and two $\pi$ bonds

10. The four C–H bonds of $CH_4$ point toward the vertices of a tetrahedron. This indicates that the hybridization of the carbon atom in methane is:
A. *sp*.
B. $sp^2$.
C. $sp^3$.
D. $sp^3d$.

11. Why is a single bond stronger than a $\pi$ bond?
I. $\pi$ bonds have greater orbital overlap.
II. *s*-orbitals have more overlap than *p*-orbitals.
III. $sp^3$ hybridization is always unstable.
A. I only
B. II only
C. I and III only
D. II and III only

12. The *p* character of the bonds formed by the carbon atom in HCN is:
A. 25%.
B. 50%.
C. 67%.
D. 75%.

13. A resonance structure describes:
I. the hybrid of all possible structures that contribute to electron distribution.
II. a potential arrangement of electrons in a molecule.
III. the single form that the molecule most often takes.
A. I only
B. II only
C. I and II only
D. I, II, and III

14. An electron is known to be in the $n = 4$ shell and the $l = 2$ subshell. How many possible combinations of quantum numbers could this electron have?
A. 1
B. 2
C. 5
D. 10

15. Compared to single bonds, triple bonds are:
A. weaker.
B. longer.
C. made up of fewer $\sigma$ bonds.
D. more rigid.

## Answer Key

1. **A** (See section 3.1)
2. **D** (See section 3.3)
3. **B** (See section 3.2)
4. **D** (See section 3.3)
5. **A** (See section 3.3)
6. **D** (See section 3.2)
7. **B** (See section 3.2)
8. **B** (See section 3.2)
9. **A** (See section 3.3)
10. **C** (See section 3.3)
11. **B** (See section 3.3)
12. **B** (See section 3.3)
13. **B** (See section 3.3)
14. **D** (See section 3.1)
15. **D** (See section 3.3)

*The relevant section of the chapter to review for each question is given in parentheses after the correct answer. Detailed explanations can be found at the end of the chapter.*

CHAPTER 3

# BONDING

## In This Chapter



### CHAPTER PROFILE

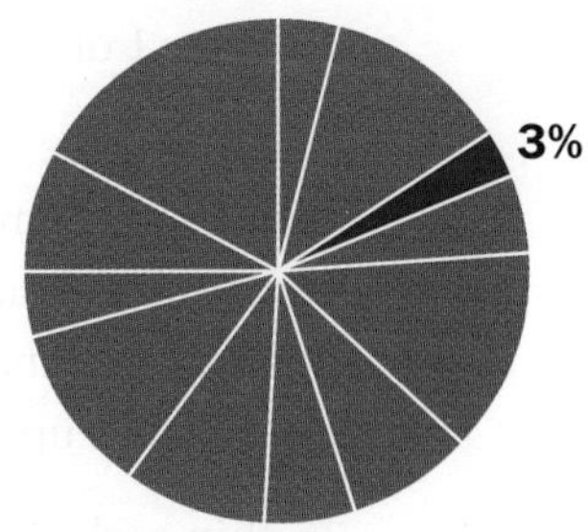


The content in this chapter should be relevant to about 3% of all questions about organic chemistry on the MCAT.

This chapter covers material from the following AAMC content categories:

**4E:** Atoms, nuclear decay, electronic structure, and atomic chemical behavior

**5B:** Nature of molecules and intermolecular interactions

## Introduction

Now that we have an understanding of nomenclature and how compounds are related, we are ready to start examining the real nature of chemical bonding. Bonding determines how atoms come together to form molecules. It also governs the ways those molecules interact with the other molecules in their environment.

Organic chemistry is the study of carbon and carbon-containing compounds. What makes carbon so special? The simple answer is that carbon has unique bonding properties. Carbon is tetravalent, which means that it can form bonds with up to four other atoms, allowing for the massive versatility required to form the foundation of biomolecules and life itself. This versatility is compounded by the fact that carbon, located near the center of the periodic table, can form bonds with many different elements because of its moderate electronegativity. In addition, because carbon atoms are fairly small, the bonds that they form are strong and stable.

Remember that there are two types of chemical bonds. The first is **ionic**, in which electrons are transferred from one atom to another and the resulting ions are held together by electrostatic interactions; the second is **covalent**, in which electrons are shared between atoms. Organic chemistry is deeply rooted in covalent bonding.

# 3.1 Atomic Orbitals and Quantum Numbers

## LEARNING OBJECTIVES

After Chapter 3.1, you will be able to:

- Describe the four quantum numbers, $n$, $l$, $m_l$, and $m_s$
- Provide ranges of possible values for each quantum number

Bonding occurs in the outermost electron shell of atoms, so an understanding of bonding is contingent on understanding the organization of electrons in an atom. Quantum numbers are discussed in detail in Chapter 1 of *MCAT General Chemistry Review*, and are briefly summarized here.

The first three quantum numbers, $n$, $l$, and $m_l$, describe the size, shape, number, and orientation of atomic orbitals an element possesses. The **principal quantum number**, $\boldsymbol{n}$, corresponds to the energy level of a given electron in an atom and is essentially a measure of size. The smaller the number, the closer the shell is to the nucleus, and the lower its energy. The possible values of $n$ range from 1 to $\infty$, although the MCAT only tests on $n$-values up to 7.

Within each electron shell, there can be several subshells. Subshells are described by the **azimuthal quantum number**, $\boldsymbol{l}$, which ranges from 0 to $n - 1$ for a given energy shell. The $l$-values 0, 1, 2, and 3 correspond to the $s$, $p$, $d$, and $f$ subshells, respectively. Just as with the principal quantum number, energy increases as the azimuthal quantum number increases.

Within each subshell, there may be several orbitals. Orbitals are described by the **magnetic quantum number**, $\boldsymbol{m_l}$, which ranges from $-l$ to $+l$ for a given subshell. Each type of atomic orbital has a specific shape, which describes the probability of finding an electron in a given region of space. An ***s*-orbital** is spherical and symmetrical, centered around the nucleus. A ***p*-orbital** is composed of two lobes located symmetrically about the nucleus and contains a **node**—an area where the probability of finding an electron is zero—at the nucleus. Picture the $p$-orbital as a dumbbell that can be positioned in three different orientations, along the $x$-, $y$-, or $z$-axis. It should make sense that there are three $p$-orbitals; the $p$ subshell has the $l$-value of 1, so there are three possible values for $m_l$: $-1$, 0, and 1. The shapes of the first five $s$- and $p$-orbitals are shown in Figure 3.1. A ***d*-orbital** is composed of four symmetrical lobes and contains two nodes. Four of the $d$-orbitals are clover-shaped, and the fifth looks like a donut wrapped around the center of a $p$-orbital. Thankfully, the multiple complex shapes of $d$- and $f$-orbitals are rarely encountered in organic chemistry. Each orbital can hold two electrons, which are distinguished by the **spin quantum number**, $\boldsymbol{m_s}$. The only values of $m_s$ are $\pm\frac{1}{2}$.

**BRIDGE**

Recall from Chapter 1 of *MCAT General Chemistry Review* that quantum numbers describe the location of an electron within an atom and that each electron has a unique combination of quantum numbers according to the Pauli exclusion principle.

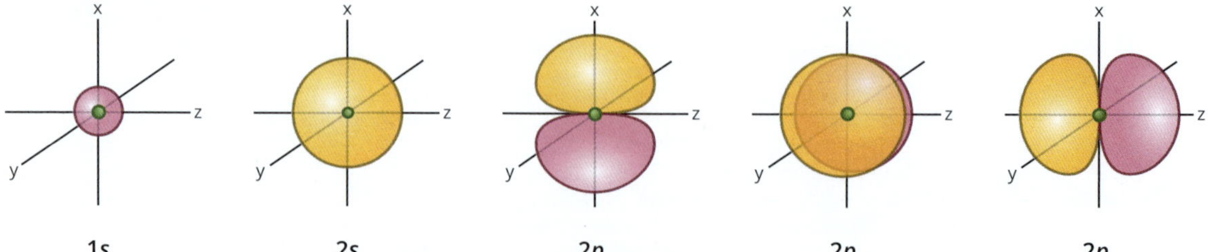


**Figure 3.1** The First Five Atomic Orbitals

## MCAT CONCEPT CHECK 3.1

Before you move on, assess your understanding of the material with this question.

1. Summarize the quantum numbers below. The first entry has been completed for clarification.

| Symbol | Name | Describes... | Organizational Level | Possible Values |
|---|---|---|---|---|
| $n$ | Principal QN | Size | Shell | 1 to $\infty$ |
| $l$ | | | | |
| $m_l$ | | | | |
| $m_s$ | | | | |

## 3.2 Molecular Orbitals

### LEARNING OBJECTIVES

After Chapter 3.2, you will be able to:

- Describe the stability and energy of bonding and antibonding orbitals
- Explain how the addition of a double or triple bond affects the electron density and molecular orbitals within a molecule
- Order the different orbital types based on strength

When two atomic orbitals combine, they form **molecular orbitals**. Molecular orbitals are obtained mathematically by adding or subtracting the wave functions of the atomic orbitals. While the mathematics of combining wave functions is outside the scope of the MCAT, some questions may ask for the visualization of molecular orbitals, as shown in Figure 3.2. If the signs of the wave functions are the same, a lower-energy (more stable) **bonding orbital** is produced. If the signs are different, a higher-energy (less stable) **antibonding orbital** is produced.

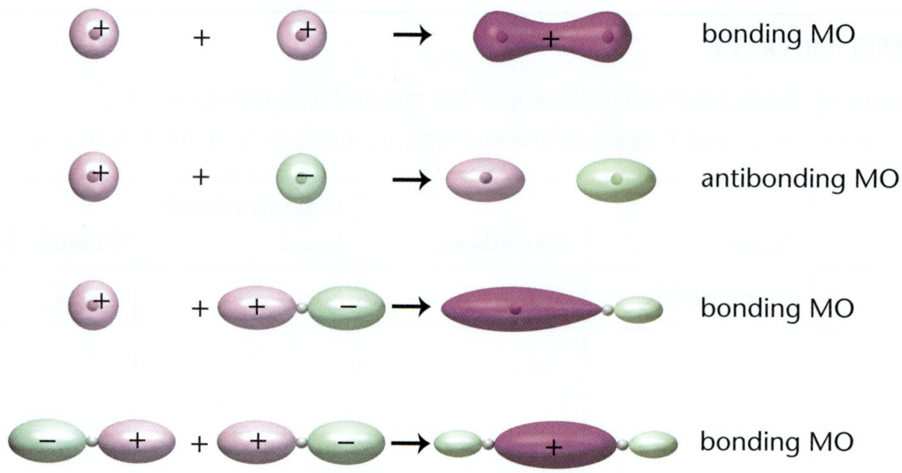


**Figure 3.2** Molecular Orbitals
*Molecular orbitals can be bonding or antibonding, depending on the signs of the atomic orbitals used to form them; head-to-head or tail-to-tail overlap of atomic orbitals results in a σ bond.*

## σ and π Bonds

When a molecular orbital is formed by head-to-head or tail-to-tail overlap, as in Figure 3.2, the resulting bond is called a **sigma (σ) bond**. All **single bonds** are σ bonds, accommodating two electrons.

When two *p*-orbitals line up in a parallel (side-by-side) fashion, their electron clouds overlap, and a bonding molecular orbital, called a **pi (π) bond**, is formed. This is demonstrated in Figure 3.3. One π bond on top of an existing σ bond is a **double bond**. A σ bond and two π bonds form a **triple bond**. Unlike single bonds, which allow free rotation of atoms around the bond axis, double and triple bonds hinder rotation and, in effect, lock the atoms into position.

**KEY CONCEPT**

Sigma (σ) bonds are formed by head-to-head or tail-to-tail overlap of atomic orbitals. These bonds are by far the most common in organic compounds and on the MCAT.

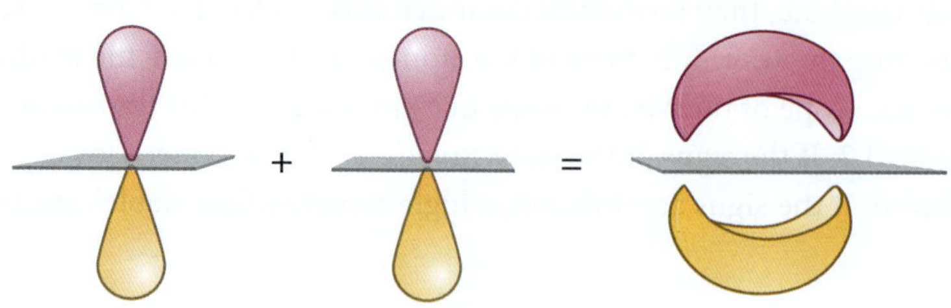


**Figure 3.3** Pi (π) Bond
*Electron density exists above and below the plane of the molecule, restricting rotation about a double bond.*

It is important to remember that a π bond cannot exist independently of a σ bond. Only after the formation of a σ bond will the *p*-orbitals of adjacent carbons be parallel and in position to form the π bond. The more bonds that are formed between atoms, the shorter the overall bond length. Therefore, a double bond is shorter than a single bond, and a triple bond is shorter than a double bond. Shorter bonds hold atoms more closely together and are stronger than longer bonds; shorter bonds require more energy to break.

While double bonds are stronger than single bonds overall, individual $\pi$ bonds are weaker than $\sigma$ bonds. Therefore, it is possible to break only one of the bonds in a double bond, leaving a single bond intact. This happens often in organic chemistry, such as when *cis–trans* isomers are interconverted between conformations. Breaking a single bond requires far more energy.

As discussed previously, double and triple bonds do not freely rotate like single bonds. As such, double bonds in compounds make for stiffer molecules. Partial double-bond character in structures with resonance also restricts free rotation, resulting in more rigid structures. Proteins exhibit this kind of limited rotation because there is resonance in the amide linkages between adjacent amino acids.

**KEY CONCEPT**

A double bond consists of both a $\sigma$ bond and a $\pi$ bond; a triple bond consists of a $\sigma$ bond and two $\pi$ bonds. $\pi$ bonds are weaker than $\sigma$ bonds, but the strength is additive, making double and triple bonds stronger overall than single bonds.

## MCAT CONCEPT CHECK 3.2

Before you move on, assess your understanding of the material with these questions.

1. Which is more stable: a bonding orbital or an antibonding orbital? Which has higher energy?
   - More stable:

     ________________________________________
   - Higher energy:

     ________________________________________
2. What differences would be observed in a molecule containing a double bond compared to the same molecule containing only single bonds?

   ________________________________________
3. Rank the following orbitals in decreasing order of strength: $\sigma$ bond, $\pi$ bond, double bond, triple bond.

   ____________ > ____________ > ____________ > ____________.

# 3.3 Hybridization

## LEARNING OBJECTIVES

After Chapter 3.3, you will be able to:

- Recall the percentage of *s* character present in a given hybridization level, such as $sp^2$
- Describe the relationship between electron density and resonance structures
- Identify the hybridization of an atom within a complex molecule:

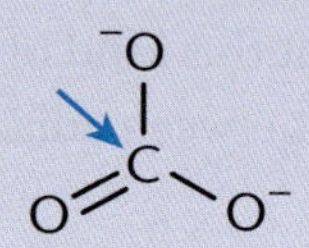

Carbon has the electron configuration $1s^22s^22p^2$ and therefore needs four electrons to complete its octet ($2s^22p^6$). A typical molecule formed by carbon is methane, $CH_4$. Experimentation shows that the four $\sigma$ bonds in methane are equivalent. This may seem inconsistent with what we know about the asymmetrical distribution of carbon's valence electrons: two electrons in the 2*s*-orbital, one in the $p_x$-orbital, one in the $p_y$-orbital, and none in the $p_z$-orbital. This apparent discrepancy is accounted for by the theory of orbital **hybridization.**

## $sp^3$

**Hybrid orbitals** are formed by mixing different types of orbitals. Just as with molecular orbitals, we can use advanced mathematics to merge three *p*-orbitals and one *s*-orbital. The result? As shown in Figure 3.4, this forms four identical $sp^3$ orbitals with new, hybridized shapes.

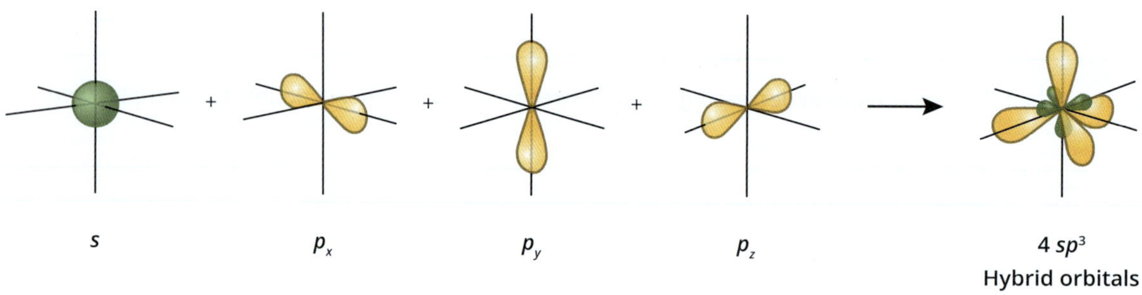


**Figure 3.4** $sp^3$-Hybridized Orbitals
*An atom with these orbitals has tetrahedral geometry, and there are no unhybridized* p*-orbitals to form* $\pi$ *bonds.*

All four of these orbitals point toward the vertices of a tetrahedron to minimize repulsion, which explains why carbon prefers tetrahedral geometry. The hybridization is accomplished by promoting one of the 2*s* electrons into the $2p_z$-orbital, as shown in Figure 3.5. This produces four valence orbitals, each with one electron, which can be mathematically mixed to model the hybrid orbitals.

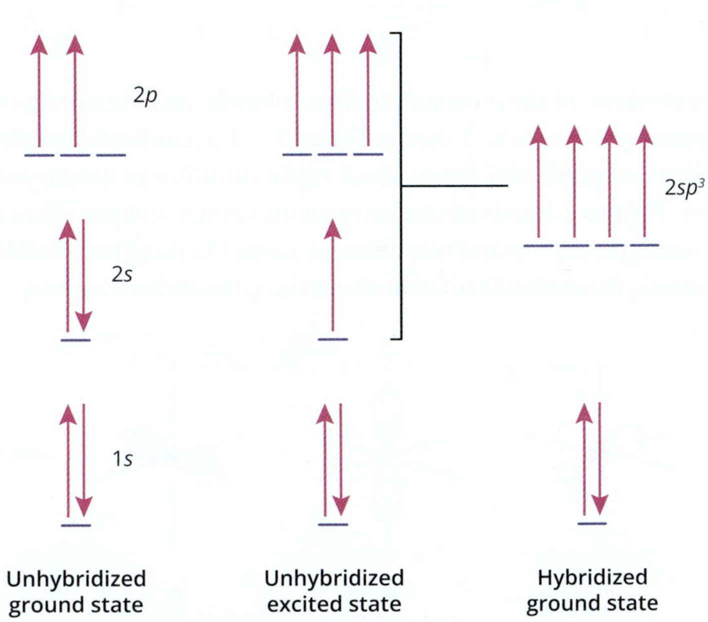


**Figure 3.5** Hybridization of Carbon Orbitals

#### KEY CONCEPT

Hybridization is a way of making all of the bonds to a central atom equivalent to each other. The $sp^3$ orbitals are the reason for the tetrahedral shape that is a hallmark of carbon-containing compounds.

The MCAT sometimes tests how much "*s* character" a certain hybrid orbital has. To answer such questions, we simply need to determine what type of hybridization exists and use the name to solve the problem. For example, in $sp^3$ orbitals, we have one *s*- and three *p*-orbitals, so the bond has 25% *s* character and 75% *p* character.

## $sp^2$

Although carbon is most often bonded with $sp^3$ hybridization, there are two other possibilities. When one *s*-orbital is mixed with two *p*-orbitals, three $sp^2$-hybridized orbitals are formed, as shown in Figure 3.6. These orbitals have 33% *s* character and 67% *p* character.

This is the hybridization seen in alkenes. The third *p*-orbital of each carbon is left unhybridized. This is the orbital that participates in the $\pi$ bond. The three $sp^2$ orbitals are oriented 120° apart, which allows for maximum separation. We know that the unhybridized *p*-orbital is involved in the $\pi$ component of the double bond, but what about the hybrid orbitals? In ethene, two of the $sp^2$ hybridized orbitals will participate in C—H bonds, and the other hybrid orbital will line up with the $\pi$ bond and form the $\sigma$ component of the C=C double bond.

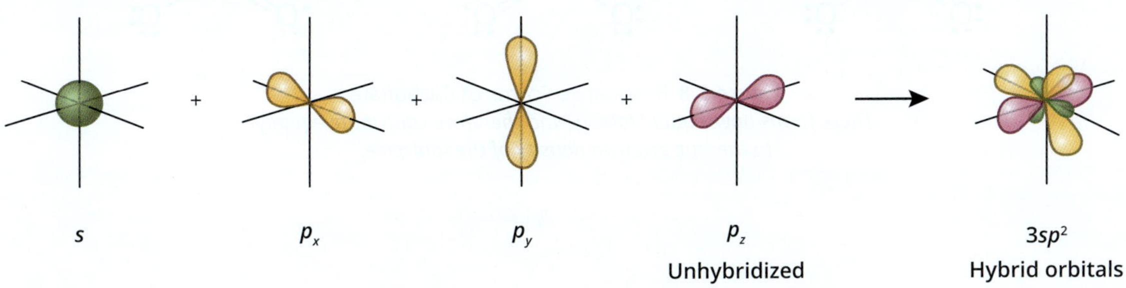


**Figure 3.6** $sp^2$-Hybridized Orbitals
*A molecule with these orbitals has trigonal planar geometry, and the one unhybridized* p*-orbital can be used to form a* $\pi$ *bond.*

### *sp*

To form a triple bond, we need two of the *p*-orbitals to form $\pi$ bonds, and the third *p*-orbital will combine with the *s*-orbital to form two *sp*-orbitals, as shown in Figure 3.7. These orbitals have 50% *s* character and 50% *p* character. These orbitals are oriented 180° apart, which explains the linear structure of molecules containing *sp*-hybridized carbons. The two $\pi$ bonds can be between the carbon and one other atom (forming a triple bond, like ethyne), or between the carbon and two different atoms (forming two double bonds in a row, like carbon dioxide). In both cases, the molecule is linear about the *sp*-hybridized carbon.

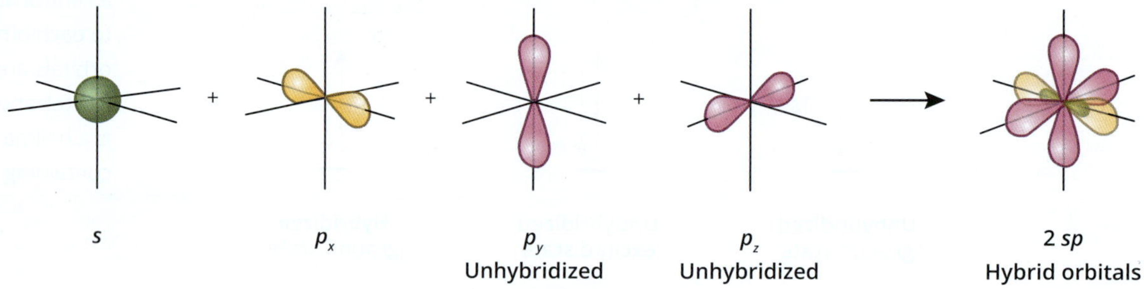


**Figure 3.7** *sp*-Hybridized Orbitals
*A molecule with these orbitals has linear geometry, and the two unhybridized* p-orbitals *can be used to form $\pi$ bonds.*

## Resonance

Resonance delocalization of electrons occurs in molecules that have conjugated bonds. **Conjugation** requires alternating single and multiple bonds because this pattern aligns a number of unhybridized *p*-orbitals down the backbone of the molecule. $\pi$ electrons can then delocalize through this *p*-orbital system, adding stability to the molecule. Resonance structures are drawn as the various transient forms the molecule takes, as shown in Figure 3.8.

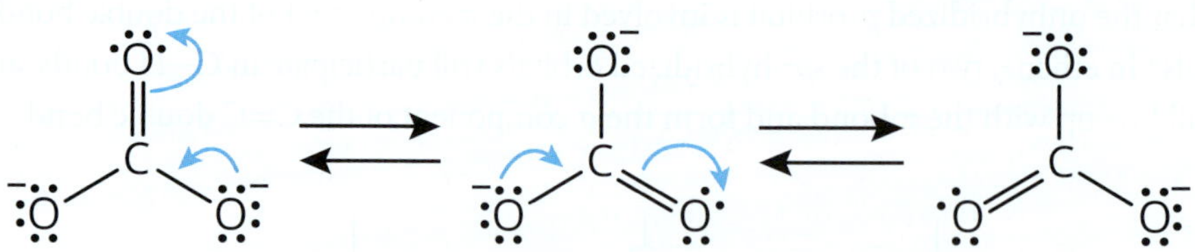

**Figure 3.8** Resonance Forms of Carbonate
*These forms have equal stability and therefore contribute equally to the true electron density of the molecule.*

However, these forms aren't in any sort of equilibrium—the electron density is distributed throughout, making the true form a hybrid of the resonance structures, as shown with ozone in Figure 3.9.

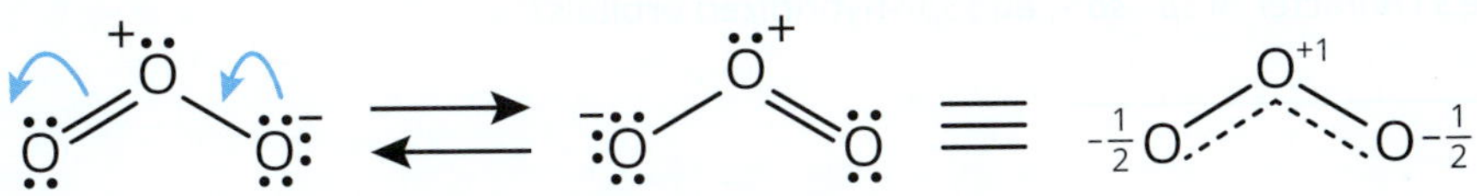

**Figure 3.9** Structure of Ozone
*The true electron density of ozone is somewhere between the two resonance forms, creating 1.5 bonds between each oxygen, and leaving each oxygen with a $-\frac{1}{2}$ charge.*

If the stabilities of the various resonance forms differ, then the true electron density will favor the most stable form. As demonstrated in Figure 3.10, particular resonance structures can be favored because they lack formal charges or form full octets on highly electronegative atoms like oxygen and nitrogen. Stabilization of positive and negative charges through induction and aromaticity can also favor certain resonance structures.

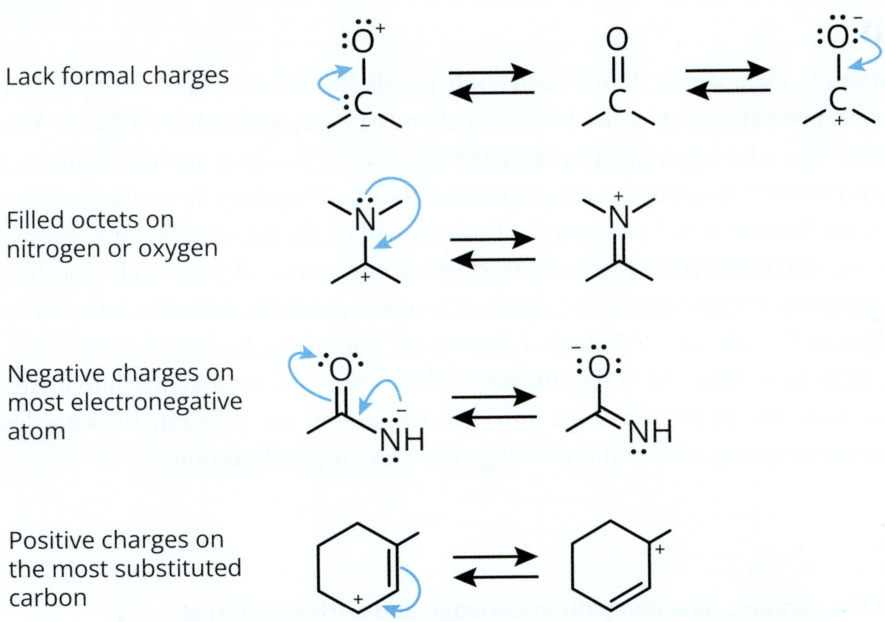


**Figure 3.10** Stabilization of Charges Favors Various Resonance Forms
*Moving from left to right, the second molecule in each row is more stable.*

## MCAT CONCEPT CHECK 3.3

Before you move on, assess your understanding of the material with these questions.

1. What is the *s* character of *sp*-, $sp^2$-, and $sp^3$-hybridized orbitals?
   - *sp*: ______________________
   - $sp^2$: ______________________
   - $sp^3$: ______________________
2. What are resonance structures? How does the true electron density of a compound relate to its resonance structures?

   ______________________________________________

## Conclusion

The ability of carbon to form single, double, and triple bonds (or to form $\sigma$ and multiple $\pi$ bonds) and to form hybrid orbitals gives rise to an entire branch of chemistry—as well as life on Earth. You may have thought this chapter was a bit brief; that's because the specifics of bonding fall mostly under the domain of general chemistry. However, without a solid grasp of orbitals and bonding, it would be difficult to explain the organic reactions that are tested on the MCAT, which will be the focus of the next seven chapters. Avoid compartmentalizing the information you learn throughout the course of your studies, as bonding plays a role in general chemistry, organic chemistry, and biochemistry, and can therefore be tested in either the *Chemical and Physical Foundations of Biological Systems* section or the *Biological and Biochemical Foundations of Living Systems* section. All of the subjects within science blend together into a seemingly complicated, yet beautifully simple, picture of the universe. The sooner you integrate the knowledge you're accumulating, the more manageable and rewarding your studying will become.

### GO ONLINE

**You've reviewed the content, now test your knowledge and critical thinking skills by completing a test-like passage set in your online resources!**

# CONCEPT SUMMARY

## Atomic Orbitals and Quantum Numbers

- **Quantum numbers** describe the size, shape, orientation, and number of **atomic orbitals** an element possesses.
- The **principal quantum number, *n***, describes the energy level (shell) in which an electron resides and indicates the distance from the nucleus to the electron. Its possible values range from 1 to $\infty$.
- The **azimuthal quantum number, *l***, determines the subshell in which an electron resides. Its possible values range from 0 to $n - 1$. The subshell is often indicated with a letter: $l = 0$ corresponds to *s*, 1 is *p*, 2 is *d*, and 3 is *f*.
- The **magnetic quantum number, $m_l$**, determines the orbital in which an electron resides. Its possible values range from $-l$ to $+l$. Different orbitals have different shapes: *s*-orbitals are spherical, while *p*-orbitals are dumbbell-shaped and located on the *x*-, *y*-, or *z*-axis.
- The **spin quantum number, $m_s$**, describes the spin of an electron. Its possible values are $\pm\frac{1}{2}$.

## Molecular Orbitals

- **Bonding orbitals** are created by head-to-head or tail-to-tail overlap of atomic orbitals of the same sign and are energetically favorable.
- **Antibonding orbitals** are created by head-to-head or tail-to-tail overlap of atomic orbitals that have opposite signs and are energetically unfavorable.
- **Single bonds** are **sigma ($\sigma$) bonds**, which contain two electrons.
- **Double bonds** contain one $\sigma$ bond and one **pi ($\pi$) bond**. $\pi$ bonds are created by sharing of electrons between two unhybridized *p*-orbitals that align side-by-side.
- **Triple bonds** contain one $\sigma$ bond and two $\pi$ bonds.
- Multiple bonds are less flexible than single bonds because rotation is not permitted in the presence of a $\pi$ bond. Multiple bonds are shorter and stronger than single bonds, although individual $\pi$ bonds are weaker than $\sigma$ bonds.

## Hybridization

- ***sp*$^3$-hybridized orbitals** have 25% *s* character and 75% *p* character. They form tetrahedral geometry with 109.5° bond angles. Carbons with all single bonds are *sp*$^3$-hybridized.
- ***sp*$^2$-hybridized orbitals** have 33% *s* character and 67% *p* character. They form trigonal planar geometry with 120° bond angles. Carbons with one double bond are *sp*$^2$-hybridized.
- ***sp*-hybridized orbitals** have 50% *s* character and 50% *p* character. They form linear geometry with 180° bond angles. Carbons with a triple bond, or with two double bonds, are *sp*-hybridized.
- **Resonance** describes the delocalization of electrons in molecules that have conjugated bonds.
  - **Conjugation** occurs when single and multiple bonds alternate, creating a system of unhybridized *p*-orbitals down the backbone of the molecule through which $\pi$ electrons can delocalize.
  - Resonance increases the stability of a molecule.
  - The various resonance forms all contribute to the true electron density of the molecule; the more stable the resonance form, the more it contributes. Resonance forms are favored if they lack formal charge, form full octets on electronegative atoms, or stabilize charges through induction and aromaticity.

## ANSWERS TO CONCEPT CHECKS

### 3.1

1.

| Symbol | Name | Describes... | Organizational Level | Possible Values |
|---|---|---|---|---|
| $n$ | Principal QN | Size | Shell | 1 to $\infty$ |
| $l$ | Azimuthal QN | Shape | Subshell | 0 to $n - 1$ |
| $m_l$ | Magnetic QN | Orientation | Orbital | $-l$ to $+l$ |
| $m_s$ | Spin QN | Spin | — | $\pm\frac{1}{2}$ |

### 3.2

1. Bonding orbitals are more stable than antibonding orbitals. Therefore, antibonding orbitals have higher energy than bonding orbitals.
2. The differences would be in bond length (shorter in double bond than single), bond energy (higher in double bond than single), and molecular rigidity (higher in double bond than single).
3. Triple bond > double bond > $\sigma$ bond > $\pi$ bond. Remember that while an individual $\pi$ bond is weaker than a $\sigma$ bond, bond strength is additive. Therefore, double bonds are stronger than single, and triple bonds are stronger still.

### 3.3

1. *sp* orbitals have 50% *s* character and 50% *p* character, $sp^2$ orbitals have 33% *s* character and 67% *p* character, and $sp^3$ orbitals have 25% *s* character and 75% *p* character.
2. Resonance structures differ in their placement of electrons in hybridized *p*-orbitals and require bond conjugation to delocalize electrons in a molecule. The true electron density is a weighted average of the resonance structures of a given compound, favoring the most stable structures.

# SCIENCE MASTERY ASSESSMENT EXPLANATIONS

1. **A**

The energies of the subshells within a principal quantum number are as follows: $s < p < d < f$

2. **D**

All single bonds are $\sigma$ bonds; double and triple bonds each contain one $\sigma$ bond and one or two $\pi$ bonds, respectively. The compounds $CH_4$, $C_2H_2$, and $C_2H_4$ all contain at least one single bond and therefore contain at least one $\sigma$ bond.

3. **B**

In a carbon with one double bond, $sp^2$ hybridization occurs—that is, one *s*-orbital hybridizes with two *p*-orbitals to form three $sp^2$-hybridized orbitals. The third *p*-orbital of the carbon atom remains unhybridized and takes part in the formation of the $\pi$ bond of the double bond. Although there is an unhybridized *p*-orbital, there are no unhybridized *s*-orbitals, eliminating **(D)**.

4. **D**

The carbon and nitrogen atoms are connected by a triple bond in $CN^-$ (:C≡N:$^-$). A triple-bonded atom is *sp* hybridized; one *s*-orbital hybridizes with one *p*-orbital to form two *sp*-hybridized orbitals. The two remaining unhybridized *p*-orbitals take part in the formation of two $\pi$ bonds.

5. **A**

Beryllium has only two electrons in its valence shell. When it bonds to two hydrogens, it requires two hybridized orbitals, meaning that its hybridization must be *sp*. Note that the presence of only single bonds does not mean that the hybridization must be $sp^3$; this is a useful assumption for carbon, but does not apply to beryllium because of its smaller number of valence electrons. The two unhybridized *p*-orbitals around beryllium are empty in $BeH_2$, which takes on the linear geometry characteristic of *sp*-hybridized orbitals.

6. **D**

When atomic orbitals combine, they form molecular orbitals. When two atomic orbitals with the same sign are added head-to-head or tail-to-tail, they form bonding molecular orbitals. When two atomic orbitals with opposite signs are added head-to-head or tail-to-tail, they form antibonding molecular orbitals. Atomic orbitals can also hybridize, forming $sp^3$, $sp^2$, or *sp* orbitals.

7. **B**

Like atomic orbitals, molecular orbitals each can contain a maximum of two electrons with opposite spins. The $2n^2$ rule in **(D)** refers to the total number of electrons that can exist in a given energy shell, not in a molecular orbital.

8. **B**

$\pi$ bonds are formed by the parallel overlap of unhybridized *p*-orbitals. The electron density is concentrated above and below the bonding axis. A $\sigma$ bond, on the other hand, can be formed by the head-to-head overlap of two *s*-orbitals or hybridized orbitals. In a $\sigma$ bond, the density of the electrons is concentrated between the two nuclei of the bonding atoms.

9. **A**

Each single bond has one $\sigma$ bond, and each double bond has one $\sigma$ and one $\pi$ bond. In this question, there are five single bonds (five $\sigma$ bonds) and one double bond (one $\sigma$ bond and one $\pi$ bond), which gives a total of six $\sigma$ bonds and one $\pi$ bond. Thus, the correct answer is **(A)**.

10. **C**

The four bonds point to the vertices of a tetrahedron, which means that the angle between two bonds is 109.5°, a characteristic of $sp^3$ orbitals. Hence, the carbon atom of $CH_4$ is $sp^3$-hybridized.

11. **B**

Bond strength is determined by the degree of orbital overlap; the greater the overlap, the greater the bond strength. A $\pi$ bond is weaker than a single bond because there is significantly less overlap between the unhybridized *p*-orbitals of a $\pi$ bond (due to their parallel orientation) than between the *s*-orbitals or hybrid orbitals of a $\sigma$ bond. $sp^3$-hybridized orbitals can be quite stable, as evidenced by the number of carbon atoms with this hybridization forming stable compounds.

12. **B**

The carbon bond in hydrogen cyanide ($H{-}C{\equiv}N{:}$) is triple-bonded, and because triple bonds require two unhybridized *p*-orbitals, the carbon must be *sp*-hybridized; *sp*-hybridized orbitals have 50% *s* character and 50% *p* character.

13. **B**

A resonance structure describes an arrangement of electrons in a molecule. Different resonance structures can be derived by moving electrons in unhybridized *p*-orbitals throughout a molecule containing conjugated bonds. In molecules that contain multiple resonance structures, some are usually more stable than others; however, each resonance structure is not necessarily the most common form a molecule takes, eliminating statement III. Statement I has reversed the terminology for resonance structures: the electron density in a molecule is the weighted average of all possible resonance structures, not the other way around.

14. **D**

An electron in the $n = 4$ shell and the $l = 2$ subshell can have five different values for $m_l$: $-2, -1, 0, 1$, or 2. In each of these orbitals, electrons can have positive or negative spin. Thus, there are $5 \times 2 = 10$ possible combinations of quantum numbers for this electron.

15. **D**

$\pi$ bonds do not permit free rotation, unlike $\sigma$ bonds; this makes triple bonds more rigid than single bonds. Triple bonds are stronger and shorter bonds than single bonds, eliminating **(A)** and **(B)**. Both single and triple bonds contain one $\sigma$ bond, eliminating **(C)**.

**GO ONLINE**

**Consult your online resources for additional practice.**

## SHARED CONCEPTS

**Biochemistry Chapter 1**
Amino Acids, Peptides, and Proteins

**General Chemistry Chapter 1**
Atomic Structure

**General Chemistry Chapter 3**
Bonding and Chemical Interactions

**General Chemistry Chapter 4**
Compounds and Stoichiometry

**Organic Chemistry Chapter 2**
Isomers

**Organic Chemistry Chapter 11**
Spectroscopy

CHAPTER 4

# ANALYZING ORGANIC REACTIONS

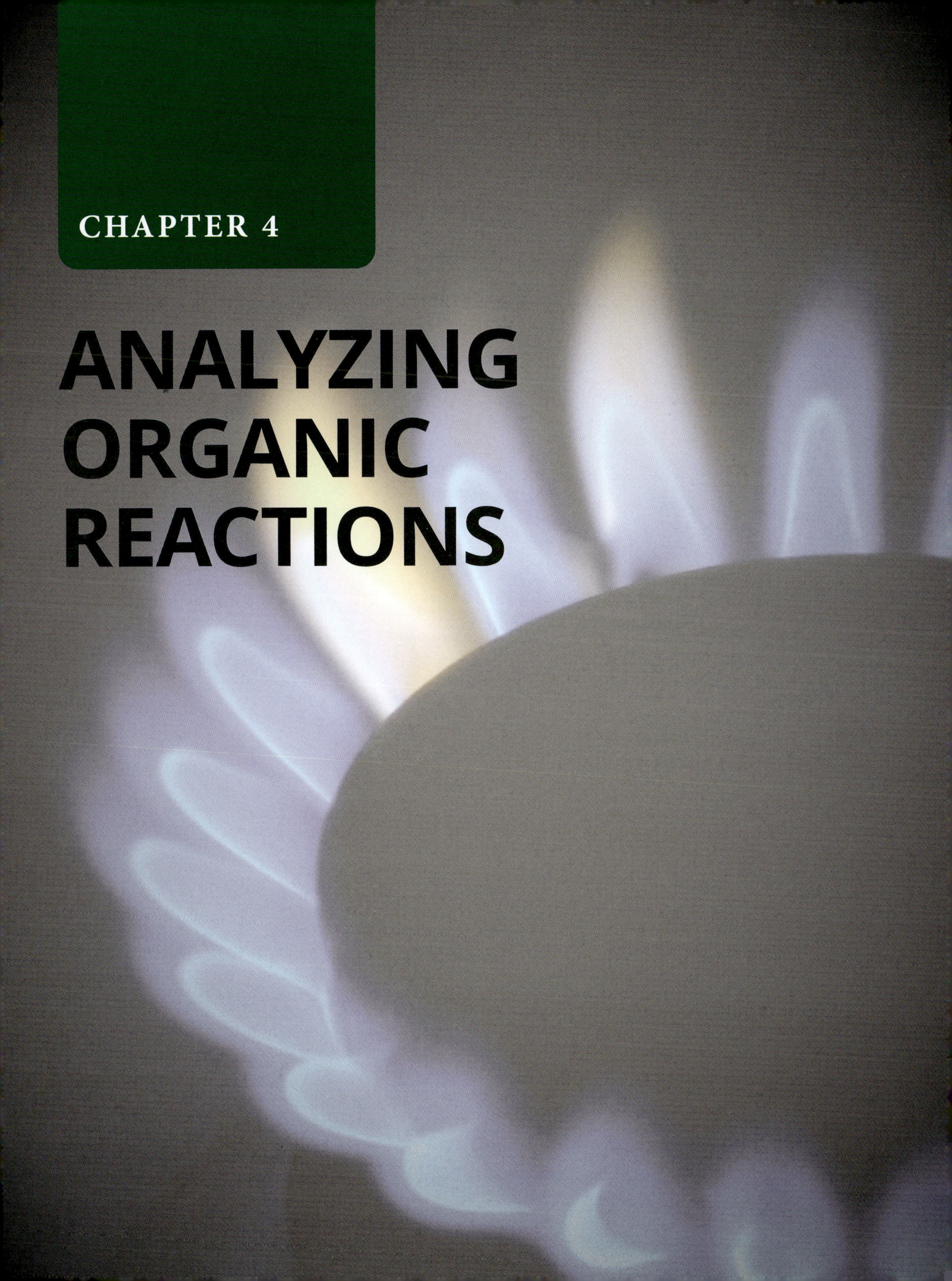

# SCIENCE MASTERY ASSESSMENT

Every pre-med knows this feeling: there is so much content I have to know for the MCAT! How do I know what to do first or what's important?

While the high-yield badges throughout this book will help you identify the most important topics, this Science Mastery Assessment is another tool in your MCAT prep arsenal. This quiz (which can also be taken in your online resources) and the guidance below will help ensure that you are spending the appropriate amount of time on this chapter based on your personal strengths and weaknesses. Don't worry though—skipping something now does not mean you'll never study it. Later on in your prep, as you complete full-length tests, you'll uncover specific pieces of content that you need to review and can come back to these chapters as appropriate.

## How to Use This Assessment

### If you answer 0–7 questions correctly:

Spend about 1 hour to read this chapter in full and take limited notes throughout. Follow up by reviewing **all** quiz questions to ensure that you now understand how to solve each one.

### If you answer 8–11 questions correctly:

Spend 20–40 minutes reviewing the quiz questions. Beginning with the questions you missed, read and take notes on the corresponding subchapters. For questions you answered correctly, ensure your thinking matches that of the explanation and you understand why each choice was correct or incorrect.

### If you answer 12–15 questions correctly:

Spend less than 20 minutes reviewing all questions from the quiz. If you missed any, then include a quick read-through of the corresponding subchapters, or even just the relevant content within a subchapter, as part of your question review. For questions you got correct, ensure your thinking matches that of the explanation and review the Concept Summary at the end of the chapter.

1. Which of the following are Lewis bases?
   I. $Ag^+$
   II. $H_2O$
   III. $NH_3$
   A. I only
   B. I and II only
   C. II and III only
   D. I, II, and III

2. Rank the following in order of decreasing nucleophilicity in an aprotic solvent: $RO^-$, RCOOH, ROH, $HO^-$
   A. RCOOH > ROH > $RO^-$ > $HO^-$
   B. $HO^-$ > ROH > $RO^-$ > RCOOH
   C. $RO^-$ > $HO^-$ > ROH > RCOOH
   D. RCOOH > $RO^-$ > $HO^-$ > ROH

3. Rank the following in order of decreasing electrophilicity: $CR_3^+$, $CH_3OH$, $CH_3OCH_3$, $CH_3Cl$
   A. $CH_3OCH_3 > CR_3^+ > CH_3OH > CH_3Cl$
   B. $CR_3^+ > CH_3OH > CH_3OCH_3 > CH_3Cl$
   C. $CH_3OCH_3 > CH_3Cl > CR_3^+ > CH_3OH$
   D. $CR_3^+ > CH_3Cl > CH_3OH > CH_3OCH_3$

4. Rank the following in order of decreasing leaving group ability: $H_2O$, $HO^-$, $Br^-$, $H^-$
   A. $H_2O > Br^- > HO^- > H^-$
   B. $H_2O > HO^- > Br^- > H^-$
   C. $HO^- > Br^- > H_2O > H^-$
   D. $HO^- > H^- > H_2O > Br^-$

5. Rank the following in order of decreasing oxidation state: amine, carboxylic acid, aldehyde, alkane
   A. Aldehyde, amine, alkane, carboxylic acid
   B. Carboxylic acid, aldehyde, amine, alkane
   C. Carboxylic acid, amine, aldehyde, alkane
   D. Alkane, amine, aldehyde, carboxylic acid

6. The last step in the Grignard reaction is acidification, in which the alkoxide ion is protonated to form the final alcohol product. During this reaction, the alkoxide ion acts as a:
   A. Lewis base only
   B. Brønsted–Lowry base and Lewis base
   C. Brønsted–Lowry base and Lewis acid
   D. Brønsted–Lowry base only

7. If 2-butanol was treated with dichromate, what reaction would occur?
   A. Reduction, resulting in the formation of butene
   B. Oxidation, resulting in the formation of butanoic acid
   C. Oxidation, resulting in the formation of butanone
   D. No reaction would occur.

8. If 1-hexanol was treated with pyridinium chlorochromate, what would the end product be?
   A. 2-Hexanol
   B. 2-Hexanone
   C. Hexanal
   D. Hexanoic acid

9. $S_N1$ reactions show first-order kinetics because:
   A. the rate-limiting step is the first step to occur in the reaction.
   B. the rate-limiting step involves only one molecule.
   C. there is only one rate-limiting step.
   D. the reaction involves only one molecule.

10. In a protic solvent, which of the following halogens would be the best nucleophile?
   A. $Br^-$
   B. $Cl^-$
   C. $F^-$
   D. $I^-$

11. Which of the compounds below can undergo oxidation by PCC?

A. 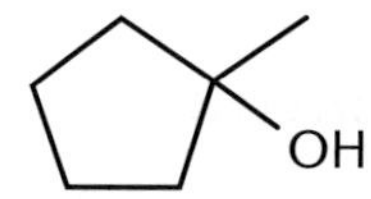


B. 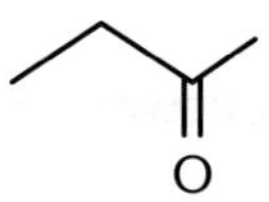


C. 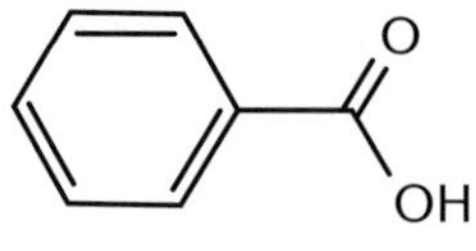


D. 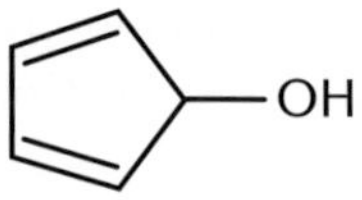

12. Which of the following substrates would most rapidly undergo an $S_N2$ reaction when paired with an appropriate nucleophile?

A.
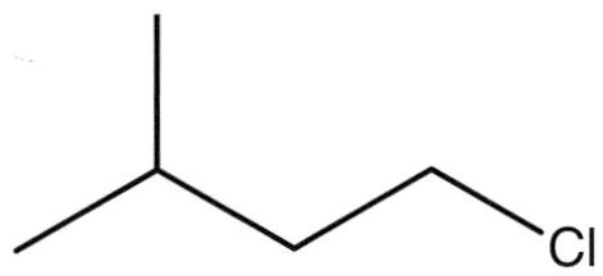


B.
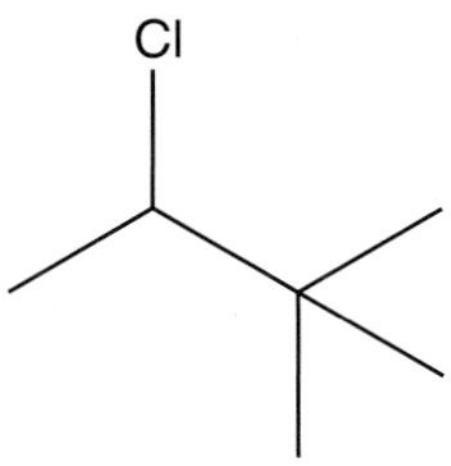


C.
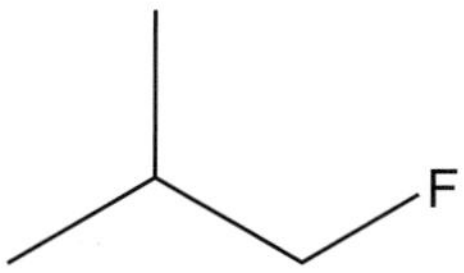


D.
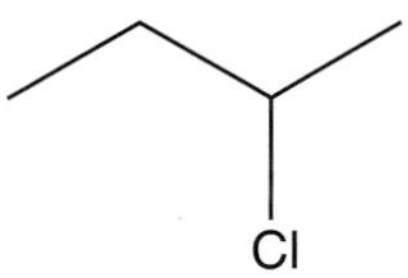


13. Which of the following solvents would be LEAST useful for a nucleophile–electrophile reaction?
   - **A.** $H_2O$
   - **B.** $CH_3CH_2OH$
   - **C.** $CH_3SOCH_3$
   - **D.** $CH_3CH_2CH_2CH_2CH_2CH_3$

14. Aldehydes are generally more reactive than equivalent ketones to nucleophiles. This is likely due to differences in:
   - **A.** steric hindrance.
   - **B.** leaving group ability.
   - **C.** resonance stabilization.
   - **D.** electron-withdrawing character.

15. Which conversion between carboxylic acid derivatives is NOT possible by a nucleophilic reaction?
   - **A.** Carboxylic acid to ester
   - **B.** Ester to carboxylic acid
   - **C.** Anhydride to amide
   - **D.** Ester to anhydride

## Answer Key

1. **C** (See section 4.1)
2. **C** (See section 4.2)
3. **D** (See section 4.2)
4. **A** (See section 4.2)
5. **B** (See section 4.3)
6. **B** (See section 4.1)
7. **C** (See section 4.3)
8. **C** (See section 4.5)
9. **B** (See section 4.4)
10. **D** (See section 4.2)
11. **D** (See section 4.3)
12. **A** (See section 4.4)
13. **D** (See section 4.2)
14. **A** (See section 4.2)
15. **D** (See section 4.5)

*The relevant section of the chapter to review for each question is given in parentheses after the correct answer. Detailed explanations can be found at the end of the chapter.*

CHAPTER 4

# ANALYZING ORGANIC REACTIONS

## In This Chapter



### CHAPTER PROFILE

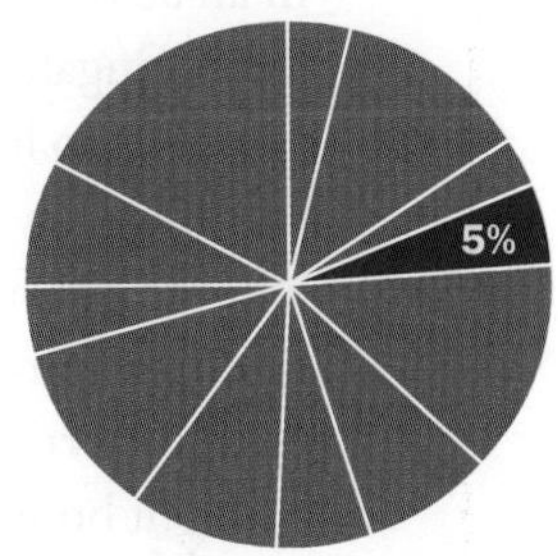


The content in this chapter should be relevant to about 5% of all questions about organic chemistry on the MCAT.

This chapter covers material from the following AAMC content categories:

**1A:** Structure and function of proteins and their constituent amino acids

**4E:** Atoms, nuclear decay, electronic structure, and atomic chemical behavior

**5A:** Unique nature of water and its solutions

**5D:** Structure, function, and reactivity of biologically-relevant molecules

## Introduction

Sitting down to solve MCAT organic chemistry problems can be overwhelming at first, particularly if the reactants or reagents are new to you. The reactions on the page may seem like stage magic—fun to watch, but controlled by forces outside of our knowledge. The good news, however, is that organic chemistry isn't magic—and it is governed by sets of rules that make understanding what will happen much simpler.

In this chapter, we will go over several of the aspects that determine how a complex reaction proceeds and take a brief look at functional group reactivity. Then, armed with this knowledge, we lay out the simple, sequential steps that we can use to determine which reactions will take place. Chapters 5 through 10 of *MCAT Organic Chemistry Review* focus on applications of these principles with different functional groups, so look for patterns between these reactions as you continue preparing for Test Day. With these tools in hand, you can show the MCAT that you know how the trick is done—it isn't magic.

### MCAT EXPERTISE

This chapter is vital for understanding all the reactions you'll see in the next six chapters of this book (Chapters 5–10). On top of that, this material is directly tested on the MCAT as often as any other topic in organic chemistry. Make sure you know all of it!

# 4.1 Acids and Bases

## LEARNING OBJECTIVES

After Chapter 4.1, you will be able to:

- Recall the importance of amphoteric species and common amphoteric molecules
- Describe the meaning of p$K_a$ and p$K_b$ values in relation to acid and base strength
- Recall common functional groups that act as acids or bases

In an acid–base reaction, an acid and a base react, resulting in the formation of the conjugate base of the acid and the conjugate acid of the base. This reaction proceeds so long as the reactants are more reactive, or stronger, than the products that they form. We will discuss acid and base definitions and strength in the following section. For the MCAT, we will concern ourselves with the broader Lewis and Brønsted–Lowry definitions of acids and bases. The Lewis definition concerns itself with the transfer of electrons in the formation of coordinate covalent bonds; the Brønsted–Lowry definition focuses on proton transfer.

### KEY CONCEPT

An acid–base reaction will only proceed if the products that will be formed (the conjugate base of the acid and the conjugate acid of the base) are weaker than the original reactants.

## Definitions

A **Lewis acid** is defined as an **electron acceptor** in the formation of a covalent bond. Lewis acids also tend to be electrophiles, which we will touch on in the next section. Lewis acids have vacant *p*-orbitals into which they can accept an electron pair, or are positively polarized atoms.

A **Lewis base** is defined as an **electron donor** in the formation of a covalent bond. Lewis bases also tend to be nucleophiles, which we will touch on in the next section. Lewis bases have a lone pair of electrons that can be donated, and are often anions, carrying a negative charge.

When Lewis acids and bases interact, they form **coordinate covalent bonds**—covalent bonds in which both electrons in the bond came from the same starting atom (the Lewis base), as shown in Figure 4.1.

### BRIDGE

Acids and bases are critically important material in organic chemistry, biochemistry, and general chemistry. The most extensive coverage of acids and bases is in Chapter 10 of *MCAT General Chemistry Review.*

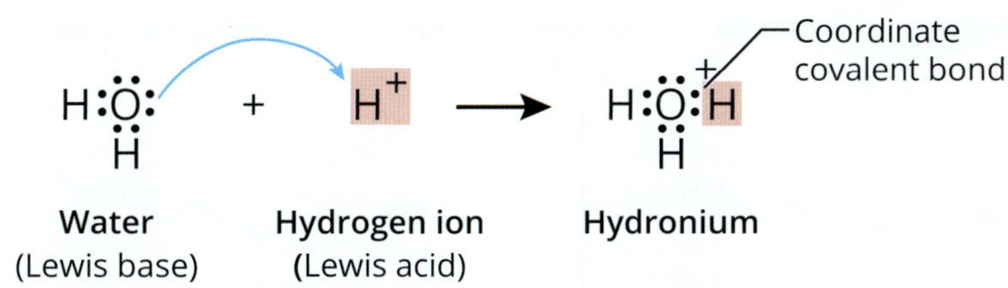


**Figure 4.1** Lewis Acid–Base Reactions
*Water acts as a Lewis base and forms a coordinate covalent bond with the hydrogen ion.*

In the **Brønsted–Lowry** definition, an acid is a species that can donate a proton ($H^+$); a base is a species that can accept a proton. Some molecules, like water, have the ability to act as either Brønsted–Lowry acids or bases, making them **amphoteric**. Water can act as an acid by donating its proton to a base, and thus becoming its conjugate base, $OH^-$. However, water can also act as a base by accepting a proton from an acid to become its conjugate acid, $H_3O^+$. The degree to which a molecule acts as an acid or a base is dependent upon the properties of the solution—water can only act as a base in an acidic solution, and only as an acid in a basic solution. Other examples of amphoteric molecules include $Al(OH)_3$, $HCO_3^-$ (see Figure 4.2), and $HSO_4^-$.

### BRIDGE

The amphoteric properties of bicarbonate, $HCO_3^-$, allow the body to maintain homeostasis. This buffer system works with the respiratory system to control $CO_2$ levels through respiration, as well as with the kidneys to regulate bicarbonate levels and hydrogen ion excretion, allowing the body to neutralize acids and bases and maintain physiological pH. More on homeostasis appears in Chapter 10 of *MCAT Biology Review*.

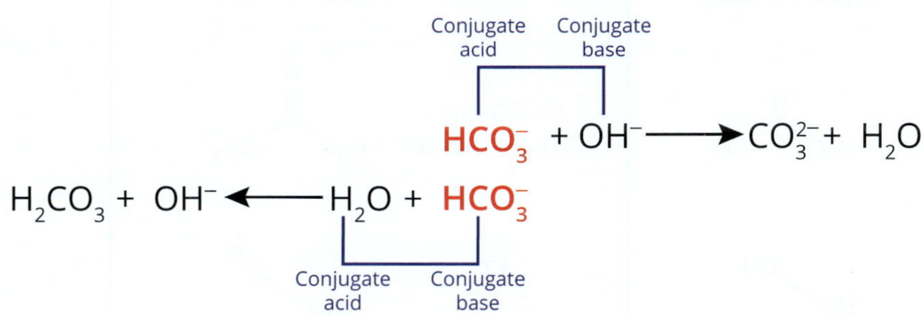


**Figure 4.2** Amphoteric Bicarbonate

## Acid and Base Strength

The **acid dissociation constant**, or $K_a$, measures the strength of an acid in solution. In the dissociation of an acid HA ($HA \rightleftharpoons H^+ + A^-$), the equilibrium constant is given by:

$$K_a = \frac{[H^+][A^-]}{[HA]}$$

**Equation 4.1**

and the p$K_a$ can be calculated as:

$$pK_a = -\log K_a$$

**Equation 4.2**

Thus, more acidic molecules will have a smaller (or even negative) p$K_a$; more basic molecules will have a larger p$K_a$. Acids with a p$K_a$ below $-2$ are considered strong acids, which almost always dissociate completely in aqueous solution. Weak organic acids often have p*K*a values between $-2$ and 20. p$K_a$ values for common functional groups are shown in Table 4.1.

| Functional group | Example | p$K_a$ (Weaker acid → Stronger acid) | Conjugate base (Stronger base → Weaker base) |
|---|---|---|---|
| Alkane | $H_3C-CH_2-CH_2-CH_3$ | ~50 | $H_3C-CH_2-CH_2-CH_2^{\ominus}$ |
| Alkene | $CH_2=CH-CH_3$ | ~43 | $CH_2=CH-CH_2^{\ominus}$ |
| Hydrogen | H– H | 42 | $H^{\ominus}$ |
| Amine | $NH_3$ | ~35 | $NH_2^{\ominus}$ |
| Alkyne | $R-C\equiv C-H$ | 25 | $R-C\equiv C^{\ominus}$ |
| Ester | $H_3CO-C(=O)-CH_3$ | 25 | $H_3CO-C(=O)-CH_2^{\ominus}$ |
| Ketone/ Aldehyde | $H_3C-C(=O)-CH_3$ | 17–20 (ald.) 20–24 (ket.) | $H_3C-C(=O)-CH_2^{\ominus}$ |
| Alcohol | $H_3C-OH$ | 17 | $H_3C-O^{\ominus}$ |
| Water | HO— H | 16 | $HO^{\ominus}$ |
| Carboxylic acid | $H_3C-C(=O)-OH$ | 4 | $H_3C-C(=O)-O^{\ominus}$ |
| Hydronium ion | $H_3O^{\oplus}$ | −1.7 | $H_2O$ |

**Table 4.1** p$K_a$ Values for Common Functional Groups

Generally, bond strength decreases down the periodic table, and acidity therefore increases. Also, the more electronegative an atom, the higher the acidity. When these two trends oppose each other, low bond strength takes precedence.

For the common functional groups on the MCAT, the $\alpha$-hydrogens of carbonyl compounds deserve special note. **$\alpha$-hydrogens** are connected to the **$\alpha$-carbon**, which is a carbon adjacent to the carbonyl. Because the *enol* form of carbonyl-containing carbanions is stabilized by resonance, these are acidic hydrogens that are easily lost. We will go into greater depth about enolate chemistry in Chapters 7 through 9 of *MCAT Organic Chemistry Review*.

## Common Functional Groups

We can also apply these acid and base rules directly to the functional groups that appear on the MCAT. Functional groups that act as acids include alcohols, aldehydes and ketones (at the $\alpha$-carbon), carboxylic acids, and most carboxylic acid derivatives. These compounds are therefore easier to target with basic (or nucleophilic) reactants because they readily accept a lone pair.

Amines and amides are the main functional groups that act as bases—keep an eye out for these compounds in the formation of peptide bonds. The nitrogen atom of an amine can form coordinate covalent bonds by donating a lone pair to a Lewis acid.

### MCAT CONCEPT CHECK 4.1

Before you move on, assess your understanding of the material with these questions.

1. When will an acid–base reaction proceed, based on the strength of the reactants and products?

    ______________________________

2. What does it mean for a molecule to be amphoteric? What biologically relevant molecules are also characteristically amphoteric?

    ______________________________

3. How is p$K_a$ defined, and what does a low p$K_a$ indicate?

    ______________________________

4. What are some functional groups that classically act as acids? As bases?

    - Acids:

    ______________________________

    - Bases:

    ______________________________

# 4.2 Nucleophiles, Electrophiles, and Leaving Groups

## LEARNING OBJECTIVES

After Chapter 4.2, you will be able to:

- Distinguish nucleophiles and electrophiles from Lewis acids and bases
- Compare nucleophilicity using the four main trends
- Describe the relationship between electrophile and leaving group in a substitution reaction
- Identify the traits that increase electrophilicity
- Recall the traits of a good leaving group

Almost all reactions in organic chemistry can be divided into one of two groups: oxidation–reduction reactions or nucleophile–electrophile reactions. Nucleophiles, electrophiles, and leaving groups are particularly important to the reactions of alcohols and carbonyl-containing compounds, which we will look at in depth in later chapters. Let's take a look at how each of these terms is defined.

## Nucleophiles

**Nucleophiles** are defined as "nucleus-loving" species with either lone pairs or $\pi$ bonds that can form new bonds to electrophiles. You may have noted that nucleophilicity and basicity appear to have similar definitions—and this is true! Good nucleophiles tend to be good bases. There is, however, a distinction between the two. Nucleophile strength is based on relative rates of reaction with a common electrophile—and is therefore a kinetic property. Base strength is related to the equilibrium position of a reaction—and is therefore a thermodynamic property. Some common examples of nucleophiles are shown in Figure 4.3.

### KEY CONCEPT

Nucleophiles tend to have lone pairs or $\pi$ bonds that can be used to form covalent bonds to electrophiles. On Test Day, look for carbon, hydrogen, oxygen, or nitrogen (CHON) with a minus sign or lone pair to identify most nucleophiles.

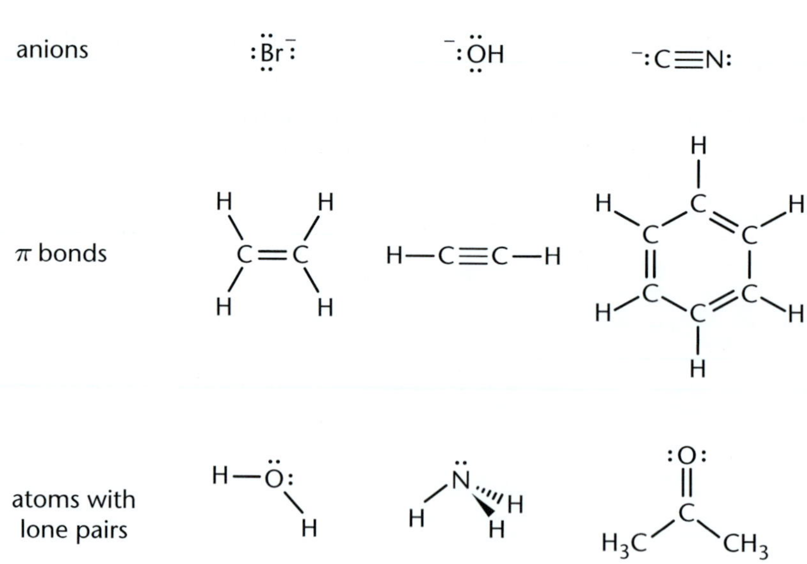


**Figure 4.3** Examples of Nucleophiles

As long as the nucleophilic atom is the same, the more basic the nucleophile, the more reactive it is. This also holds when comparing atoms in the same row of the periodic table, but *not* when proceeding down a column in the periodic table. Nucleophilicity is determined by four major factors:

- **Charge:** Nucleophilicity increases with increasing electron density (more negative charge)
- **Electronegativity:** Nucleophilicity decreases as electronegativity increases because these atoms are less likely to share electron density
- **Steric hindrance:** Bulkier molecules are less nucleophilic
- **Solvent:** Protic solvents can hinder nucleophilicity by protonating the nucleophile or through hydrogen bonding

## Solvent Effects

The solvent consideration is worth spending a bit more time on. In polar protic solvents, nucleophilicity increases *down* the periodic table. In polar aprotic solvents, nucleophilicity increases *up* the periodic table, as shown in Figure 4.4.

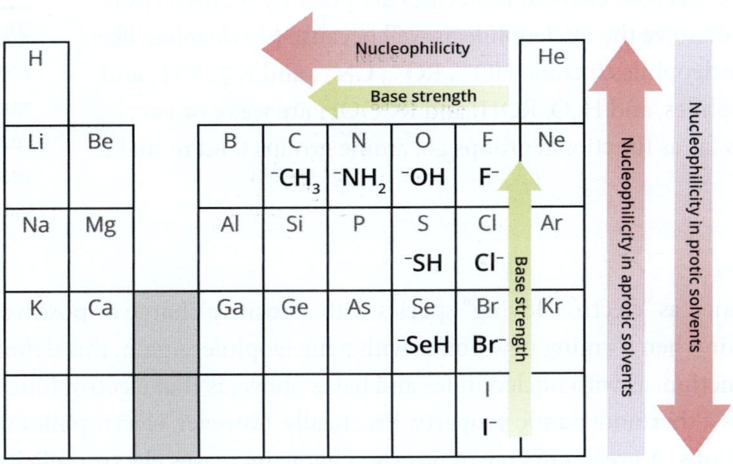


**Figure 4.4** Nucleophilicity Trends

Examples of both types of solvents are shown in Figure 4.5.

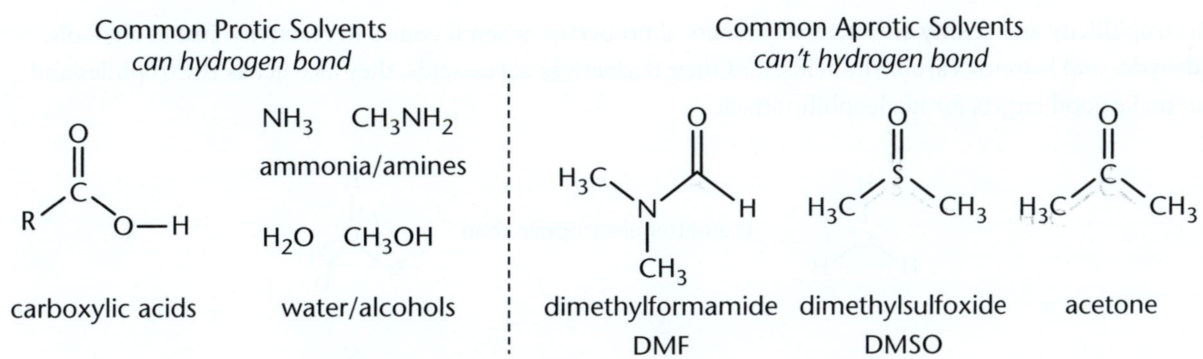


**Figure 4.5** Examples of Polar Protic and Polar Aprotic Solvents

The halogens are good examples of the effects of the solvent on nucleophilicity. In protic solvents, nucleophilicity decreases in the order:

$$I^- > Br^- > Cl^- > F^-$$

This is because the protons in solution will be attracted to the nucleophile. $F^-$ is the conjugate base of HF, a weak acid. As such, it will form bonds with the protons in solution and be less able to access the electrophile to react. $I^-$, on the other hand, is the conjugate base of HI, a strong acid. As such, it is less affected by the protons in solution and can react with the electrophile.

In aprotic solvents, on the other hand, nucleophilicity decreases in the order:

$$F^- > Cl^- > Br^- > I^-$$

This is because there are no protons to get in the way of the attacking nucleophile. In aprotic solvents, nucleophilicity relates directly to basicity.

We won't use nonpolar solvents with this type of reaction because we need our nucleophile to dissolve. Because charged molecules are polar by nature, a polar solvent is required to dissolve the nucleophile as well because *like dissolves like.* Examples of strong nucleophiles include $HO^-$, $RO^-$, $CN^-$, and $N_3^-$. $NH_3$ and $RCO_2^-$ are fair nucleophiles, and $H_2O$, ROH, and RCOOH are weak or very weak nucleophiles. As far as functional groups go, amine groups tend to make good nucleophiles.

**MCAT EXPERTISE**

If a solvent is not given on Test Day, assume that the reaction occurs in a polar solvent. Polar solvents—whether protic or aprotic—can dissolve nucleophiles and assist in any reaction in which electrons are moved. Organic chemistry is all about moving electrons, so it's less common for these reactions to be performed in nonpolar solvents.

**KEY CONCEPT**

We can't use nonpolar solvents in these nucleophile–electrophile reactions because our reactants are polar—they wouldn't dissolve!

## Electrophiles

**Electrophiles** are defined as "electron-loving" species with a positive charge or positively polarized atom that accepts an electron pair when forming new bonds with a nucleophile. Again, this definition brings to mind Lewis acids. The distinction, as with nucleophiles and bases above, is that electrophilicity is a kinetic property, whereas acidity is a thermodynamic property. Practically, however, electrophiles will almost always act as Lewis acids in reactions. A greater degree of positive charge increases electrophilicity, so a carbocation is more electrophilic than a carbonyl carbon. Some comparisons between electrophiles are drawn in Figure 4.6. Additionally, the nature of the leaving group influences electrophilicity in species without empty orbitals; better leaving groups make it more likely that a reaction will happen. If empty orbitals are present, an incoming nucleophile can make a bond with the electrophile without displacing the leaving group.

Electrophilicity and acidity are effectively identical properties when it comes to reactivity. Just as alcohols, aldehydes and ketones, carboxylic acids, and their derivatives act as acids, they also act as electrophiles and can make good targets for nucleophilic attack.

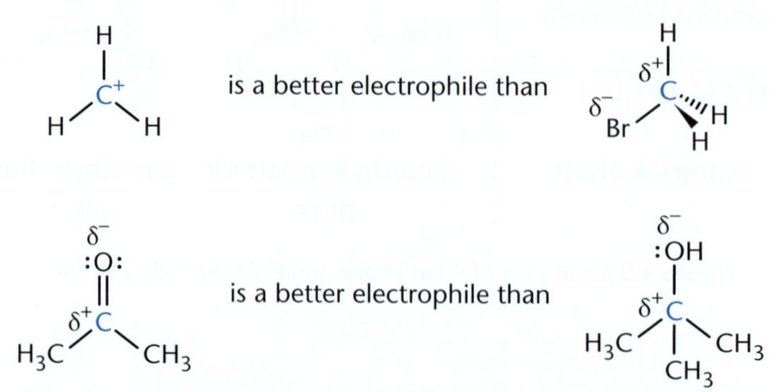


**Figure 4.6** Comparisons of Electrophilicity

The carboxylic acid derivatives are often ranked by electrophilicity. Acyl halides are the most reactive, followed by anhydrides, carboxylic acids and esters, and then amides, as shown in Figure 4.7. In practical terms, this means that derivatives of higher reactivity can form derivatives of lower reactivity but not vice versa, similar to the acid–base reactions described previously.

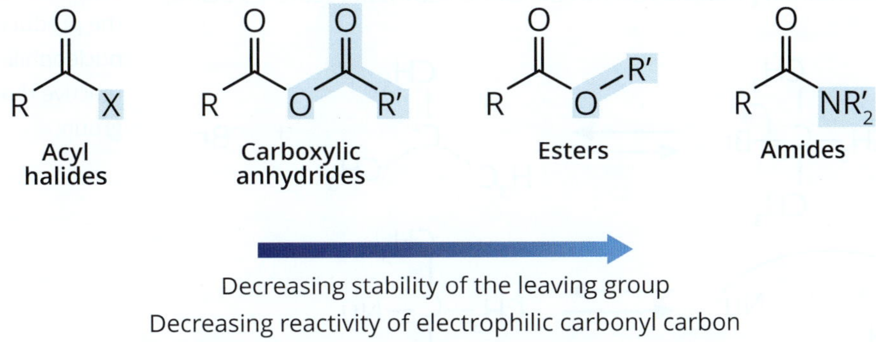


**Figure 4.7** Reactivity of Carboxylic Acid Derivatives

## Leaving Groups

**Leaving groups** are the molecular fragments that retain the electrons after heterolysis. **Heterolytic reactions** are essentially the opposite of coordinate covalent bond formation: a bond is broken and both electrons are given to one of the two products. The best leaving groups will be able to stabilize the extra electrons. Weak bases are more stable with an extra set of electrons and therefore make good leaving groups. By this logic, the conjugate bases of strong acids (like $I^-$, $Br^-$, and $Cl^-$) tend to make good leaving groups, as seen in Figure 4.8. Leaving group ability can be augmented by resonance and by inductive effects from electron-withdrawing groups: these help delocalize and stabilize negative charge.

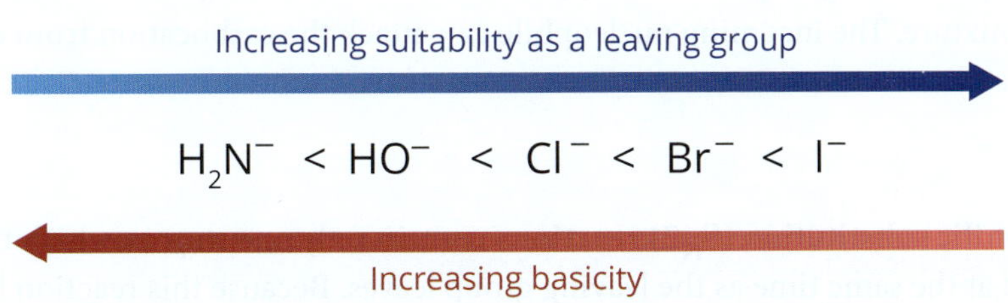


**Figure 4.8** Relative Basicity and Leaving Group Stability

Alkanes and hydrogen ions will almost never serve as leaving groups because they form very reactive, strongly basic anions. We can think of leaving groups and nucleophiles as serving opposite functions. In substitution reactions, the weaker base (the leaving group) is replaced by the stronger base (the nucleophile).

## Nucleophilic Substitution Reactions

**Nucleophilic substitution reactions** are perfect examples for demonstrating nucleophile–electrophile reactions. In both $S_N1$ and $S_N2$ reactions, a nucleophile forms a bond with a substrate carbon and a leaving group leaves.

## $S_N1$ Reactions

**Unimolecular nucleophilic substitution ($S_N1$) reactions** contain two steps. The first step is the rate-limiting step in which the leaving group leaves, generating a positively charged **carbocation**. The nucleophile then attacks the carbocation, resulting in the substitution product. This mechanism is shown in Figure 4.9 below.

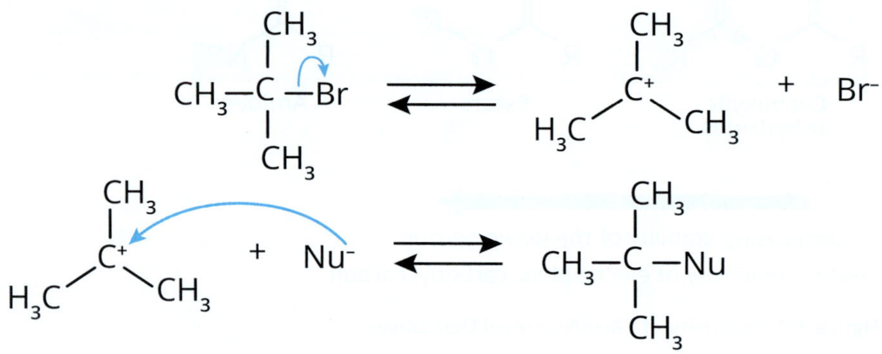


**Figure 4.9** Mechanism of $S_N1$ Reaction
*Step 1: Formation of the carbocation (rate-limiting);*
*Step 2: Nucleophilic attack.*

### KEY CONCEPT

Just like acid–base reactions, nucleophilic attack will only occur if the reactants are more reactive than the products. Thus, the nucleophile must be more reactive than the leaving group.

The more substituted the carbocation, the more stable it is because the alkyl groups act as electron donors, stabilizing the positive charge. Because the formation of the carbocation is the rate-limiting step, the rate of the reaction depends only on the concentration of the substrate: rate $= k[\text{R}-\text{L}]$, where R—L is an alkyl group containing a leaving group. This is a first-order reaction; anything that accelerates the formation of the carbocation will increase the rate of an $S_N1$ reaction.

Because $S_N1$ reactions pass through a planar intermediate before the nucleophile attacks, the product will usually be a racemic mixture. The incoming nucleophile can attack the carbocation from either side, resulting in varied stereochemistry.

## $S_N2$ Reactions

**Bimolecular nucleophilic substitution ($S_N2$) reactions** contain only one step, in which the nucleophile attacks the compound at the same time as the leaving group leaves. Because this reaction has only one step, we call it a **concerted** reaction. The reaction is called bimolecular because this single rate-limiting step involves two molecules.

In $S_N2$ reactions, the nucleophile actively displaces the leaving group in a **backside attack**. For this to occur, the nucleophile must be strong, and the substrate cannot be sterically hindered. Therefore, the less substituted the carbon, the more reactive it is in $S_N2$ reactions. Note that this is the opposite of the trend for $S_N1$ reactions. The one-step mechanism is shown in Figure 4.10.

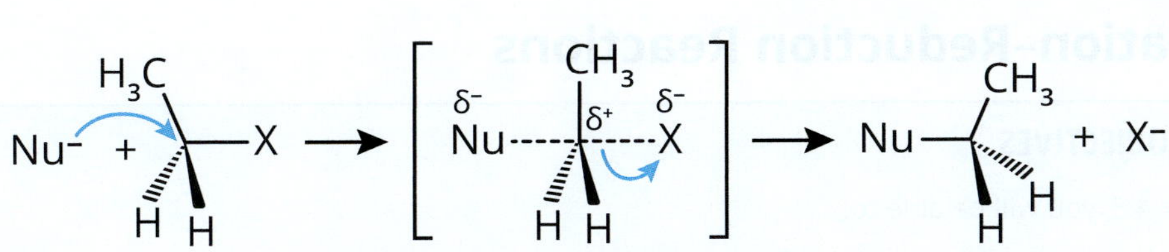


**Figure 4.10** Mechanism of $S_N2$ Reaction

The single step of an $S_N2$ reaction involves two reacting species: the substrate (often an alkyl halide, tosylate, or mesylate) and the nucleophile. Therefore, the concentrations of both have a role in determining the rate: rate $= k[\text{Nu:}][\text{R}-\text{L}]$

$S_N2$ reactions are accompanied by an inversion of relative configuration. Much like an umbrella being turned inside out on a blustery day, the position of substituents around the substrate carbon will be inverted. If the nucleophile and leaving group have the same priority in their respective molecules, this inversion will also correspond to a change in absolute configuration from (*R*) to (*S*) or vice-versa. This is an example of a **stereospecific** reaction, one in which the configuration of the reactant determines the configuration of the product due to the reaction mechanism.

## MCAT CONCEPT CHECK 4.2

Before you move on, assess your understanding of the material with these questions.

1. How do the definitions of nucleophile and electrophile differ from those of Lewis base and acid?

   ________________________________

2. Rank the following molecules in order of increasing nucleophilicity: methoxide, *t*-butoxide, isopropanolate, ethoxide.

   ________ < ________ < ________ < ________.

3. How must the nucleophile and leaving group be related in order for a substitution reaction to proceed?

   ________________________________

4. What trends increase electrophilicity?

   ________________________________

5. What are some features of good leaving groups?

   ________________________________

## 4.3 Oxidation–Reduction Reactions

**LEARNING OBJECTIVES**

After Chapter 4.3, you will be able to:

- Recall common oxidizing agents and the characteristics of a good oxidizing agent
- Recall common reducing agents and the characteristics of a good reducing agent
- Order a given list of molecules from most oxidized to least oxidized:

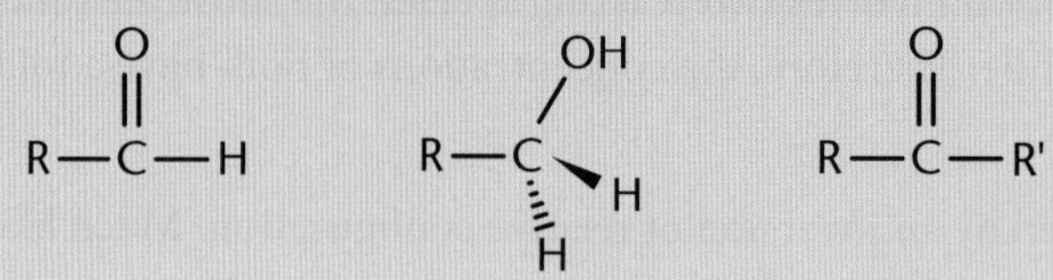

Another important class of reactions are **oxidation–reduction (redox) reactions**, in which the oxidation states of the reactants change. **Oxidation state** is an indicator of the hypothetical charge that an atom would have if all bonds were completely ionic. Oxidation state can be calculated from the molecular formula for a molecule. For example, the carbon in methane ($CH_4$) has an oxidation state of $-4$ because the hydrogens each have an oxidation state of $+1$. This is the most reduced form of carbon. In carbon dioxide ($CO_2$), each of the oxygen atoms has an oxidation state of $-2$, and the carbon has an oxidation state of $+4$. This is the most oxidized form of carbon. For an ion, the oxidation state is simply the charge—so $Na^+$ and $S^{2-}$ would have oxidation states of $+1$ and $-2$, respectively. Carboxylic acids are more oxidized than aldehydes, ketones, and imines, which in turn are more oxidized than alcohols, alkyl halides, and amines.

We won't need to know too much about how to assign oxidation states in organic chemistry, but should know the definitions of oxidation and reduction. **Oxidation** refers to an increase in oxidation state, which means a loss of electrons. In organic chemistry, it is often easier to view oxidation as increasing the number of bonds to oxygen or other heteroatoms (atoms besides carbon and hydrogen). **Reduction** refers to a decrease in oxidation state, or a gain in electrons. In organic chemistry, it is often easier to view reduction as increasing the number of bonds to hydrogen.

### Oxidizing Agents and Reactions

As we mentioned above, oxidation refers to an increase in oxidation state. Oxidation of a carbon atom occurs when a bond between a carbon atom and an atom that is less electronegative than carbon is replaced by a bond to an atom that is more electronegative than carbon. In practice, this usually means decreasing the number of bonds to hydrogen and increasing the number of bonds to other carbons, nitrogen, oxygen, or halides.

The **oxidizing agent** is the element or compound in an oxidation–reduction reaction that accepts an electron from another species. Because the oxidizing agent is gaining electrons, it is said to be reduced. Good oxidizing agents have a high affinity for electrons (such as $O_2$, $O_3$, and $Cl_2$) or unusually high oxidation states (like $Mn^{7+}$ in permanganate, $MnO_4^-$, and $Cr^{6+}$ in chromate, $CrO_4^{2-}$).

**KEY CONCEPT**

One can organize the different functional groups by "levels" of oxidation:

- Level 0 (no bonds to heteroatoms): alkanes
- Level 1: alcohols, alkyl halides, amines
- Level 2: aldehydes, ketones, imines
- Level 3: carboxylic acids, anhydrides, esters, amides
- Level 4 (four bonds to heteroatoms): carbon dioxide

Primary alcohols can be oxidized by one level to become aldehydes, or can be further oxidized to form carboxylic acids. This reaction commonly proceeds all the way to the carboxylic acid when using strong oxidizing agents such as chromium trioxide ($CrO_3$) or sodium or potassium dichromate ($Na_2Cr_2O_7$ or $K_2Cr_2O_7$), but can be made to stop at the aldehyde level using specific reagents such as pyridinium chlorochromate (PCC). Secondary alcohols can be oxidized to ketones.

A number of oxidation reactions and the relevant oxidizing agents are shown in Figure 4.11. Note that the goal at this point should not be memorization of these reactions, but recognition of two themes: oxidation reactions tend to feature an increase in the number of bonds to oxygen, and oxidizing agents often contain metals bonded to a large number of oxygen atoms.

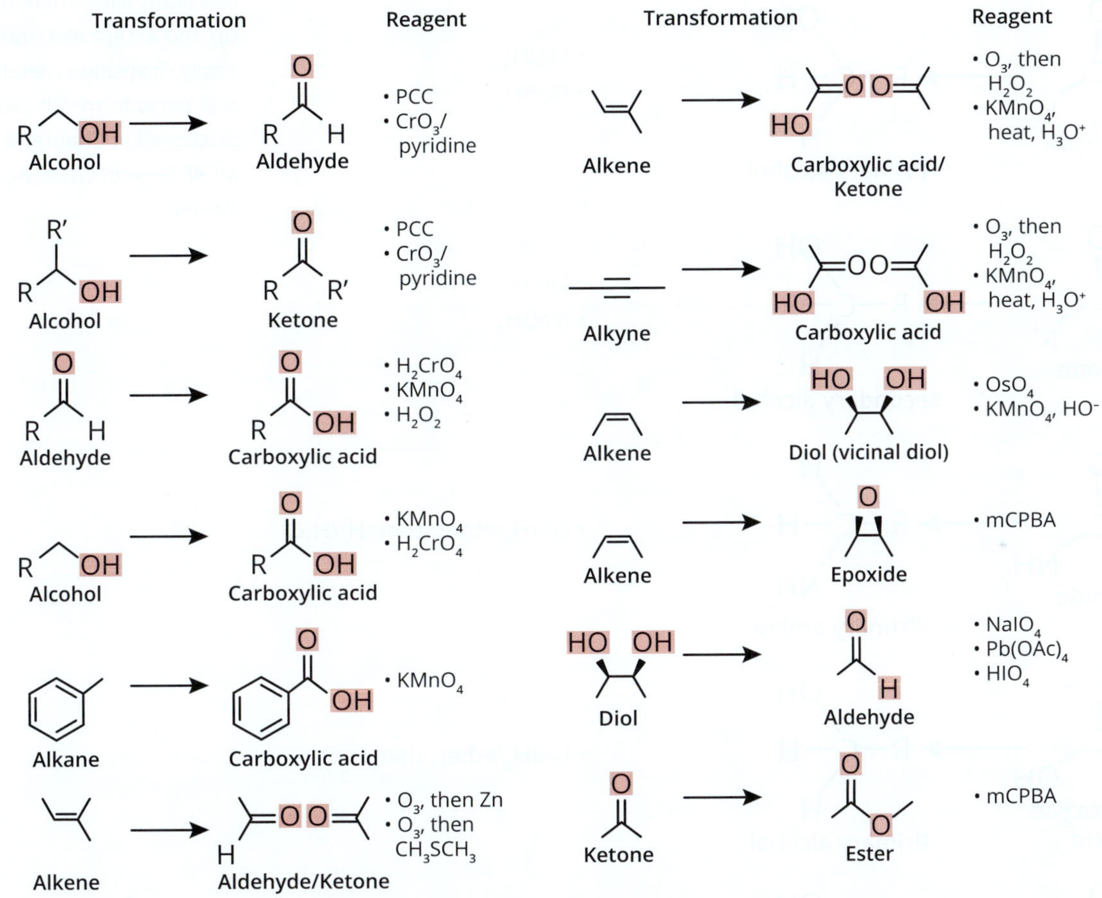


**Figure 4.11** Oxidation Reactions and Common Oxidizing Agents

## Reducing Agents and Reactions

Conversely, reduction refers to a decrease in oxidation state. Reduction of a carbon occurs when a bond between a carbon atom and an atom that is more electronegative than carbon is replaced by a bond to an atom that is less electronegative than carbon. In practice, this usually means increasing the number of bonds to hydrogen and decreasing the number of bonds to other carbons, nitrogen, oxygen, or halides.

Good reducing agents include sodium, magnesium, aluminum, and zinc, which have low electronegativities and ionization energies. Metal hydrides, such as NaH, $CaH_2$, $LiAlH_4$, and $NaBH_4$, are also good reducing agents because they contain the $H^-$ ion.

Aldehydes and ketones will be reduced to primary and secondary alcohols, respectively. This reaction is exergonic, but exceedingly slow without a catalyst. Amides can be reduced to amines using $LiAlH_4$. This same reducing agent will reduce carboxylic acids to primary alcohols and esters to a pair of alcohols. Examples of reduction reactions are shown in Figure 4.12. Again, the focus is not on memorization, but on recognizing that reduction reactions tend to feature an increase in the number of bonds to hydrogen, and reducing agents often contain metals bonded to a large number of hydrides.

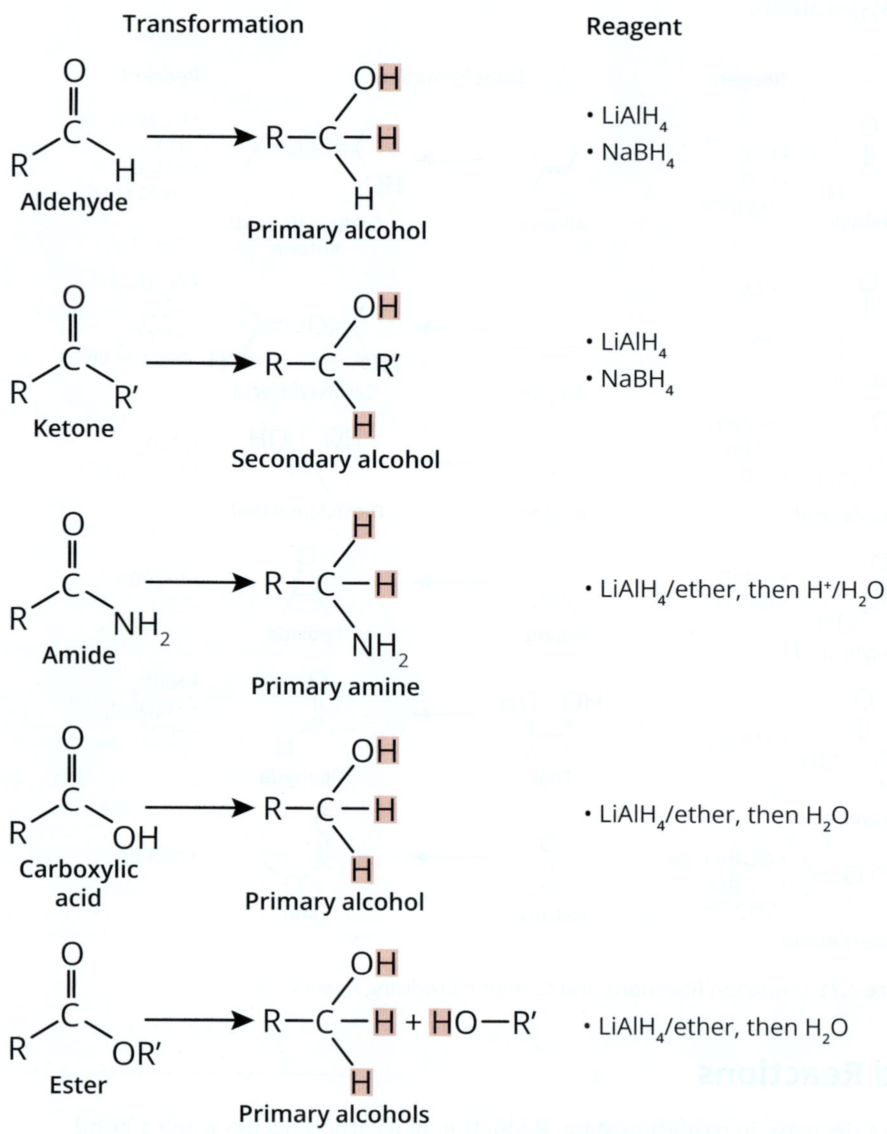


**Figure 4.12** Reduction Reactions and Common Reducing Agents

## BRIDGE

Note that many of the common oxidizing and reducing agents include transition metals. This is because transition metals can often take on many different oxidation states. Their low ionization energies and presence of *d*-orbitals allow them to give up and accept electrons easily. Transition metals and periodic trends are discussed in Chapter 2 of *MCAT General Chemistry Review.*

### MCAT CONCEPT CHECK 4.3

Before you move on, assess your understanding of the material with these questions.

1. What are some characteristics of good oxidizing agents? List some examples of common oxidizing agents.
   - Characteristics: ___
   - Examples: ___
2. What are some characteristics of good reducing agents? List some examples of common reducing agents.
   - Characteristics: ___
   - Examples: ___
3. List the following carbon-containing compounds from most oxidized carbon to most reduced: methane, carbon dioxide, ketone, alcohol, carboxylic acid
   - Most oxidized: ___
   - ___
   - ___
   - ___
   - Most reduced: ___

## 4.4 Chemoselectivity

### LEARNING OBJECTIVES

After Chapter 4.4, you will be able to:

- Describe the types of compounds that are most likely to undergo $S_N1$ and $S_N2$ reactions
- Identify the two reactive centers of a carbonyl-containing compound:

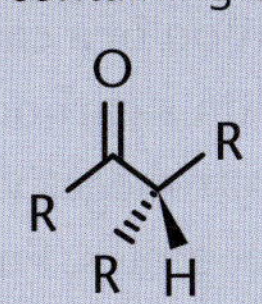


A key skill in recognizing which reactions will occur is recognizing the reactive regions within a molecule. The preferential reaction of one functional group in the presence of other functional groups is termed **chemoselectivity**.

## Reactive Locations

Which site is the reactive site of a molecule depends on the type of chemistry that's occurring. A redox reagent, as described earlier, will tend to act on the highest-priority functional group. Thus, in a molecule with an alcohol and a carboxylic acid, a reducing agent is more likely to act on the carboxylic acid than on the alcohol, as shown in Figure 4.13.

**KEY CONCEPT**

The more oxidized the functional group, the more reactive it is in both nucleophile–electrophile and oxidation–reduction reactions.

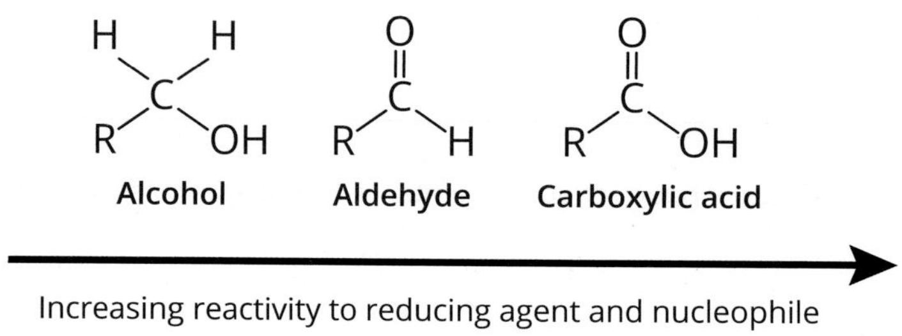


**Figure 4.13** Reducibility of Functional Groups

For a reaction involving nucleophiles and electrophiles, reactions also tend to occur at the highest-priority functional group because it contains the most oxidized carbon. A nucleophile is looking for a good electrophile; the more oxidized the carbon, the more electronegative groups around it, and the larger partial positive charge it will experience. Thus, carboxylic acids and their derivatives are the first to be targeted by a nucleophile, followed by an aldehyde or ketone, followed by an alcohol or amine, as demonstrated in Figure 4.14. Aldehydes are generally more reactive toward nucleophiles than ketones because they have less steric hindrance.

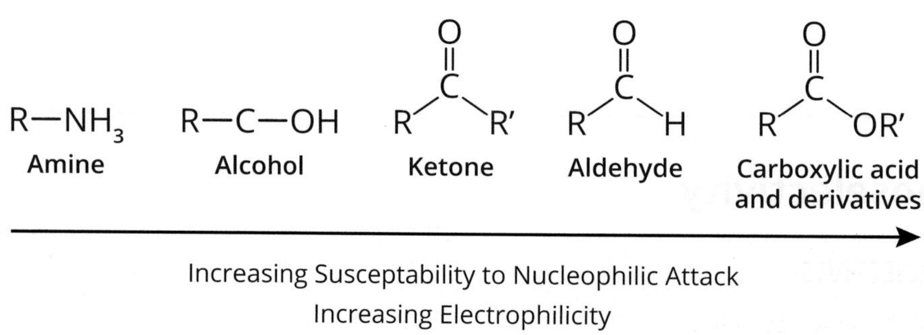


**Figure 4.14** Chemoselectivity Trends

One common reactive site on the MCAT is the carbon of a carbonyl, which can be found in carboxylic acids and their derivatives, aldehydes, and ketones. Within a carbonyl-containing compound, the carbon of the carbonyl acquires a positive polarity due to the electronegativity of the oxygen. Thus, the carbonyl carbon becomes electrophilic and can be a target for nucleophiles. Further, the $\alpha$-hydrogens are much more acidic than in a regular C—H bond due to the resonance stabilization of the enol form. These can be deprotonated easily with a strong base, forming an enolate, as shown in Figure 4.15. The enolate then becomes a strong nucleophile, and alkylation can result if good electrophiles are available.

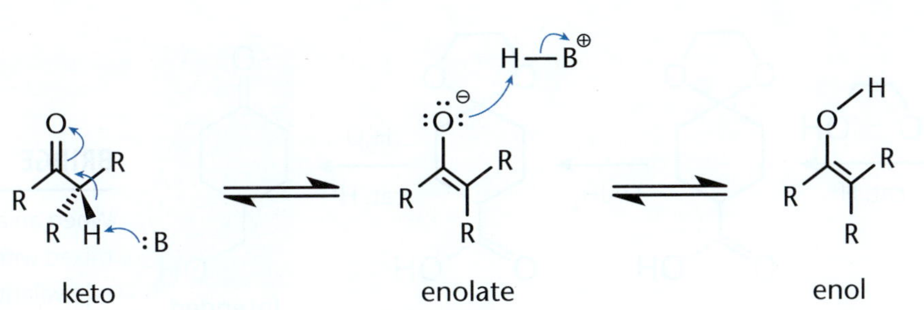


**Figure 4.15** Enol and Enolate Forms of a Ketone

A second reactive site for consideration is the substrate carbon in substitution reactions. $S_N1$ reactions, which have to overcome the barrier of carbocation stability, prefer tertiary to secondary carbons as reactive sites, and secondary to primary. For $S_N2$ reactions, which have a bigger barrier in steric hindrance, methyl and primary carbons are preferred over secondary, and tertiary carbons won't react. This is all because of the mechanism of these two reactions.

## Steric Protection

**Steric hindrance** describes the prevention of reactions at a particular location within a molecule due to the size of substituent groups. For example, $S_N2$ reactions won't occur with tertiary substrates, as depicted in Figure 4.16. This characteristic of **steric protection** can be a useful tool in the synthesis of desired molecules and the prevention of the formation of alternative products. Effectively, bulky groups make it impossible for the nucleophile to reach the most reactive electrophile, making the nucleophile more likely to attack another region.

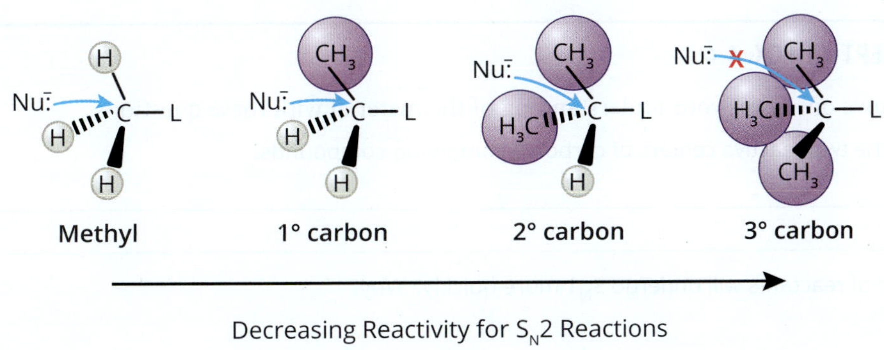


**Figure 4.16** Steric Effects on $S_N2$ Reactivity

Another way that sterics come into play is in the protection of leaving groups. One can temporarily mask a reactive leaving group with a sterically bulky group during synthesis. For example, reduction of a molecule containing both carboxylic acids and aldehydes or ketones can result in reduction of all of the functional groups. To prevent this, the aldehyde or ketone is first converted to a nonreactive acetal or ketal, which serves as the **protecting group**, and the reaction can proceed. This reaction is shown in Figure 4.17. Another protective reaction is the reversible reduction of alcohols to *tert*-butyl ethers.

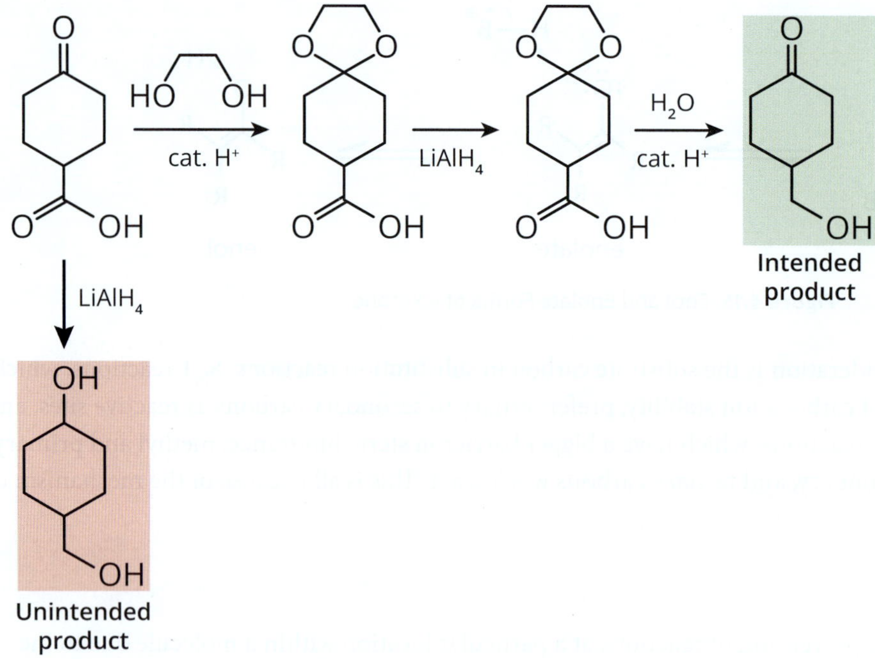


**Figure 4.17** Protection of a Ketone by Conversion to an Acetal

## BRIDGE

When an aldehyde is mixed with a diol (or two equivalents of alcohol), it forms an acetal. When a ketone is mixed with a diol (or two equivalents of alcohol), it forms a ketal. Acetal and ketal chemistry is discussed in Chapter 6 of *MCAT Organic Chemistry Review.*

Don't worry if this seems overwhelming—this is just a preview of what we will see in later chapters, along with a set of rules that will make it easier to understand how chemical reactions will proceed! Feel free to come back to this chapter later to remind yourself of the rules that apply across the board after reading further chapters.

### MCAT CONCEPT CHECK 4.4

Before you move on, assess your understanding of the material with these questions.

1. What are the two reactive centers of carbonyl-containing compounds?

   - ______________________________
   - ______________________________

2. Which pair of reactants will undergo $S_N1$ more quickly? Why?

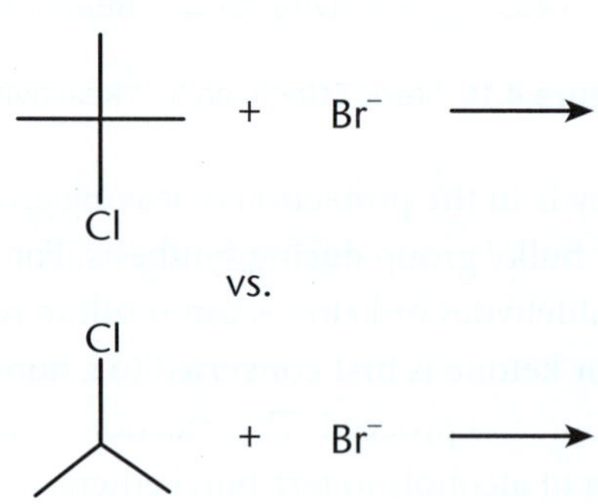


______________________________

3. Which of the following electrophiles will be more favorable to an $S_N2$ reaction? Why?

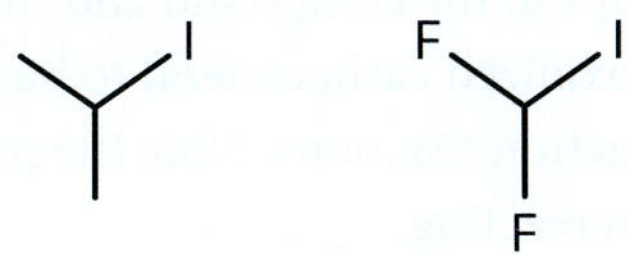

______________________________________________

## 4.5 Steps to Problem Solving **High Yield**

### LEARNING OBJECTIVES

After Chapter 4.5, you will be able to:

- List the six steps for solving organic chemistry reactions
- Predict how a reaction will proceed if you are not given reaction conditions

With all of these rules in hand, we can now apply our knowledge in a systematic way to simplify organic chemistry reactions that appear on the MCAT. These steps are described below.

### Step 1: Know Your Nomenclature

Before you can even start to understand what reactions will occur and what products will form, it is vital to know which compounds IUPAC and common names refer to! If you're still having trouble with nomenclature, be sure to review Chapter 1 of *MCAT Organic Chemistry Review.*

### Step 2: Identify the Functional Groups

Look at the organic molecules in the reaction. What functional groups are in the molecules? Do these functional groups act as acids or bases? How oxidized is the carbon? Are there functional groups that act as good nucleophiles, electrophiles, or leaving groups? This step will help define a category of reactions that can occur with the given functional groups.

### Step 3: Identify the Other Reagents

In this step, determine the properties of the other reagents in the reaction. Are they acidic or basic? Are they suggestive of a particular reaction? Are they good nucleophiles or a specific solvent? Are they good oxidizing or reducing agents?

**MCAT EXPERTISE**

While studying organic chemistry for the MCAT, don't permit yourself to simply nod along with the reaction mechanisms—get involved! During each step of a mechanism, ask yourself how the trends and problem-solving steps in this chapter play out.

### Step 4: Identify the Most Reactive Functional Group(s)

Once you've identified the functional groups in the compound and the other reagents present, this step should be relatively quick. Remember that more oxidized carbons tend to be more reactive to both nucleophile–electrophile reactions and oxidation–reduction reactions. Note the presence of protecting groups that exist to prevent a particular functional group from reacting.

### Step 5: Identify the First Step of the Reaction

If the reaction involves an acid or a base, the first step will usually be protonation or deprotonation. If the reaction involves a nucleophile, the first step is generally for the nucleophile to attack the electrophile, forming a bond with it. If the reaction involves an oxidizing or reducing agent, the most oxidized functional group will be oxidized or reduced, accordingly.

Once you know what will react, think through how the reaction will go. Did the protonation or deprotonation of a functional group increase its reactivity? When the nucleophile attacks, how does the carbon respond to avoid having five bonds? Does a leaving group leave, or does a double bond get reduced to a single bond (like the opening of a carbonyl)?

### Step 6: Consider Stereospecificity/Stereoselectivity

Though not all reactions are stereospecific or stereoselective, these possibilities should be considered when predicting products. For stereospecificity, consider whether the configuration of the reactant necessarily leads to a specific configuration in the product, as seen in $S_N2$ reactions. Stereoselectivity, on the other hand, occurs in reactions where one configuration of product is more readily formed due to product characteristics. Stereoselectivity is seen in many reactions, as different products often possess different traits which affect their relative stability. If there is more than one product, the major product will generally be determined by differences in strain or stability between the two molecules. More strained molecules (with significant angle, torsional, or nonbonded strain) are less likely to form than molecules without significant sources of strain. Products with conjugation (alternating single and multiple bonds) are significantly more stable than those without.

## Example Reactions

Now, we'll apply these rules to three novel reactions. Focus on the decision-making element of this process so that you will be able to apply the same logic to reactions that appear on Test Day.

### Reaction 1

We'll start with a series of reactions involving ethyl 5-oxohexanoate. First, it is reacted with 1,2-ethanediol and *p*-toluenesulfonic acid in benzene; second, with lithium aluminum hydride in tetrahydrofuran, followed by a heated acidic workup. What are the intermediates and final product?

Let's go through the steps:

1. First, let's draw out the reactants and reaction conditions.

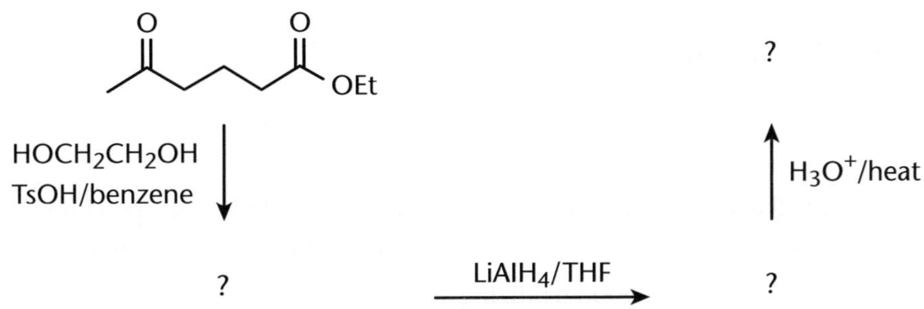


2. This molecule has an alkane backbone, a ketone, and an ester. Both of the carbonyl carbons are electrophilic targets for nucleophiles. The carbonyl oxygens can also be reduced. Acidic $\alpha$-hydrogens are also present.
3. For the first part of the reaction, we have a diol, which is commonly used as a protecting group for aldehydes or ketones. Diols are nucleophiles because of lone pairs on the oxygens in the hydroxyl groups. For the second reaction, we have a reducing agent in an organic solvent. Finally, we have an acidic workup—which is often used to remove protecting groups. We're starting to get hints as to what is happening here.
4. In the first reaction, both the ketone and ester carbonyls are highly reactive. One or both of these functional groups will react in the first step.
5. The diol is a good nucleophile because it contains lone pairs on the oxygen atoms in the hydroxyl groups. Further, the presence of a diol hints at protecting the ketone carbonyl because diols are commonly used for this function. This gives our first intermediate—the ketone carbonyl will be replaced by a protected diether. The second reaction, then, will only be able to proceed on the ester. $LiAlH_4$ is a strong reducing agent, so the next reaction will be reduction of the carbonyl all the way to an alcohol. In the final reaction, the protecting group will be removed by acidic workup, leaving us with our original ketone group.
6. The product and intermediate have no stereoselectivity, so this won't be a consideration.

Let's see what we came up with. The first intermediate will have a protective diether at the ketone carbonyl. The second will show the reduction of the ester to an alcohol, with the protecting group still present. The third will be our final product.

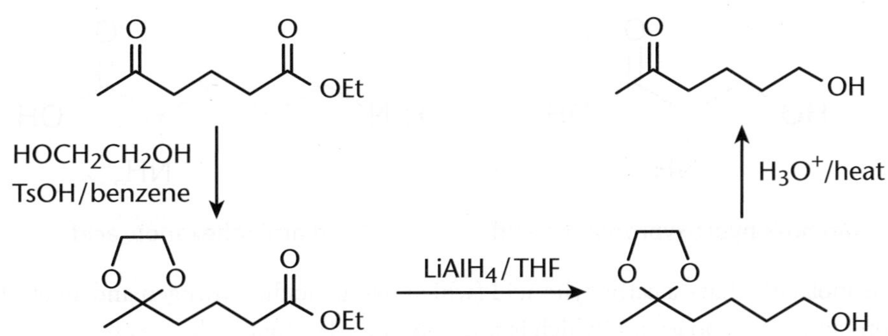

### Reaction 2

If ethanol is reacted in acidic solution with potassium dichromate, what will the end product be?

Let's go through the steps again.

1. First, let's draw out our molecules.

$$CH_3CH_2OH \xrightarrow[H_2SO_4]{K_2Cr_2O_7}$$

2. This molecule has an alkane backbone and a primary alcohol. Alcohols make good nucleophiles and can also be oxidized. The hydroxyl group can also act as a leaving group, especially if it gets protonated.
3. Next, the reagents. Dichromate is a good oxidizing agent.
4. The alcohol carbon is most likely to react because it is the most oxidized.
5. The primary product of a primary alcohol with a strong oxidant like dichromate will be a carboxylic acid. One other possible product could have been an aldehyde, so this could trip us up! Remember, however, that primary alcohols can only be oxidized to aldehydes by reagents specifically designated for this purpose, like pyridinium chlorochromate (PCC). If we start with ethanol, we'll obtain ethanoic acid (acetic acid) after reaction with dichromate.
6. Stereospecificity again isn't a consideration and won't change the outcome in this reaction.

Therefore, the primary product of this reaction will be ethanoic acid.

$$CH_3CH_2OH \xrightarrow[H_2SO_4]{K_2Cr_2O_7} CH_3COOH$$

### Reaction 3

Determine the product of a reaction between 2-amino-3-hydroxypropanoic acid and 2,6-diaminohexanoic acid in aqueous solution.

Let's go through the steps one last time.

1. First, let's draw out both molecules.

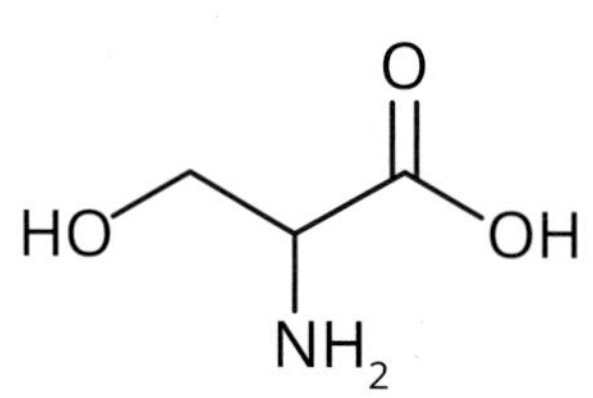


**2-amino-3-hydroxypropanoic acid**

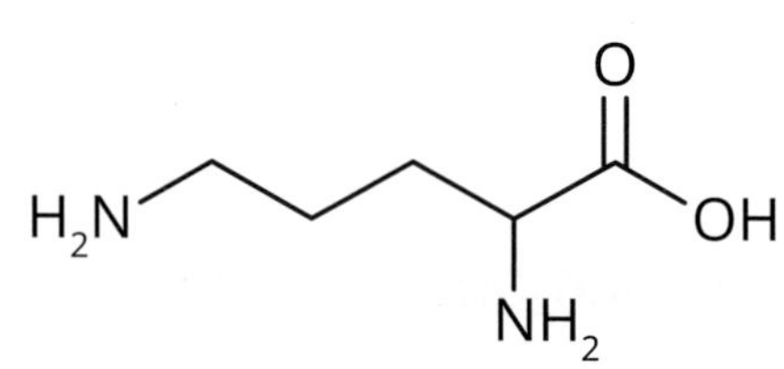


**2,6-diaminohexanoic acid**

2. Both of these molecules have a carboxylic acid (which has an acidic hydrogen and an electrophilic carbonyl carbon) and an amino group (which is nucleophilic). The first molecule also has a hydroxyl group; the second has an additional amino group and a long alkane chain.
3. There are no additional reagents listed. Therefore, it will be the properties of the two reactants alone that determine how the reaction will proceed.

4. Either of the two molecules could act as the nucleophile in this reaction, and either could be the electrophile. The most reactive species are likely the nucleophilic amino groups attacking the electrophilic carbonyl carbon.
5. The first step of this reaction will be nucleophilic attack by the amino group on the electrophilic carbonyl carbon. Carbon cannot have five bonds, so the carbonyl group will have to open up. The hydroxyl group on the carboxylic acid is a poor leaving group, but proton rearrangements in the molecule turn the hydroxyl group into water, improving its leaving group ability. Then, the carbonyl will reform, kicking off the water molecule as a leaving group.
6. We might ask why the hydroxyl group on 2-amino-3-hydroxypropanoic acid doesn't react. Remember that more oxidized groups tend to be more reactive, and the carboxylic acid is significantly more oxidized than the hydroxyl group. Another question to consider is which of the amino groups of 2,6-diaminohexanoic acid will react. This is a question that is perhaps best answered retrospectively; in this case, the amino group closer to the carbonyl will react because the resulting product will be stabilized by resonance.

Does this reaction look familiar? It should! 2-amino-3-hydroxypropanoic acid and 2,6-diaminohexanoic acid are serine and lysine, respectively—in this reaction, we are forming a peptide bond. Note that without using protecting groups, a simple reaction between two different amino acids would result in a mixture of products (Ser-Ser, Lys-Ser, Ser-Lys, and Lys-Lys) because either amino acid can act as the nucleophile or the electrophile. If we treat them as generic amino acids, this is the reaction:

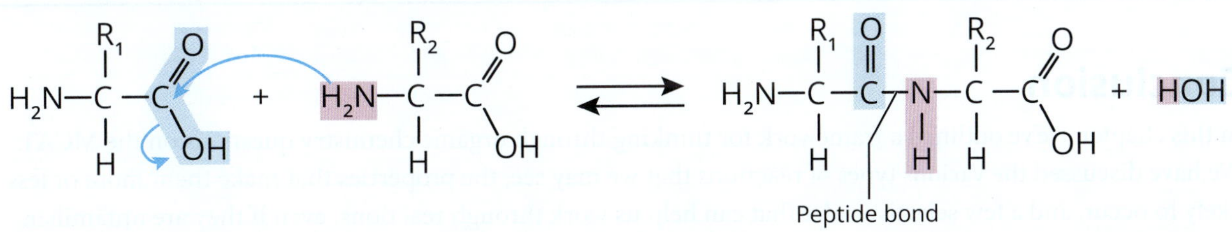


We've worked through a few problems here to get a handle on how to use this method. Once you have read further chapters and learned specific mechanisms that we did not touch on here, be sure to come back and see how these rules apply to novel reactions.

## MCAT CONCEPT CHECK 4.5

Before you move on, assess your understanding of the material with these questions.

1. What are the six steps for solving organic chemistry reactions?

   1. ____________________

   2. ____________________

   3. ____________________

   4. ____________________

   5. ____________________

   6. ____________________

2. If there are no reaction conditions listed, what determines how the reaction will proceed?

   ____________________

## Conclusion

In this chapter, we've outlined a framework for thinking through organic chemistry questions on the MCAT. We have discussed the various types of reactions that we may see, the properties that make them more or less likely to occur, and a few selective rules that can help us work through reactions, even if they are unfamiliar. Finally, we put this framework to the test on example problems in order to cement its application. With this framework in mind, there's nothing you can't tackle—revisit these rules and methods as you continue working through the different functional groups and their reactions in the next six chapters!

**GO ONLINE**

**You've reviewed the content, now test your knowledge and critical thinking skills by completing a test-like passage set in your online resources!**

# CONCEPT SUMMARY

## Acids and Bases

- **Lewis acids** are electron acceptors; they have vacant orbitals or positively polarized atoms.
- **Lewis bases** are electron donors; they have a lone pair of electrons and are often anions.
- **Brønsted–Lowry acids** are proton donors; **Brønsted–Lowry bases** are proton acceptors.
- **Amphoteric molecules** can act as either acids or bases, depending on reaction conditions. Water is a common example of an amphoteric molecule.
- The **acid dissociation constant, $K_a$**, is a measure of acidity. It is the equilibrium constant corresponding to the dissociation of an acid, HA, into a proton ($H^+$) and its conjugate base ($A^-$).
  - **p$K_a$** is the negative logarithm of $K_a$. A lower (or even negative) p$K_a$ indicates a stronger acid.
  - p$K_a$ decreases down the periodic table and as electronegativity increases.
- Alcohols, aldehydes, ketones, carboxylic acids, and carboxylic acid derivatives are common acidic functional groups. **$\alpha$-hydrogens** (hydrogens connected to an **$\alpha$-carbon**, a carbon adjacent to a carbonyl) are acidic.
- Amines and amides are common basic functional groups.

## Nucleophiles, Electrophiles, and Leaving Groups

- **Nucleophiles** are "nucleus-loving" and contain lone pairs or $\pi$ bonds. They have increased electron density and often carry a negative charge.
  - Nucleophilicity is similar to basicity; however, nucleophilicity is a kinetic property, while basicity is thermodynamic.
  - Charge, electronegativity, steric hindrance, and the solvent can all affect nucleophilicity.
  - Amino groups are common organic nucleophiles.
- **Electrophiles** are "electron-loving" and contain a positive charge or are positively polarized.
  - More positive compounds are more electrophilic.
  - Alcohols, aldehydes, ketones, carboxylic acids, and their derivatives can act as electrophiles.
- **Leaving groups** are the molecular fragments that retain the electrons after **heterolysis**.
  - The best leaving groups can stabilize additional charge through resonance or induction.
  - Weak bases (the conjugate bases of strong acids) make good leaving groups.
  - Alkanes and hydrogen ions are almost never leaving groups because they form reactive anions.
- **Unimolecular nucleophilic substitution ($S_N1$) reactions** proceed in two steps.
  - In the first step, the leaving group leaves, forming a **carbocation**, an ion with a positively charged carbon atom.
  - In the second step, the nucleophile attacks the planar carbocation from either side, leading to a racemic mixture of products.
  - $S_N1$ reactions prefer more substituted carbons because the alkyl groups can donate electron density and stabilize the positive charge of the carbocation.
  - The rate of an $S_N1$ reaction is dependent only on the concentration of the substrate: rate $= k[R{-}L]$.

- **Bimolecular nucleophilic substitution** ($S_N2$) **reactions** proceed in one **concerted** step.
  - The nucleophile attacks at the same time as the leaving group leaves.
  - The nucleophile must perform a **backside attack**, which leads to an inversion of stereochemistry.
  - The absolute configuration is changed—(*R*) to (*S*) and vice versa—if the incoming nucleophile and the leaving group have the same priority in the molecule.
  - $S_N2$ reactions prefer less-substituted carbons because the alkyl groups create steric hindrance and inhibit the nucleophile from accessing the electrophilic substrate carbon.
  - The rate of an $S_N2$ reaction is dependent on the concentrations of both the substrate and the nucleophile: rate $= k[\text{Nu:}][\text{R–L}]$.

## Oxidation–Reduction Reactions

- The **oxidation state** of an atom is the charge it would have if all its bonds were completely ionic.
  - $CH_4$ is the lowest oxidation state of carbon (most reduced); $CO_2$ is the highest (most oxidized).
  - Carboxylic acids and carboxylic acid derivatives are the most oxidized functional groups, followed by aldehydes, ketones, and imines, followed by alcohols, alkyl halides, and amines.
- **Oxidation** is an increase in oxidation state and is assisted by oxidizing agents.
  - **Oxidizing agents** accept electrons and are reduced in the process. They have a high affinity for electrons or an unusually high oxidation state. They often contain a metal and a large number of oxygens.
  - Primary alcohols can be oxidized to aldehydes by pyridinium chlorochromate (PCC) or to carboxylic acids by stronger oxidizing agents, like chromium trioxide ($CrO_3$) or sodium or potassium dichromate ($Na_2Cr_2O_7$ or $K_2Cr_2O_7$).
  - Secondary alcohols can be oxidized to ketones by most oxidizing agents.
  - Aldehydes can be oxidized to carboxylic acids by most oxidizing agents.
- **Reduction** is a decrease in oxidation state and is assisted by reducing agents.
  - **Reducing agents** donate electrons and are oxidized in the process. They have low electronegativity and ionization energy. They often contain a metal and a large number of hydrides.
  - Aldehydes, ketones, and carboxylic acids can be reduced to alcohols by lithium aluminum hydride ($LiAlH_4$).
  - Amides can be reduced to amines by $LiAlH_4$.
  - Esters can be reduced to a pair of alcohols by $LiAlH_4$.

## Chemoselectivity

- Both nucleophile–electrophile and oxidation–reduction reactions tend to act at the highest-priority (most oxidized) functional group.
- One can make use of steric hindrance properties to selectively target functional groups that might not primarily react, or to protect functional groups.
  - Diols are often used as protecting groups for aldehyde or ketone carbonyls.
  - Alcohols may be protected by conversion to *tert*-butyl ethers.

## Steps to Problem Solving

1. Know your nomenclature
2. Identify the functional groups
3. Identify the other reagents
4. Identify the most reactive functional group(s)
5. Identify the first step of the reaction
6. Consider stereoselectivity

## ANSWERS TO CONCEPT CHECKS

### 4.1

1. An acid–base reaction will proceed when the acid and base react to form conjugate products that are weaker than the reactants.
2. Amphoteric species can act as either an acid or a base. Water, bicarbonate, and dihydrogen phosphate are common amphoteric species in biological systems.
3. $pK_a = -\log K_a$, where $K_a$ is the equilibrium constant for the dissociation of an acid. $pK_a$ indicates acid strength: a stronger acid has a lower (or even negative) $pK_a$.
4. Alcohols, aldehydes and ketones, carboxylic acids, and most carboxylic acid derivatives act as acids. Amines and amides act as bases.

### 4.2

1. Nucleophilicity and electrophilicity are based on relative rates of reactions and are therefore kinetic properties. Acidity and basicity are measured by the position of equilibrium in a protonation or deprotonation reaction and are therefore thermodynamic properties.
2. *t*-Butoxide < isopropanolate < ethoxide < methoxide. The four main determinants of nucleophilicity are charge (more negative = better nucleophile), electronegativity (more electronegative = worse nucleophile), steric hindrance (larger = worse nucleophile), and the solvent (protic solvents can protonate or hydrogen bond with the nucleophile, decreasing its reactivity). Each of these nucleophiles has the same attacking atom (oxygen), but differ in their bulkiness. The molecules with the least steric hindrance will be the more effective nucleophiles.
3. A substitution reaction will proceed when the nucleophile is a stronger base (more reactive) than the leaving group.
4. Greater positive charge increases electrophilicity, and better leaving groups increase electrophilicity by making the reaction more likely to proceed.
5. Good leaving groups can stabilize the extra electrons that result from heterolysis. Weak bases (the conjugate bases of strong acids) are good leaving groups. Resonance stabilization and inductive effects from electron-withdrawing groups also improve leaving group ability.

## 4.3

1. Good oxidizing agents have a high affinity for electrons or have very high oxidation states. Examples include $O_2$, $O_3$, $Cl_2$, permanganate ($MnO_4^-$), chromate ($CrO_4^-$), dichromate ($CrO_4^{2-}$), and pyridinium chlorochromate. These compounds often contain a metal and a large number of oxygen atoms.
2. Good reducing agents have low electronegativities and ionization energies or contain a hydride ion ($H^-$). Examples include sodium, magnesium, aluminum, zinc, sodium hydride (NaH), calcium dihydride ($CaH_2$), lithium aluminum hydride ($LiAlH_4$), and sodium borohydride ($NaBH_4$). These compounds often contain a metal and a large number of hydrides.
3. Carbon dioxide, carboxylic acid, ketone, alcohol, methane

## 4.4

1. The two reactive centers are the carbonyl carbon, which is electrophilic, and the $\alpha$-hydrogens, which are acidic.
2. $S_N1$ reactions are most likely to occur on tertiary carbons where a carbocation can be most easily stabilized. The first reaction has a tertiary carbon containing a good leaving group while the second reaction has a secondary carbon containing a good leaving group. The first reaction will proceed more quickly.
3. $S_N2$ reactions are easily inhibited by steric hindrance. The fluorides are smaller than the methyls and so the difluoride molecule will be more suitable for an $S_N2$.

## 4.5

1. 1. Know your nomenclature
   2. Identify the functional groups
   3. Identify the other reagents
   4. Identify the most reactive functional group(s)
   5. Identify the first step of the reaction
   6. Consider stereoselectivity
2. If there are no reagents other than the reactants, then the properties of the functional groups on the reactants themselves (acid–base; nucleophile–electrophile) will determine the outcome.

# SCIENCE MASTERY ASSESSMENT EXPLANATIONS

1. **C**

$NH_3$ and $H_2O$ are Lewis bases because nitrogen and oxygen can donate lone pairs. $Ag^+$ is a Lewis acid because it can accept a lone pair into an unoccupied orbital.

2. **C**

Remember, good nucleophiles tend to have lone pairs or $\pi$ bonds and are negatively charged or polarized. Alkoxide ($OR^-$) and hydroxide ($OH^-$) anions are strong nucleophiles. Alcohols (ROH) and carboxylic acids (RCOOH) are weak nucleophiles. The alkyl group of an alkoxide anion donates additional electron density, making it more reactive than the hydroxide ion. The carboxylic acid contains more electron-withdrawing oxygen atoms than the alcohol, making it less nucleophilic.

3. **D**

Good electrophiles are positively charged or polarized. $CR_3^+$ is a tertiary carbocation; it has a positive charge, which makes it very electrophilic. $CH_3Cl$ and $CH_3OH$ are both polarized; however, the leaving groups differ between these two. $Cl^-$ is a weaker base than $OH^-$ (HCl is a stronger acid than $H_2O$). As such, $Cl^-$ will be more stable in solution than $OH^-$, which increases the electrophilic reactivity of $CH_3Cl$ above $CH_3OH$. $CH_3OCH_3$ has a much less stable leaving group, $CH_3O^-$, and is therefore significantly less electrophilic.

4. **A**

Good leaving groups are weak bases, which are the conjugates of strong acids. Leaving groups must also be stable once they leave the molecule. $H_2O$ is, by far, the most stable leaving group and will be extremely unreactive once it leaves the molecule through heterolysis. $Br^-$ is the conjugate base of HBr; $HO^-$ is the conjugate base of water. HBr is a much stronger acid than water, so $Br^-$ is a better leaving group than $HO^-$. Finally, hydride ($H^-$) is a very poor leaving group because it is extremely unstable in solution.

5. **B**

Carboxylic acids are the second most oxidized form of carbon (only carbon dioxide is more oxidized). In carboxylic acids, the carbon atom has three bonds to oxygen. In aldehydes, the carbon atom has two bonds to oxygen. In amines, the carbon atom has one bond to nitrogen. In an alkane, the carbon only has bonds to other carbons and hydrogens.

6. **B**

During this reaction, the alkoxide anion accepts a proton, meaning this molecule acts as a Brønsted-Lowry base. Also, in accepting the proton, the alkoxide anion donates a lone pair of electrons to form a coordinate covalent bond with the incoming hydrogen ion. In this way, the alkoxide anion is also acting as a Lewis base. Together, these observations support **(B)**.

7. **C**

Because 2-butanol is a secondary alcohol, oxidation by a strong oxidizing agent like dichromate will result in a ketone, butanone.

8. **C**

Pyridinium chlorochromate is a weak oxidizing agent, and will oxidize an alcohol to an aldehyde. Stronger oxidizing agents are required to convert a primary alcohol to a carboxylic acid.

9. **B**

An $S_N1$ reaction is a first-order nucleophilic substitution reaction. It is called first-order because the rate-limiting step involves only one molecule. **(A)** is true, but does not explain why $S_N1$ reactions have first-order kinetics; the rate-limiting step of an $S_N2$ reaction is also the first (and only) step of that reaction, but $S_N2$ reactions have second-order kinetics, not first-order. **(C)** is a true statement as well, but again does not explain why the reaction is first-order. Finally, **(D)** is incorrect because it is the rate-limiting step, not the reaction overall, that involves only one molecule.

10. **D**

In a protic solvent, the protons in solution can attach to the nucleophile, decreasing its nucleophilicity. The larger the nucleophile, and the stronger its conjugate acid, the stronger the nucleophile will be. Of the options given, $I^-$ will therefore be the strongest nucleophile because it is least likely to associate with the protons in solution.

11. **D**

Primary and secondary alcohols can be oxidized by PCC because the central carbon atom can form additional bonds with oxygen while losing bonds to hydrogen, justifying **(D)** as the right answer. Choices **(A)**, a tertiary alcohol; **(B)**, a ketone; and **(C)**, a carboxylic acid, cannot be oxidized by PCC because the central carbon in these molecules is already making four bonds to other carbon or oxygen atoms, and therefore cannot readily form more bonds to oxygen.

12. **A**

Steric hindrance slows $S_N2$ pathways, so the molecule that is fastest to react will be the one that is least sterically hindered. The reactivity trend based on steric hindrance is methyl > primary > secondary (note that tertiary substrates are too hindered to react via $S_N2$ at all). The molecule in **(A)** is a primary substrate, that is, the least sterically hindered, and will therefore react rapidly by an $S_N2$ pathway. Additionally, the molecule in **(A)** has a good leaving group. Together, these trends make **(A)** the best substrate for rapid $S_N2$. Note that while **(C)** also depicts a primary substrate, this molecule does not have a good leaving group, so **(C)** can be eliminated. Choices **(B)** and **(D)** can be eliminated because these molecules are secondary substrates.

13. **D**

To carry out a nucleophile–electrophile reaction, the nucleophile must be able to dissolve in the solvent. Nucleophiles are nearly always polar, and often carry a charge. Polar solvents are therefore preferred for these reactions. Hexane is a nonpolar solvent and will not be useful for a nucleophile–electrophile reaction.

14. **A**

Aldehydes have one alkyl group connected to the carbonyl carbon, whereas ketones have two. This creates more steric hindrance in ketones, which lowers their reactivity to nucleophiles. Ketones are also less reactive because their carbonyl carbon has less positive charge character; the additional alkyl group can donate electron density—the opposite of **(D)**—which decreases the electrophilicity of the compound.

15. **D**

Remember, there is a hierarchy to the reactivity of carboxylic acid derivatives that dictates how reactive they are toward nucleophilic attack. In order from highest to lowest, this is anhydrides > carboxylic acids and esters > amides. In practical terms, this means that derivatives of higher reactivity can form derivatives of lower reactivity but not vice versa. Nucleophilic attack of an ester cannot result in the corresponding anhydride because anhydrides are more reactive than esters.

**GO ONLINE**

**Consult your online resources for additional practice.**

## EQUATIONS TO REMEMBER

(4.1) **Acid dissociation constant:** $K_a = \frac{[H^+][A^-]}{[HA]}$

(4.2) **Definition of p$K_a$:** $pK_a = -\log K_a$

## SHARED CONCEPTS

**General Chemistry Chapter 5**
Chemical Kinetics

**General Chemistry Chapter 10**
Acids and Bases

**General Chemistry Chapter 11**
Oxidation–Reduction Reactions

**Organic Chemistry Chapter 1**
Nomenclature

**Organic Chemistry Chapter 5**
Alcohols

**Organic Chemistry Chapter 7**
Aldehydes and Ketones II

CHAPTER 5

# ALCOHOLS

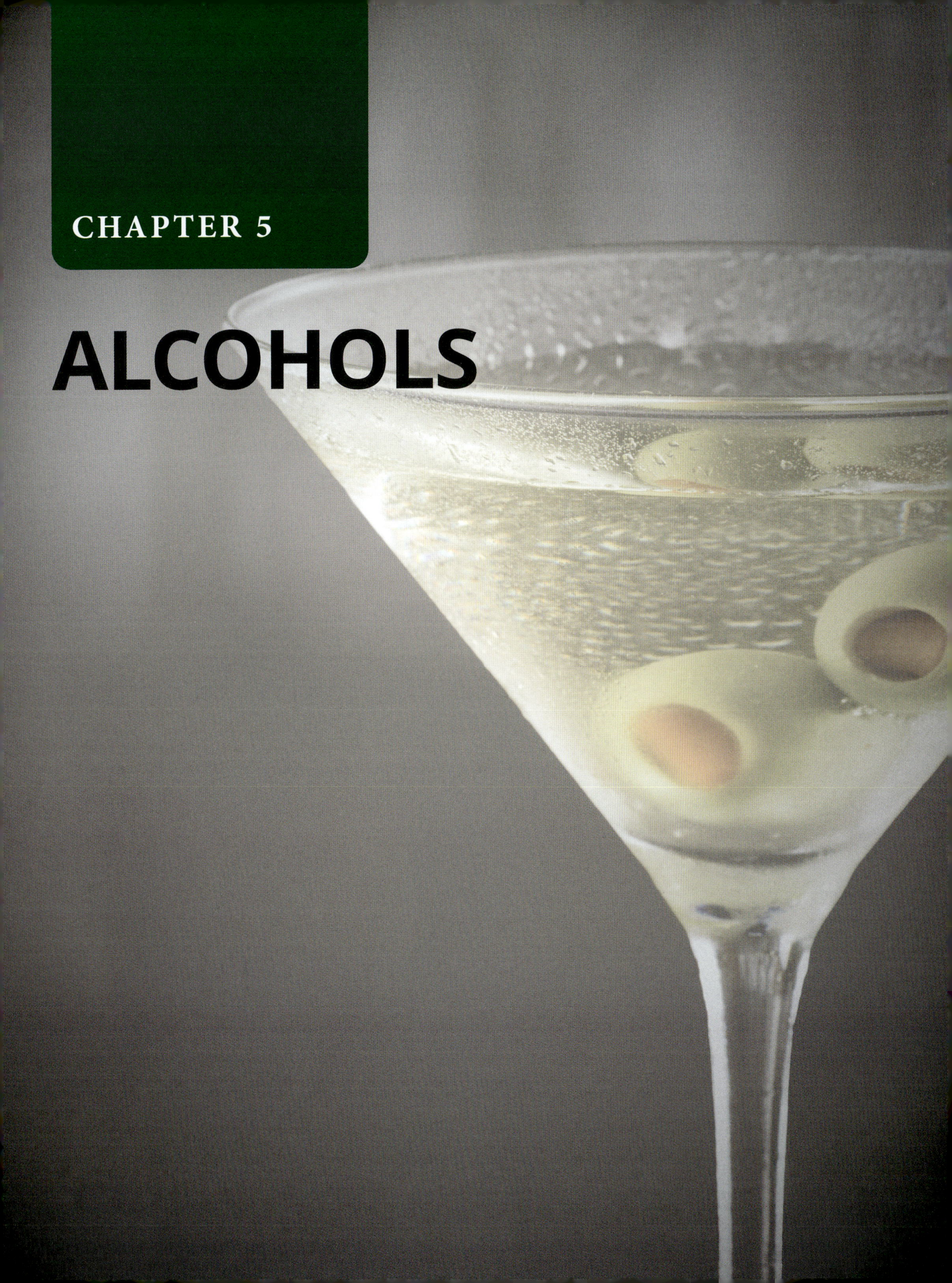

# SCIENCE MASTERY ASSESSMENT

Every pre-med knows this feeling: there is so much content I have to know for the MCAT! How do I know what to do first or what's important?

While the high-yield badges throughout this book will help you identify the most important topics, this Science Mastery Assessment is another tool in your MCAT prep arsenal. This quiz (which can also be taken in your online resources) and the guidance below will help ensure that you are spending the appropriate amount of time on this chapter based on your personal strengths and weaknesses. Don't worry though—skipping something now does not mean you'll never study it. Later on in your prep, as you complete full-length tests, you'll uncover specific pieces of content that you need to review and can come back to these chapters as appropriate.

## How to Use This Assessment

### If you answer 0–7 questions correctly:

Spend about 1 hour to read this chapter in full and take limited notes throughout. Follow up by reviewing **all** quiz questions to ensure that you now understand how to solve each one.

### If you answer 8–11 questions correctly:

Spend 20–40 minutes reviewing the quiz questions. Beginning with the questions you missed, read and take notes on the corresponding subchapters. For questions you answered correctly, ensure your thinking matches that of the explanation and you understand why each choice was correct or incorrect.

### If you answer 12–15 questions correctly:

Spend less than 20 minutes reviewing all questions from the quiz. If you missed any, then include a quick read-through of the corresponding subchapters, or even just the relevant content within a subchapter, as part of your question review. For questions you got correct, ensure your thinking matches that of the explanation and review the Concept Summary at the end of the chapter.

1. Alcohols have higher boiling points than their analogous hydrocarbons because:
   - **A.** the oxygen atoms in alcohols have shorter bond lengths.
   - **B.** hydrogen bonding is present in alcohols.
   - **C.** alcohols are more acidic than their analogous hydrocarbons.
   - **D.** alcohols can be oxidized to ketones.

2. Tertiary alcohols are oxidized with difficulty because:
   - **A.** there is no hydrogen attached to the carbon with the hydroxyl group.
   - **B.** there is no hydrogen attached to the $\alpha$-carbon of the carbonyl.
   - **C.** tertiary alcohols contain hydroxyl groups with no polarization.
   - **D.** they are relatively inert.

3. The IUPAC name of this molecule is:

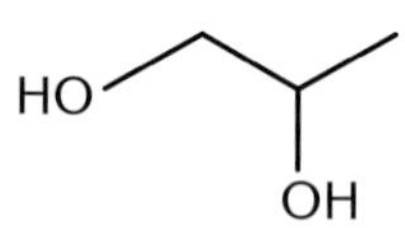


   - **A.** ethane-1,2-diol.
   - **B.** propane-1,2-diol.
   - **C.** dimethanol.
   - **D.** dipropanol.

4. The IUPAC name of this molecule is:

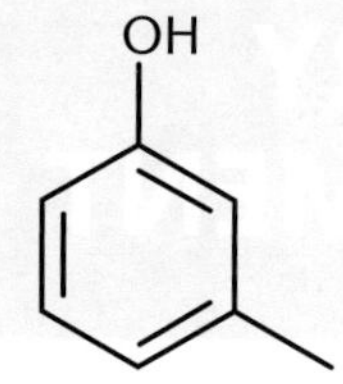


   - **A.** 2-methylcyclohexanol.
   - **B.** *m*-methylphenol.
   - **C.** *p*-methylphenol.
   - **D.** 3-methylcyclohexanol.

5. Which of the following correctly lists methanol, isobutyl alcohol, and propanol by decreasing boiling point?
   - **A.** Methanol > isobutyl alcohol > propanol
   - **B.** Isobutyl alcohol > methanol > propanol
   - **C.** Isobutyl alcohol > propanol > methanol
   - **D.** Methanol > propanol > isobutyl alcohol

6. Which of the following correctly lists hexanol, phenol, and cyclohexanol by increasing acidity of the hydroxyl hydrogen?
   - **A.** Phenol < hexanol < cyclohexanol
   - **B.** Cyclohexanol < hexanol < phenol
   - **C.** Cyclohexanol < phenol < hexanol
   - **D.** Phenol < cyclohexanol < hexanol

7. Which of the following will convert $CH_3CH_2CH_2OH$ to $CH_3CH_2CHO$?
   I. $CrO_3$
   II. PCC
   III. $K_2Cr_2O_7$
   A. I only
   B. II only
   C. I and III only
   D. I, II, and III

8. Which of the following will convert cyclohexanol to cyclohexanone?
   I. Chromium trioxide
   II. Pyridinium chlorochromate
   III. Sodium dichromate
   A. I only
   B. II only
   C. I and III only
   D. I, II, and III

9. Successfully converting 3-phenylpropanol to 3-phenylpropanoic acid by the Jones oxidation requires the oxidizing agent, the solvent, and:
   A. dilute sulfuric acid.
   B. dilute sodium hydroxide.
   C. anhydrous conditions.
   D. high temperature.

10. Treating 2-methyl-1-propanol with methylsulfonyl chloride in base, followed by reaction with pyridinium chlorochromate, and a final step in strong acid, will give an end product of:
   A. 2-methyl-1-propanol.
   B. 2-methylpropanal.
   C. 2-methylpropanoic acid.
   D. 2-methyl-1-propane.

11. Reaction of 1-phenylethanone with ethylene glycol, also known as ethane-1,2-diol, in aqueous $H_2SO_4$ will result in the formation of:
   A. a ketal.
   B. a carboxylic acid.
   C. an aldehyde.
   D. a hemiacetal.

12. Treatment of this molecule with $CrO_3$ under appropriate reaction conditions will yield which of the following molecules?

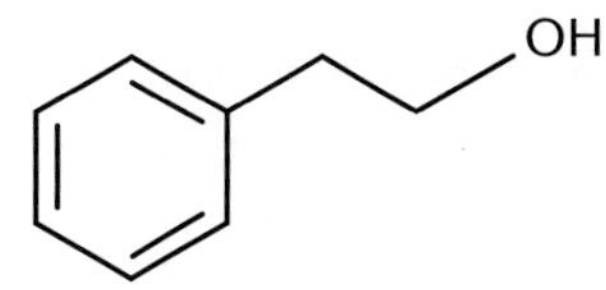


   A. 2-Phenylethanol
   B. Phenylacetaldehyde
   C. Phenylacetone
   D. 2-Phenylethanoic acid

13. In order to convert phenols into hydroxyquinones, how many steps of oxidation or reduction are required?
   A. 1 oxidation step
   B. 2 oxidation steps
   C. 1 reduction step
   D. 2 reduction steps

14. The conversion of ubiquinone to ubiquinol requires what type of reaction?
   A. Condensation
   B. Oxidation
   C. Reduction
   D. Hydrolysis

15. Which of the following will convert a cyclic acetal to a carbonyl and a dialcohol?
   A. Aqueous acid
   B. $LiAlH_4$
   C. $CrO_3$
   D. Acetone

## Answer Key

1. **B** (See section 5.1)
2. **A** (See section 5.2)
3. **B** (See section 5.1)
4. **B** (See section 5.1)
5. **C** (See section 5.1)
6. **B** (See section 5.1)
7. **B** (See section 5.2)
8. **D** (See section 5.2)
9. **A** (See section 5.3)
10. **A** (See section 5.2)
11. **A** (See section 5.3)
12. **D** (See section 5.3)
13. **B** (See section 5.3)
14. **C** (See section 5.2)
15. **A** (See section 5.2)

*The relevant section of the chapter to review for each question is given in parentheses after the correct answer. Detailed explanations can be found at the end of the chapter.*

CHAPTER 5

# ALCOHOLS

## In This Chapter



**CHAPTER PROFILE**

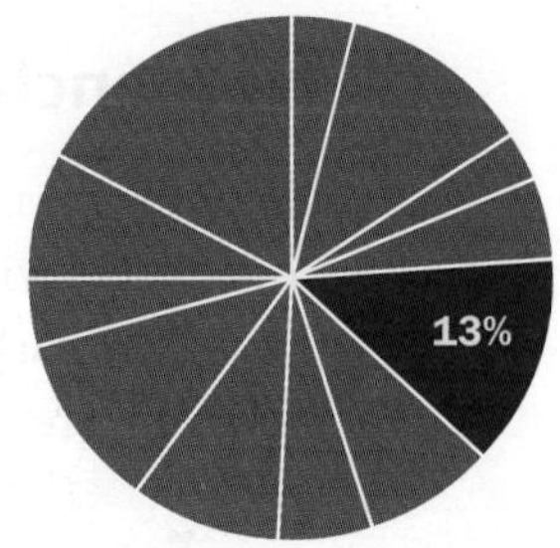


The content in this chapter should be relevant to about 13% of all questions about organic chemistry on the MCAT.

This chapter covers material from the following AAMC content category:

**5D:** Structure, function, and reactivity of biologically-relevant molecules

## Introduction

Alcohols are probably the most popular chemicals you'll encounter in organic chemistry. Ethanol has been popular with humans for more than 10,000 years. It's not just humans, either: many animals are known to seek out rotten fruits that have fermented enough to contain moderate levels of ethanol. Note that when we talk about consuming "alcohol," we are referring exclusively to ethanol (grain alcohol). In fact, consuming other alcohols can have drastically negative effects. Methanol (wood alcohol), for example, is oxidized by the body to formic acid, which is extremely toxic to the optic nerve and retina and can cause blindness when ingested. Isopropyl alcohol, commonly used as an antiseptic, can cause severe central nervous system depression. For organic chemistry purposes, of course, we do not restrict ourselves to only one type of alcohol—many are used synthetically and in analytic techniques.

## 5.1 Description and Properties

**LEARNING OBJECTIVES**

After Chapter 5.1, you will be able to:

- Predict the relative $pK_a$ values of two given alcohols
- Order alcohols based on boiling point

Alcohols have the general formula ROH, with the functional group —OH referred to as a **hydroxyl** group.

**MCAT EXPERTISE**

Alcohols are an important group of compounds. They will be seen on the MCAT as protic solvents, reactants, products, and prime examples of hydrogen bonding.

### Nomenclature

Alcohols are named in the IUPAC system by replacing the –e ending of the root alkane with the ending **–ol**. If the alcohol is the highest-priority functional group, the carbon atom attached to it receives the lowest possible number. Some examples are shown in Figure 5.1.

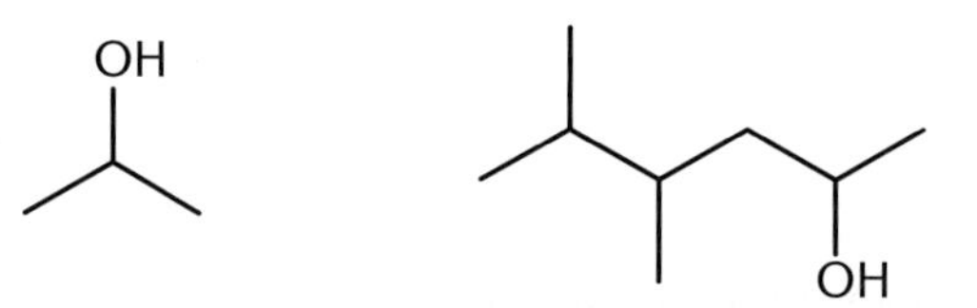


2-propanol     4,5-dimethyl-2-hexanol

**Figure 5.1** IUPAC Names of Alcohols

Alternatively, the common naming practice is to name the alkyl group as a derivative, followed by **alcohol**, as shown in Figure 5.2.

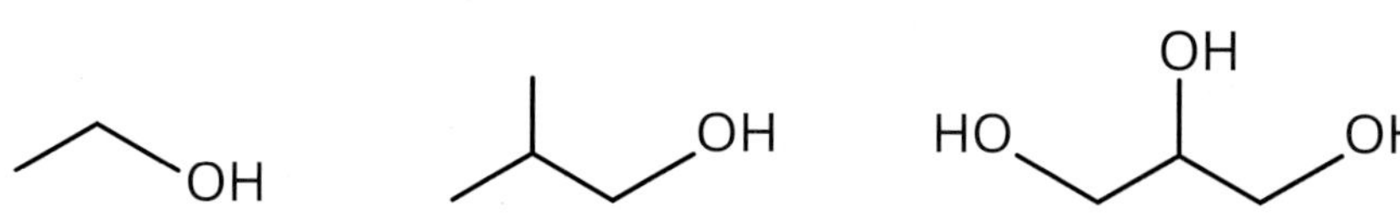


**ethyl alcohol** (ethanol)     **isobutyl alcohol** (2-methylpropan-1-ol)     **glycerol** (propane-1,2,3-triol)

**Figure 5.2** Common Names of Alcohols

When the alcohol is not the highest-priority group, it is named as a substituent, with the prefix **hydroxy–**, as shown in Figure 5.3. In 3-hydroxybutanoic acid, the hydroxyl group on carbon 3 is named using the prefix hydroxy– because the carboxylic acid functional group (C1) has higher naming priority. Similarly, in 1,3-dihydroxypropan-2-one, the hydroxyl groups on carbons 1 and 3 are named using the prefix hydroxy– because the ketone functional group (C2) has higher naming priority.

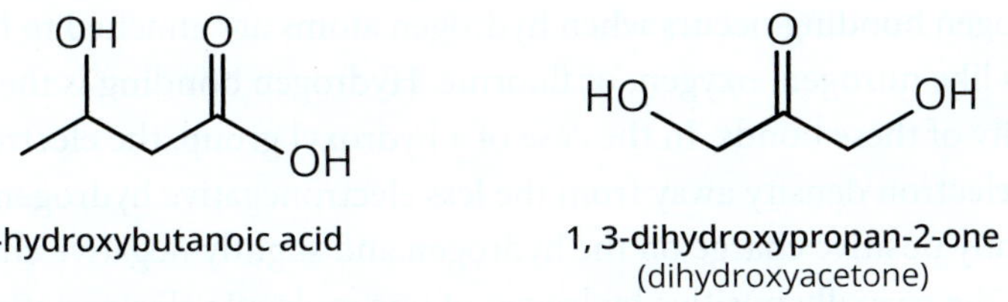


**Figure 5.3** Naming Alcohols as Substituents

Finally, we will also see that hydroxyl groups can be attached to aromatic rings, as shown in Figure 5.4. These compounds are called **phenols**. The hydroxyl hydrogens of phenols are particularly acidic due to resonance within the phenol ring. When benzene rings contain two substituents, their relative positions must be indicated. Two groups on adjacent carbons are called ***ortho***–, or simply ***o***–. Two groups separated by a carbon are called ***meta***–, or ***m***–. Two groups on opposite sides of the ring are called ***para***–, or ***p***–.

### KEY CONCEPT

Aromatic alcohols are called phenols. The possible resonance between the ring and the lone pairs of the oxygen atom in the hydroxyl group make the hydrogen of the alcohol more acidic than other alcohols.

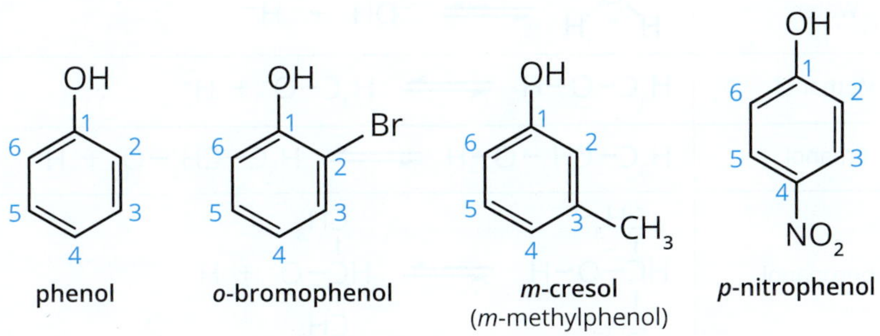


**Figure 5.4** Phenols: Aromatic Alcohols

## Physical Properties

One of the prominent properties of alcohols is that they are capable of intermolecular hydrogen bonding, which results in significantly higher melting and boiling points than those of analogous hydrocarbons, as shown in Figure 5.5.

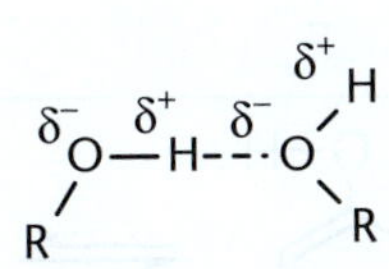


**Figure 5.5** Intermolecular Hydrogen Bonding in Alcohols

Molecules with more than one hydroxyl group show greater degrees of hydrogen bonding. This is evident from the boiling points shown in Figure 5.6.

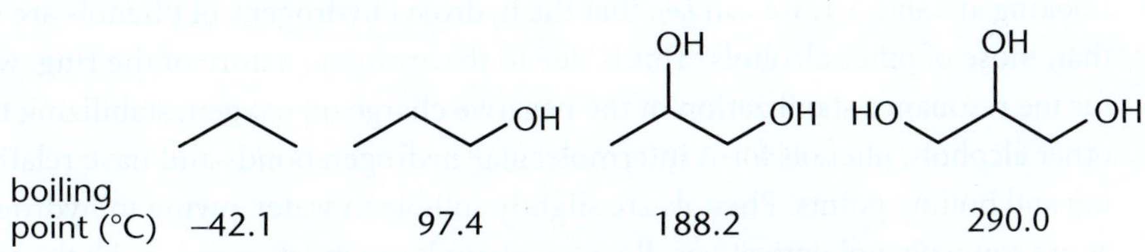


**Figure 5.6** Effect of Hydroxyl Groups on Boiling Point
*Boiling point increases significantly with additional hydroxyl groups, which permit more hydrogen bonding.*

### MCAT EXPERTISE

Hydrogen bonding causes increased melting points, boiling points, and solubility in water.

Hydrogen bonding occurs when hydrogen atoms are attached to highly electronegative atoms like nitrogen, oxygen, or fluorine. Hydrogen bonding is the result of the extreme polarity of these bonds. In the case of a hydroxyl group, the electronegative oxygen atom pulls electron density away from the less electronegative hydrogen atom. This generates a slightly positive charge on the hydrogen and slightly negative charge on the oxygen. Then, the partially positive hydrogen of one molecule electrostatically attracts the partially negative oxygen of another molecule, generating a noncovalent bonding force known as a **hydrogen bond**.

The hydroxyl hydrogen is weakly acidic, and alcohols can dissociate into protons and alkoxide ions in the same way that water dissociates into protons and hydroxide ions. Table 5.1 gives p$K_a$ values of several hydroxyl-containing compounds.

### BRIDGE

Remember from Chapter 10 of *MCAT General Chemistry Review* that p$K_a = -\log K_a$. Strong acids have high $K_a$ values and low p$K_a$ values. Thus, phenol, which has the smallest p$K_a$, is the most acidic of the alcohols listed in Table 5.1.

| Compound | Dissociation | p$K_a$ |
|---|---|---|
| Water | $H-O-H \rightleftharpoons {}^-OH + H^+$ | 14.0 |
| Methanol | $H_3C-O-H \rightleftharpoons H_3C-O^- + H^+$ | 15.5 |
| Ethanol | $H_3C-CH_2-O-H \rightleftharpoons H_3C-CH_2-O^- + H^+$ | 15.9 |
| Isopropanol | $(CH_3)_2HC-O-H \rightleftharpoons (CH_3)_2HC-O^- + H^+$ | 16.5 |
| *tert*-butanol | $H_3C-C(CH_3)_2-O-H \rightleftharpoons H_3C-C(CH_3)_2-O^- + H^+$ | 17.0 |
| 2,2,2-trifluoroethanol | $F-CF_2-CH_2-O-H \rightleftharpoons F-CF_2-CH_2-O^- + H^+$ | 12.5 |
| Phenol | 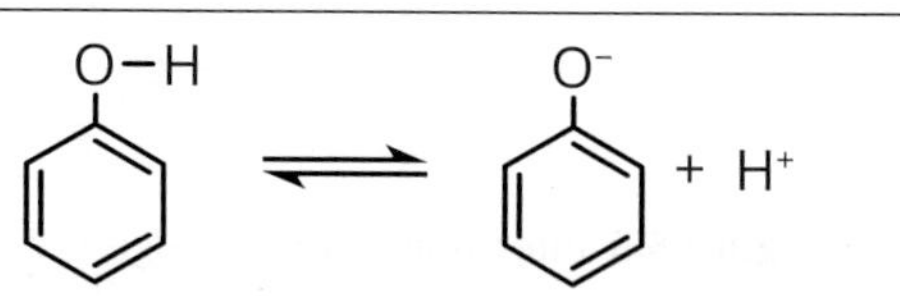 | ~10.0 |

**Table 5.1** p$K_a$ Values of Hydroxyl-Containing Compounds

Looking at Table 5.1, we can see that the hydroxyl hydrogens of phenols are more acidic than those of other alcohols. This is due to the aromatic nature of the ring, which allows for the resonance stabilization of the negative charge on oxygen, stabilizing the anion. Like other alcohols, phenols form intermolecular hydrogen bonds and have relatively high melting and boiling points. Phenols are slightly soluble in water, owing to hydrogen bonding, as are some phenol derivatives. Because phenols are much more acidic than nonaromatic alcohols, they can form salts with inorganic bases such as NaOH.

The presence of other substituents on the ring has significant effects on the acidity, boiling points, and melting points of phenols. As with other compounds, electron-withdrawing substituents increase acidity, and electron-donating groups decrease acidity. Figure 5.7 illustrates these stabilization and destabilization effects on an alkoxide anion.

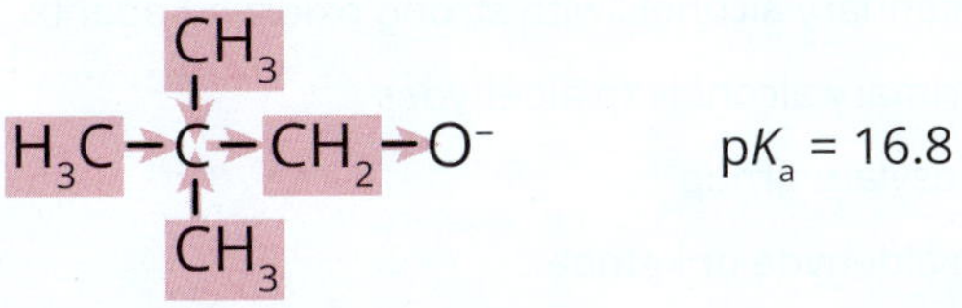


**2,2-dimethylpropanol**

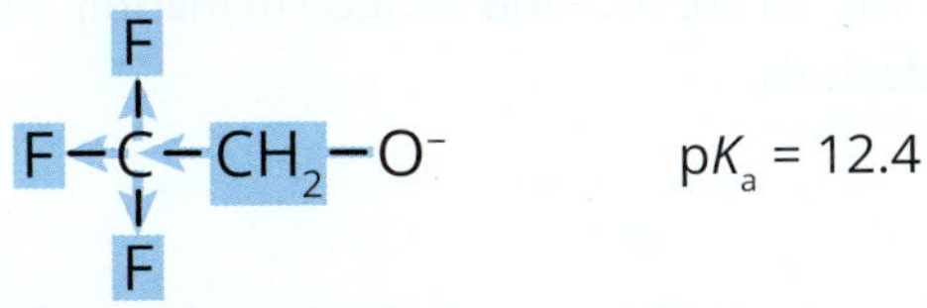


**2,2,2-trifluoroethanol**

**Figure 5.7** Influence of Electron-Donating and Electron-Withdrawing Groups on Alcohol Acidity

Another trend seen in Table 5.1 is that the presence of more alkyl groups in nonaromatic alcohols produces less acidic molecules. Because alkyl groups donate electron density, they destabilize a negative charge. Additionally, alkyl groups help stabilize positive charges, explaining why more substituted carbocations have higher stability than less substituted carbocations.

### KEY CONCEPT

Charges like to be spread out as much as possible. Acidity decreases as more alkyl groups are attached because they are electron-donating, which destabilizes the alkoxide anion. Resonance or electron-withdrawing groups stabilize the alkoxide anion, making the alcohol more acidic.

### MCAT CONCEPT CHECK 5.1

Before you move on, assess your understanding of the material with these questions.

1. Which has a lower $pK_a$: ethanol or *p*-ethylphenol? Why?

______________________________

______________________________

______________________________

2. Rank the following by decreasing boiling point: 1-pentanol, 1-hexanol, 1,6-hexanediol

1. ______________________________

2. ______________________________

3. ______________________________

## 5.2 Reactions of Alcohols

### LEARNING OBJECTIVES

After Chapter 5.2, you will be able to:

- Predict the reaction of primary and secondary alcohols with strong oxidizing agents
- Recall the reagent(s) used to oxidize primary alcohols to aldehydes
- Explain the purpose of a mesylate or tosylate group
- Describe the process for protecting an aldehyde or ketone

The main reactions that we will see on the MCAT for alcohols include oxidation, preparation of mesylates and tosylates, and protection of carbonyls by alcohols.

## Oxidation Reactions

Oxidation of alcohols can produce several products. Primary alcohols can be oxidized to aldehydes, but only by **pyridinium chlorochromate (PCC)**, a mild anhydrous oxidant. This reactant stops after the primary alcohol has been converted to an aldehyde because PCC lacks the water necessary to hydrate the otherwise easily hydrated aldehyde. With other oxidizing agents, aldehydes are rapidly hydrated to form **geminal diols** (1,1-diols), which can be easily oxidized to carboxylic acids, as shown in Figure 5.8.

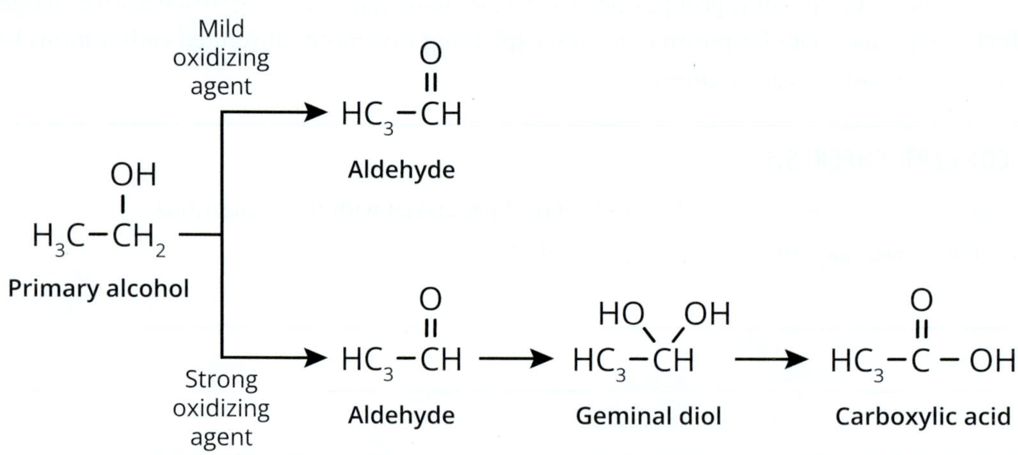


**Figure 5.8** Oxidation of a Primary Alcohol

Secondary alcohols can be oxidized to ketones by PCC or any stronger oxidizing agent. Tertiary alcohols cannot be oxidized because they are already as oxidized as they can be without breaking a carbon–carbon bond.

The oxidation of primary alcohols with a strong oxidizing agent like chromium(VI) will produce a carboxylic acid. In the process, chromium(VI) is reduced to chromium(III). Common examples of chromium-containing oxidizing agents include sodium and potassium dichromate salts ($Na_2Cr_2O_7$ and $K_2Cr_2O_7$). As with other strong oxidizing agents, these will fully oxidize primary alcohols to carboxylic acids, and secondary alcohols to ketones, as can be seen in Figure 5.9.

### KEY CONCEPT

Alcohols are readily oxidized to carboxylic acids by any oxidizing agent other than PCC (which will only oxidize primary alcohols to aldehydes).

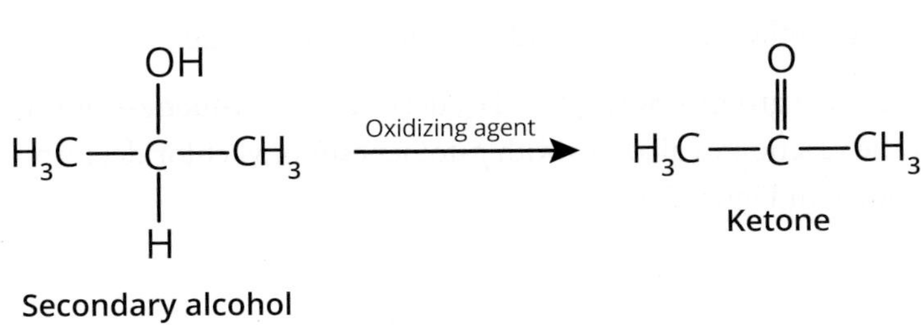


**Figure 5.9** Oxidation of a Secondary Alcohol

Tertiary alcohols, however, cannot be oxidized. Because the carbinol carbon (the carbon attached to the –OH group) has no hydrogen atoms, it cannot form a double bond with oxygen. Therefore, tertiary alcohols do not react with oxidizing agents, as shown in Figure 5.10.

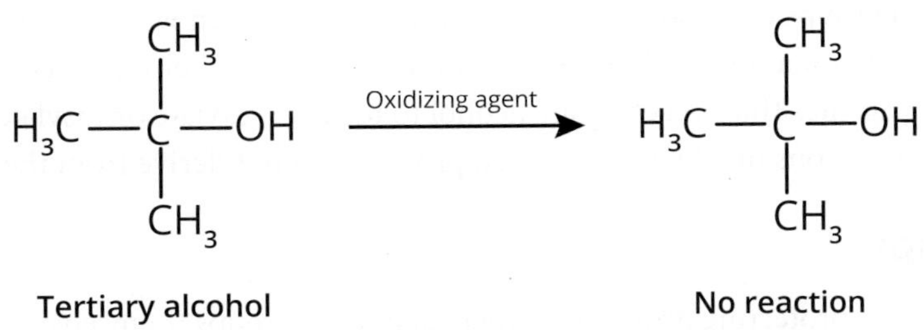


**Figure 5.10** Attempted Oxidation of a Tertiary Alcohol

Finally, an even stronger chromium-containing oxidizing agent is chromium trioxide, $CrO_3$. When dissolved with dilute sulfuric acid in acetone, this is called the **Jones oxidation**, as shown in Figure 5.11. As expected, this reaction oxidizes primary alcohols to carboxylic acids and secondary alcohols to ketones.

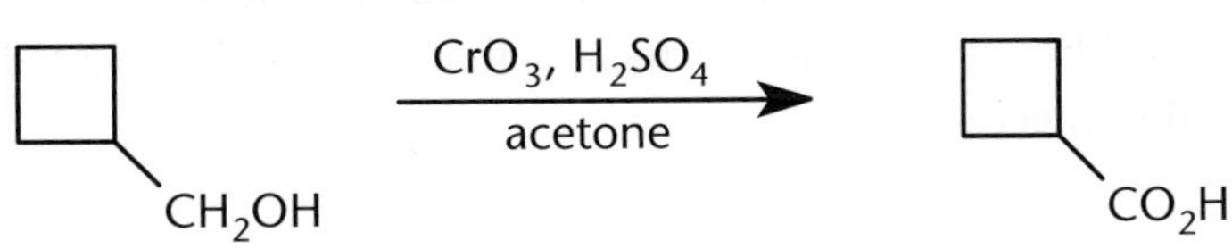


**Figure 5.11** Jones Oxidation
*A primary alcohol is oxidized to a carboxylic acid by $CrO_3$.*

## Mesylates and Tosylates

The hydroxyl groups of alcohols are fairly poor leaving groups for nucleophilic substitution reactions. However, they can be protonated, or reacted to form much better leaving groups called mesylates and tosylates. A **mesylate** is a compound containing the functional group $-SO_3CH_3$, derived from **methanesulfonic acid**; its anionic form is shown in Figure 5.12.

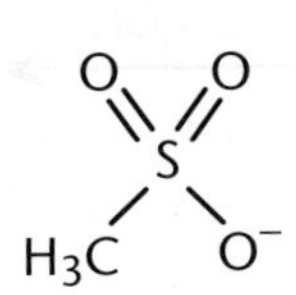


**Figure 5.12** Structure of the Mesylate Anion

Mesylates are prepared using methylsulfonyl chloride and an alcohol in the presence of a base.

**Tosylates** contain the functional group $-SO_3C_6H_4CH_3$, derived from **toluenesulfonic acid**. These compounds are produced by the reaction of alcohols with *p*-toluenesulfonyl chloride, forming esters of toluenesulfonic acid. A tosylate is shown in Figure 5.13.

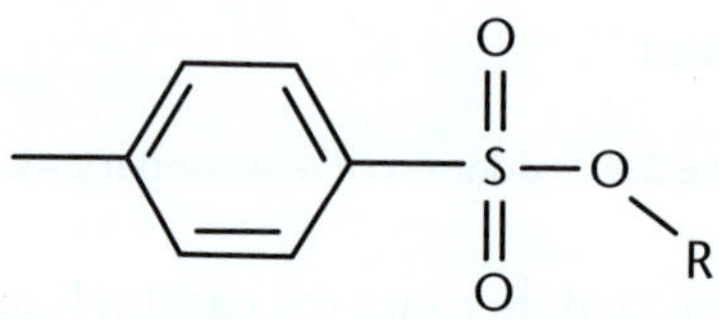


**Figure 5.13** Structure of a Tosylate

In addition to making hydroxyl groups of alcohols into better leaving groups for nucleophilic substitution reactions, mesyl and tosyl groups can also serve as protecting groups when we do not want alcohols to react. These groups are protective in that they will not react with many of the other reagents that would attack alcohols, especially oxidizing agents. Thus, reacting an alcohol to form a mesylate or tosylate is sometimes performed before multistep reactions in which the desired products do not derive from the alcohol.

## Protecting Groups

Alcohols can also be used as protecting groups for other functional groups themselves. For example, aldehydes and ketones can be reacted with two equivalents of an alcohol or a diol (dialcohol), forming **acetals** (primary carbons with two $-OR$ groups and a hydrogen atom) or **ketals** (secondary carbons with two $-OR$ groups). See Figure 5.14. Carbonyls are very reactive with strong reducing agents like lithium aluminum hydride ($LiAlH_4$). Acetals and ketals, on the other hand, do not react with $LiAlH_4$. The acetal or ketal functionality thereby protects the aldehyde or ketone from reaction. This reaction proceeds through a hemiacetal or hemiketal intermediate. The acetal or ketal functionality protects the aldehyde or ketone from reaction. After reducing other functionalities in the molecule, the acetal or ketal can be reverted back to a carbonyl with aqueous acid, a step called **deprotection**.

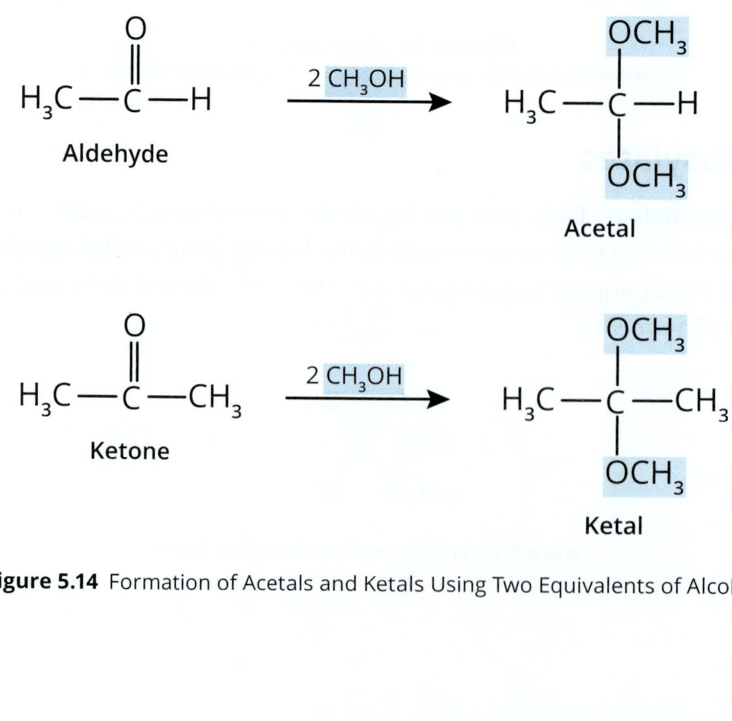


**Figure 5.14** Formation of Acetals and Ketals Using Two Equivalents of Alcohol

**MCAT CONCEPT CHECK 5.2**

Before you move on, assess your understanding of the material with these questions.

1. What will happen to primary and secondary alcohols, respectively, in the presence of strong oxidizing agents?
   - Primary alcohols:

     ______________________________

   - Secondary alcohols:

     ______________________________

2. What is the product when 1-butanol is treated with PCC? With chromium trioxide?
   - PCC:

     ______________________________

   - Chromium trioxide:

     ______________________________

3. What is the purpose of a mesylate or tosylate?

   ______________________________

4. How can aldehydes or ketones be protected using alcohols?

   ______________________________

## 5.3 Reactions of Phenols **High Yield**

**LEARNING OBJECTIVES**

After Chapter 5.3, you will be able to:

- Recall the process for production of quinones and hydroxyquinones
- Identify the properties of ubiquinone that allow it to function as an electron carrier:

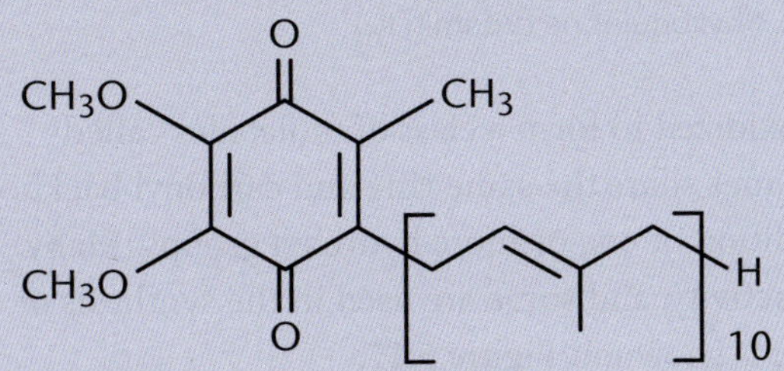


ubiquinone

Reactions of phenols proceed in similar fashion to reactions of alcohols. However, as discussed previously, the hydrogen in the hydroxyl group of phenols is particularly acidic because the oxygen-containing anion is resonance-stabilized by the ring.

## Quinones and Hydroxyquinones

Treatment of phenols with oxidizing agents produces compounds called **quinones** (2,5-cyclohexadiene-1,4-diones), as shown in Figure 5.15.

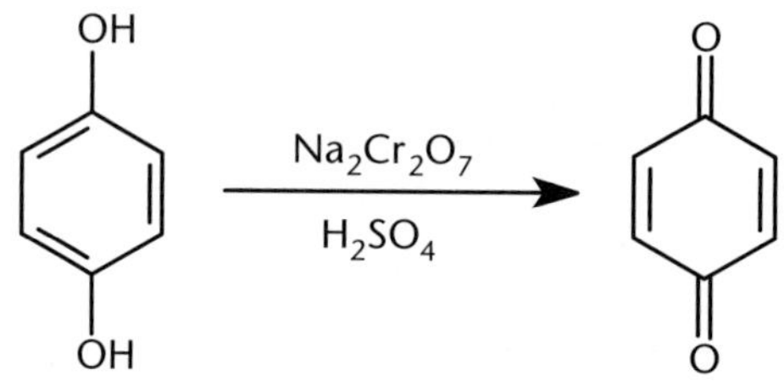


*p*-benzenediol 1,4-benzoquinone

**Figure 5.15** Oxidation of *p*-Benzenediol (a Hydroquinone) to a Quinone

Quinones are named by indicating the position of the carbonyls numerically and adding **quinone** to the name of the parent phenol. Due to the conjugated ring system, these molecules are resonance-stabilized electrophiles. Remember, however, that these are not necessarily aromatic because they lack the classic aromatic conjugated ring structure. Some quinones do have an aromatic ring, but this is not always the case. Quinones serve as electron acceptors biochemically, specifically in the electron transport chain in both photosynthesis and aerobic respiration. Vitamin $K_1$ is the common name of the quinone 2-methyl-3-[(2*E*)-3,7,11,15-tetramethylhexadec-2-en-1-yl]naphthoquinone, shown in Figure 5.16. This molecule is also called **phylloquinone** and is important for photosynthesis and the carboxylation of some of the clotting factors in blood. Vitamin $K_2$, similarly, corresponds to a class of molecules called **menaquinones**.

**BRIDGE**

Phylloquinone and menaquinone are the common names of Vitamin $K_1$ and Vitamin $K_2$, respectively. These molecules are fat-soluble vitamins that play a role in carboxylation of clotting factors II, VII, IX, and X, and proteins C and S in blood. The functions of fat-soluble vitamins are explored in Chapter 5 of *MCAT Biochemistry Review.*

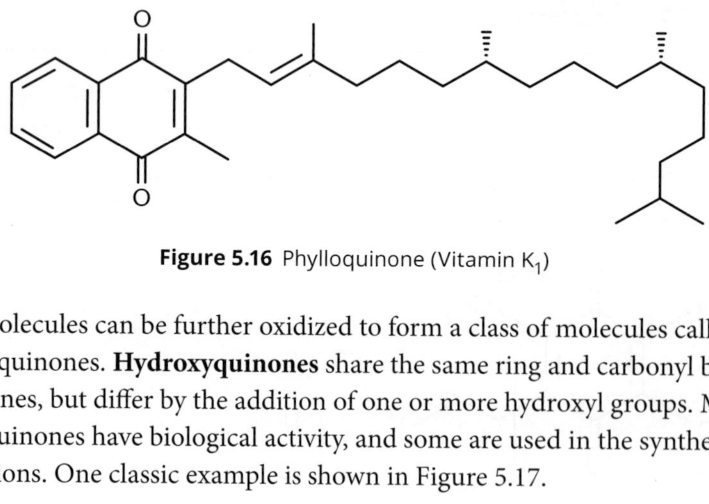


**Figure 5.16** Phylloquinone (Vitamin $K_1$)

These molecules can be further oxidized to form a class of molecules called hydroxyquinones. **Hydroxyquinones** share the same ring and carbonyl backbone as quinones, but differ by the addition of one or more hydroxyl groups. Many ydroxyquinones have biological activity, and some are used in the synthesis of medications. One classic example is shown in Figure 5.17.

**MCAT EXPERTISE**

Note the subtle difference in terminology between Figure 5.15 and Figure 5.17. A *hydroquinone* is a benzene ring with two hydroxyl groups. A *hydroxyquinone* contains two carbonyls and a variable number of hydroxyl groups.

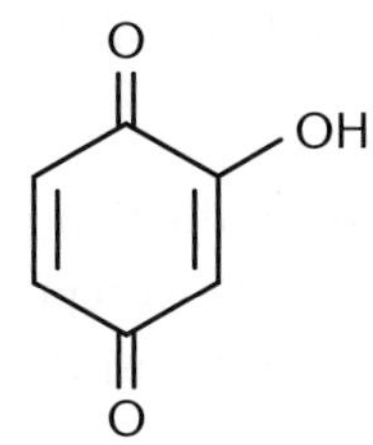


**Figure 5.17** 2-Hydroxy-1,4-Benzoquinone, a Hydroxyquinone

Because of resonance, hydroxyquinones behave like quinones with electron-donating groups, making these slightly less electrophilic (although still quite reactive). When naming these compounds, the position of the hydroxyl groups is indicated by a number, and the total number of hydroxyl groups (if there is more than one) is indicated by a prefix (such as di–, or tri–) with the substituent name hydroxy–. Several examples are shown in Figure 5.18.

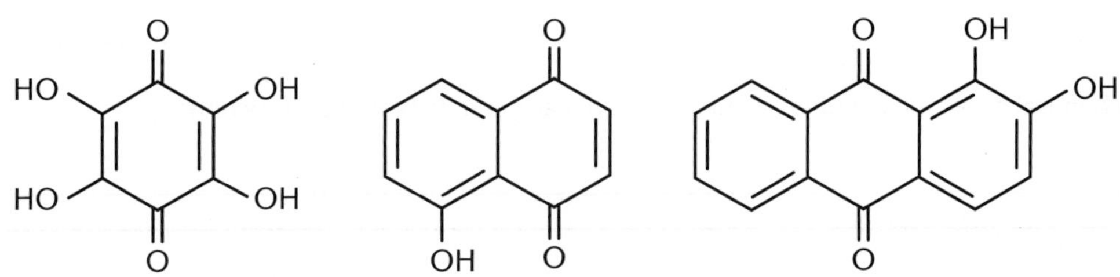


(a) (b) (c)

**Figure 5.18** Three Examples of Hydroxyquinones
*(a) Tetrahydroxybenzoquinone; (b) 5-hydroxynaphthoquinone; (c) 1,2-dihydroxyanthraquinone.*

## Ubiquinone

**Ubiquinone** is one example of a biologically active quinone. Ubiquinone is also called **coenzyme Q** and is a vital electron carrier associated with Complexes I, II, and III of the electron transport chain. Ubiquinone is the most oxidized form that this molecule takes physiologically: it can also be reduced to **ubiquinol** upon the acceptance of electrons, as shown in Figure 5.19. This oxidation–reduction capacity allows the molecule to perform its physiological function of electron transport.

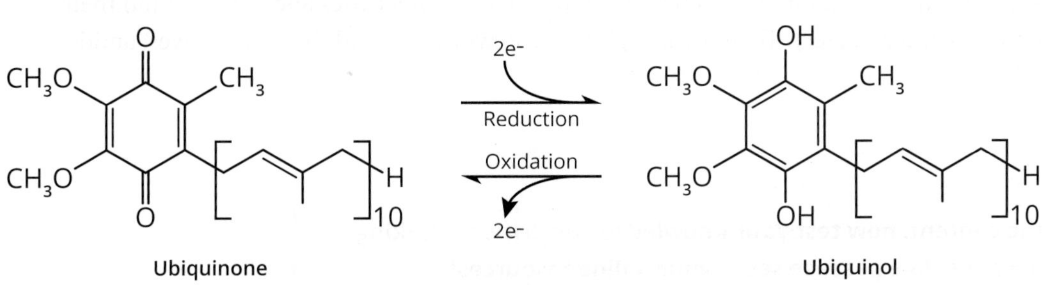


**Figure 5.19** Ubiquinone (Coenzyme Q) and Ubiquinol
*Ubiquinone is the oxidized form; when it picks up electrons, it is converted to its reduced form (ubiquinol).*

**BRIDGE**

Coenzyme Q plays a role in Complexes I, II, and III of the electron transport chain. In Complex III, it is the main player in the Q cycle, which contributes to the formation of the proton-motive force across the inner mitochondrial membrane. The respiratory complexes are discussed in Chapter 10 of *MCAT Biochemistry Review.*

The long alkyl chain of this molecule allows it to be lipid soluble, which allows it to act as an electron carrier within the phospholipid bilayer.

Other biological molecules that undergo oxidation–reduction reactions as part of their normal function include NADH, $FADH_2$, and NADPH. These molecules accept and donate electrons readily, similar to ubiquinone, and are discussed more thoroughly in Chapters 9 and 10 of *MCAT Biochemistry Review*.

**MCAT CONCEPT CHECK 5.3**

Before you move on, assess your understanding of the material with these questions.

1. How are quinones generally produced?

 ________________________________________

2. How are hydroxyquinones produced?

 ________________________________________

3. What chemical properties of ubiquinone allow it to carry out its biological functions?

 ________________________________________

## Conclusion

Alcohols are a particular favorite of the MCAT test makers. We got our first look at the unique properties that stem from hydrogen bonding, an important ability of alcohols. Alcohols can be oxidized to aldehydes, ketones, or carboxylic acids depending on the substitution of the alcohol and the strength of the oxidizing agent. From this point forward, oxidation and reduction will be important reactions with all functional groups. Alcohols can also participate in nucleophilic substitution reactions, which may be facilitated by converting the alcohol into a mesylate or tosylate. Finally, phenols (and their oxidized counterparts, quinones and hydroxyquinones) are involved in a number of biochemical pathways. In particular, their utility is seen in processes that require rapid oxidation and reduction, such as photosynthesis and the electron transport chain.

Over the next four chapters, we'll explore other oxygen-containing compounds. Recognize that these chapters are put in a specific order: as you move further along in *MCAT Organic Chemistry Review*, the functional groups will become more oxidized and more reactive. First, we'll look at aldehydes and ketones (and their deprotonated forms, enols and enolates). Then, we'll explore carboxylic acids and their derivatives: amides, esters, and anhydrides.

**GO ONLINE**

**You've reviewed the content, now test your knowledge and critical thinking skills by completing a test-like passage set in your online resources!**

# CONCEPT SUMMARY

## Description and Properties

- **Alcohols** have the general form ROH and are named with the suffix –**ol**. If they are not the highest priority, they are given the prefix **hydroxy**–.
- **Phenols** are benzene rings with hydroxyl groups. They are named for the relative positions of the hydroxyl groups: ***ortho***– (adjacent carbons), ***meta***– (separated by one carbon), or ***para***– (on opposite sides of the ring).
- Alcohols can hydrogen bond, raising their boiling and melting points relative to corresponding alkanes. Hydrogen bonding also increases the solubility of alcohols.
- Phenols are more acidic than other alcohols because the aromatic ring can delocalize the charge of the conjugate base.
- Electron-donating groups like alkyl groups decrease acidity because they destabilize negative charges. Electron-withdrawing groups, such as electronegative atoms and aromatic rings, increase acidity because they stabilize negative charges.

## Reactions of Alcohols

- Primary alcohols can be oxidized to aldehydes only by **pyridinium chlorochromate** (**PCC**); they will be oxidized all the way to carboxylic acids by any stronger oxidizing agents.
- Secondary alcohols can be oxidized to ketones by any common oxidizing agent.
- Alcohols can be converted to mesylates or tosylates to make them better leaving groups for nucleophilic substitution reactions.
  - **Mesylates** contain the functional group $-SO_3CH_3$, which is derived from methanesulfonic acid.
  - **Tosylates** contain the functional group $-SO_3C_6H_4CH_3$, which is derived from toluenesulfonic acid.
- Aldehydes or ketones can be protected by converting them into acetals or ketals.
  - Two equivalents of alcohol or a dialcohol are reacted with the carbonyl to form an **acetal** (a primary carbon with two –OR groups and a hydrogen atom) or **ketal** (a secondary carbon with two –OR groups).
  - Other functional groups in the compound can be reacted (especially by reduction) without effects on the newly formed acetal or ketal.
  - The acetal or ketal can then be converted back to a carbonyl by catalytic acid, which is called **deprotection**.

## Reactions of Phenols

- **Quinones** are synthesized through oxidation of phenols.
  - Quinones are resonance-stabilized electrophiles.
  - Vitamin $K_1$ (**phylloquinone**) and Vitamin $K_2$ (the **menaquinones**) are examples of biochemically relevant quinones.
- **Hydroxyquinones** are produced by oxidation of quinones, adding a variable number of hydroxyl groups.
- **Ubiquinone** (**coenzyme Q**) is another biologically active quinone that acts as an electron acceptor in Complexes I, II, and III of the electron transport chain. It is reduced to **ubiquinol**.

## ANSWERS TO CONCEPT CHECKS

### 5.1

1. Phenols like *p*-ethylphenol have increased acidity due to resonance and the electron-withdrawing character of the phenol aromatic ring. Because *p*-ethylphenol is a stronger acid than ethanol, it will have a lower $pK_a$.
2. 1,6-Hexanediol will have the highest boiling point; a molecule with two hydroxyl moieties can have more hydrogen bonding. The 1-hexanol boiling point will be next, with 1-pentanol having the lowest boiling point. 1-Hexanol has a higher boiling point than 1-pentanol because the longer hydrocarbon chain has increased van der Waals forces.

### 5.2

1. In the presence of strong oxidizing agents, primary alcohols are completely oxidized to carboxylic acids. Secondary alcohols can only be oxidized to ketones.
2. Reacting 1-butanol with PCC results in the aldehyde, 1-butanal. Chromium trioxide is a stronger oxidizing agent that will produce the carboxylic acid, butanoic acid.
3. Mesylates and tosylates are used to convert an alcohol into a better leaving group. This is particularly useful for nucleophilic substitution reactions because it increases the stability of the product. They can also be used as protecting groups because many reagents (especially oxidizing agents) that would react with an alcohol cannot react with these compounds.
4. Aldehydes or ketones can be reacted with two equivalents of alcohol or a diol to form an acetal or ketal. Acetals and ketals are less reactive than aldehydes and ketones (especially to reducing agents), and can thus protect the functional group from reacting. The acetal or ketal can then be reverted back to the carbonyl by catalytic acid.

### 5.3

1. Quinones are produced by oxidation of phenols.
2. Hydroxyquinones are produced by the oxidation of quinones, adding a variable number of additional hydroxyl groups.
3. Ubiquinone has conjugated rings that stabilize the molecule when accepting electrons. Additionally, the long alkyl chain in the molecule allows for lipid solubility, which allows the molecule to function in the phospholipid bilayer.

## SCIENCE MASTERY ASSESSMENT EXPLANATIONS

**1. B**

Alcohols have higher boiling points than their analogous hydrocarbons as a result of their polarized O—H bonds, in which oxygen is partially negative and hydrogen is partially positive. This enables the oxygen atoms of other alcohol molecules to be attracted to the hydrogen, forming a hydrogen bond. Heat is required to overcome these hydrogen bonds, thereby increasing the boiling point. The analogous hydrocarbons do not form hydrogen bonds and, therefore, vaporize at lower temperatures. **(A)** is irrelevant; oxygen's bond length is not a factor in determining a substance's boiling point. **(C)** and **(D)** are true statements, but are also irrelevant to boiling point determination.

2. **A**

Tertiary alcohols can be oxidized only under extreme conditions because their substrate carbons do not have spare hydrogens to give up. Alcohol oxidation involves the removal of such a hydrogen so that carbon can instead make another bond to oxygen. If no hydrogen is present, a carbon–carbon bond must be cleaved, which requires a great deal of energy and will, therefore, occur only under extreme conditions. **(B)** is incorrect because alcohols are not carbonyl-containing compounds and would more properly describe a carbonyl-containing compound that is unable to form an enolate. **(C)** is incorrect because the hydroxyl group of the tertiary carbon is still polarized. **(D)** is a false statement; tertiary alcohols are still involved in other reactions, such as $S_N1$ reactions.

3. **B**

Remember, diols are named after the parent alkane, with the position of the alcohols indicated, and ending in the suffix *-diol*. Here the carbon chain is three carbons, with a hydroxyl group on carbons 1 and 2. Thus, the name is propane-1,2-diol.

4. **B**

This molecule is a phenol, not a hexanol, because the cyclic group has aromatic double bonds rather than single bonds. The methyl group is separated from the hydroxyl carbon by one carbon in between, making this molecule *m*-methylphenol.

5. **C**

All else being equal, boiling points increase with increasing size of the alkyl chain because of increased van der Waals attractions. Isobutyl alcohol has the largest alkyl chain and will thus have the highest boiling point; methanol has the smallest chain and will thus have the lowest boiling point.

6. **B**

Phenols have significantly more acidic hydroxyl hydrogens than other alcohols because of resonance stabilization of the conjugate base, so this will be the most acidic hydroxyl hydrogen. The acidity of hexanol and cyclohexanol are close, but the hydroxyl hydrogen of hexanol is slightly more acidic because the ring structure of cyclohexanol is slightly electron-donating, which makes its hydroxyl hydrogen slightly less acidic.

7. **B**

$CH_3CH_2CH_2OH$ is 1-propanol, a primary alcohol. The desired end product, $CH_3CH_2CHO$, is propanal, an aldehyde. Of the available options, the only reactant capable of oxidizing primary alcohols to aldehydes is pyridinium chlorochromate (PCC). Chromic trioxide and dichromate salts will both oxidize primary alcohols to carboxylic acids.

8. **D**

Cyclohexanol is a secondary alcohol, so any of the oxidizing agents listed will convert it to a ketone.

9. **A**

Acidic conditions, provided by dilute sulfuric acid, are required to complete the Jones oxidation. This reaction is carried out in aqueous conditions, eliminating **(C)**. While heat may speed up the reaction, high temperatures are not required for this reaction, eliminating **(D)**.

10. **A**

Methylsulfonyl chloride serves as a protecting group for alcohols, which are converted into mesylates. Reacting with this reagent before continuing with what would normally be an oxidation reaction keeps the alcohol from reacting; when the protecting group is then removed using strong acid, the resultant product is the same as the initial reactant. Neither of the oxidation products in **(B)** or **(C)**, nor the reduction product in **(D)**, will be formed.

11. **A**

This reaction will create a ketal. This is the first step of the protection of aldehydes or ketones using dialcohols.

12. **D**

This is the Jones oxidation, which will convert a primary alcohol into a carboxylic acid. **(A)** is the original reacting molecule, and because the reaction will proceed, this is not correct. Because the reaction uses strong oxidizing agents, it won't stop at the aldehyde, **(B)**. This reaction also cannot make the ketone in **(C)** because it starts with a primary alcohol.

13. **B**

In order to convert phenols into hydroxyquinones, they must first be converted to quinones through an oxidation step; a second oxidation step is required to further oxidize quinones to hydroxyquinones.

14. **C**

The reaction that converts ubiquinone into ubiquinol is a reduction reaction in which two ketones are reduced to two hydroxyl groups.

15. **A**

An acetal can be converted to a carbonyl and a dialcohol by treatment with aqueous acid. This is the final step when using alcohols as protecting groups, called deprotection.

**GO ONLINE**

**Consult your online resources for additional practice.**

## SHARED CONCEPTS

**Biochemistry Chapter 5**
Lipid Structure and Function

**General Chemistry Chapter 8**
The Gas Phase

**Organic Chemistry Chapter 1**
Nomenclature

**Organic Chemistry Chapter 4**
Analyzing Organic Reactions

**Organic Chemistry Chapter 6**
Aldehydes and Ketones I

**Organic Chemistry Chapter 8**
Carboxylic Acids

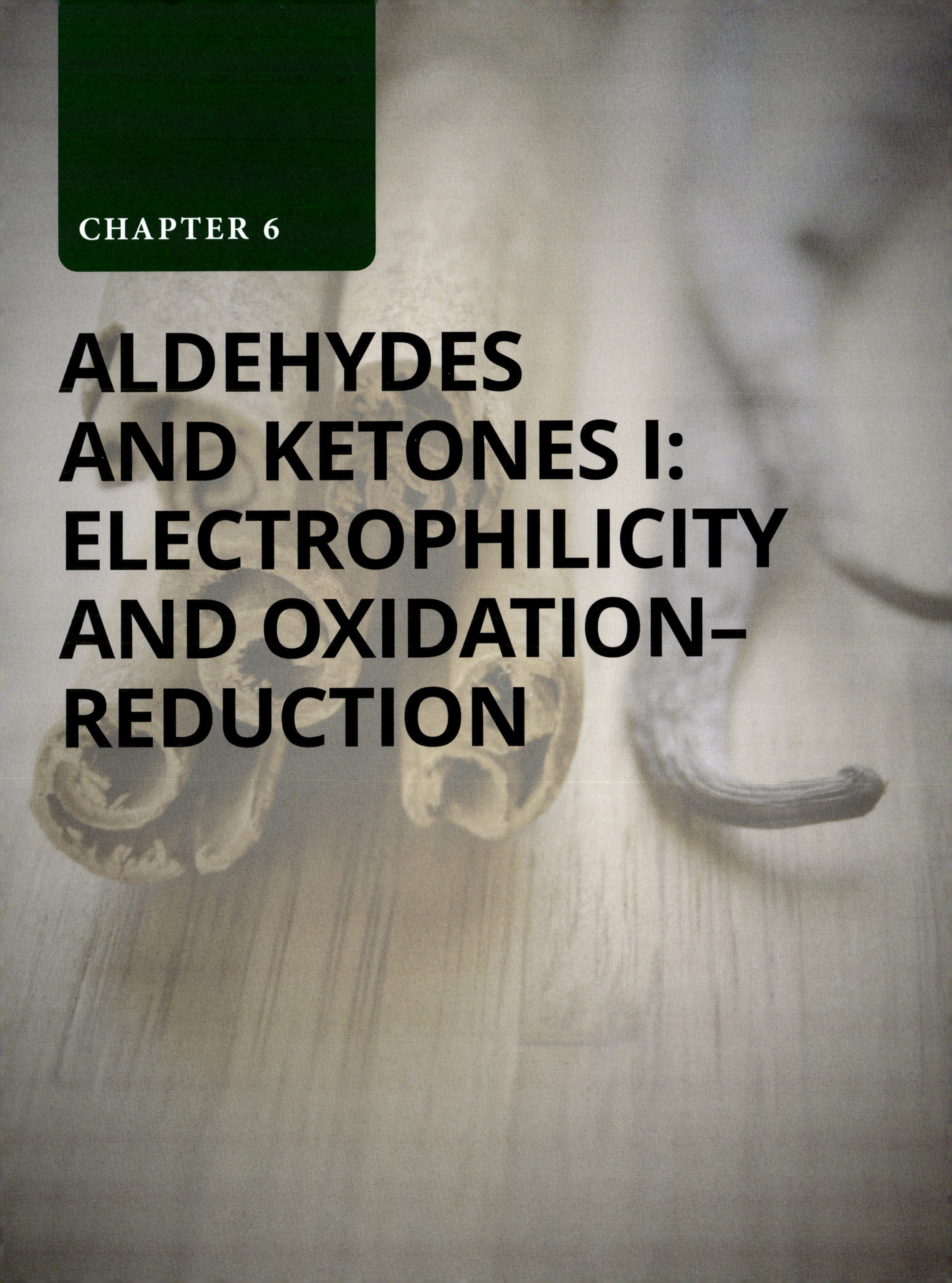

CHAPTER 6

# ALDEHYDES AND KETONES I: ELECTROPHILICITY AND OXIDATION–REDUCTION

# SCIENCE MASTERY ASSESSMENT

Every pre-med knows this feeling: there is so much content I have to know for the MCAT! How do I know what to do first or what's important?

While the high-yield badges throughout this book will help you identify the most important topics, this Science Mastery Assessment is another tool in your MCAT prep arsenal. This quiz (which can also be taken in your online resources) and the guidance below will help ensure that you are spending the appropriate amount of time on this chapter based on your personal strengths and weaknesses. Don't worry though—skipping something now does not mean you'll never study it. Later on in your prep, as you complete full-length tests, you'll uncover specific pieces of content that you need to review and can come back to these chapters as appropriate.

## How to Use This Assessment

**If you answer 0–7 questions correctly:**

Spend about 1 hour to read this chapter in full and take limited notes throughout. Follow up by reviewing **all** quiz questions to ensure that you now understand how to solve each one.

**If you answer 8–11 questions correctly:**

Spend 20–40 minutes reviewing the quiz questions. Beginning with the questions you missed, read and take notes on the corresponding subchapters. For questions you answered correctly, ensure your thinking matches that of the explanation and you understand why each choice was correct or incorrect.

**If you answer 12–15 questions correctly:**

Spend less than 20 minutes reviewing all questions from the quiz. If you missed any, then include a quick read-through of the corresponding subchapters, or even just the relevant content within a subchapter, as part of your question review. For questions you got correct, ensure your thinking matches that of the explanation and review the Concept Summary at the end of the chapter.

**1.** All of the following are true with respect to carbonyls EXCEPT:

**A.** the carbonyl carbon is electrophilic.
**B.** the carbonyl oxygen is electron-withdrawing.
**C.** a resonance structure of the functional group places a positive charge on the carbonyl carbon.
**D.** the $\pi$ electrons are mobile and are pulled toward the carbonyl carbon.

**2.** Order the following compounds by increasing boiling point: butane, butanol, butanone

**A.** Butanol < butane < butanone
**B.** Butane < butanone < butanol
**C.** Butanone < butane < butanol
**D.** Butane < butanol < butanone

**3.** What is the product of the reaction below?

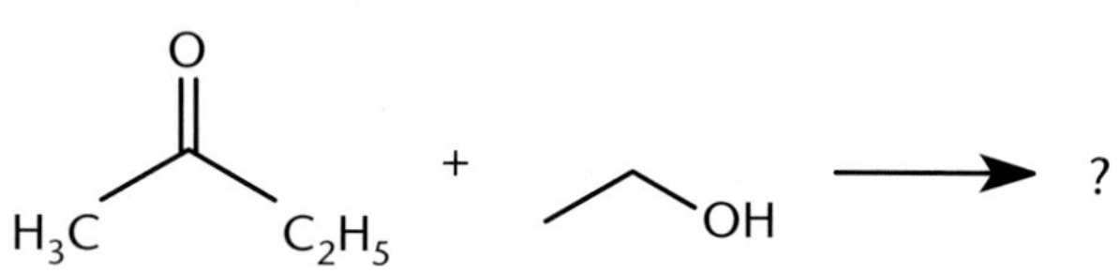


**A.**
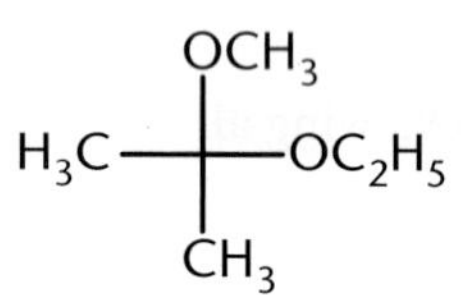


**B.**
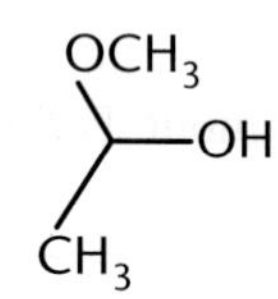


**C.**
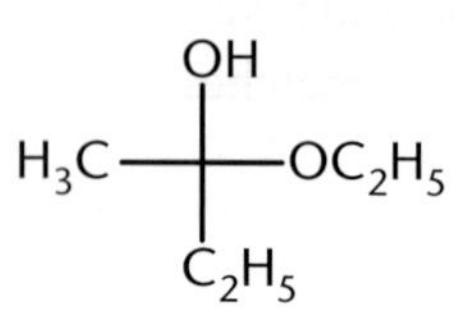


**D.**
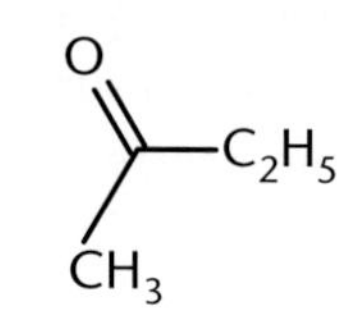


**4.** What is the product of the reaction below?

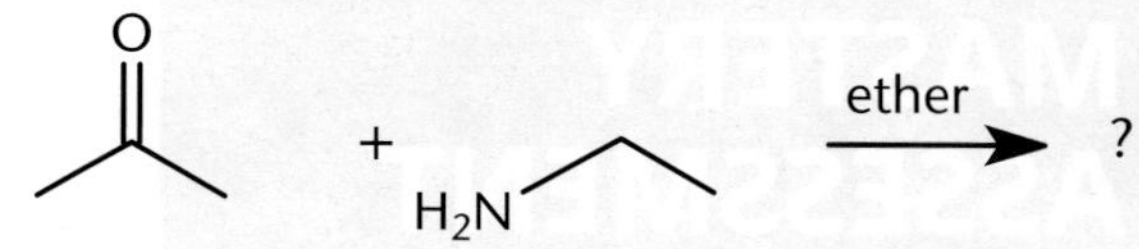


**A.**
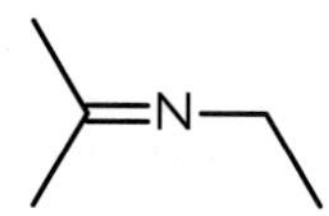


**B.**
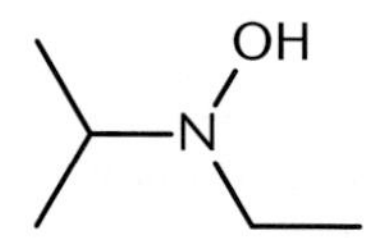


**C.**
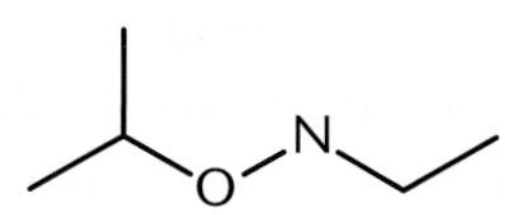


**D.**
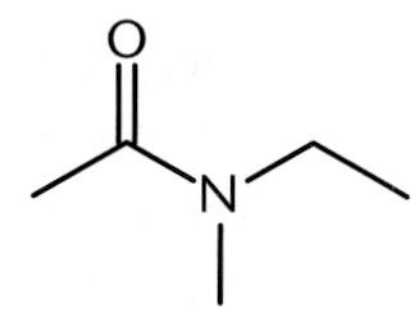


**5.** What is the product of the reaction below?

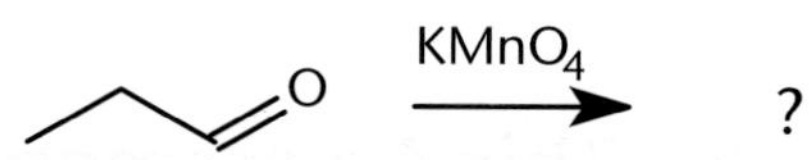


**A.** $C_3H_7OH$
**B.** $C_2H_5COOH$
**C.** $C_2H_5CHO$
**D.** $CH_3COOH$

6. What is the product of the reaction below?

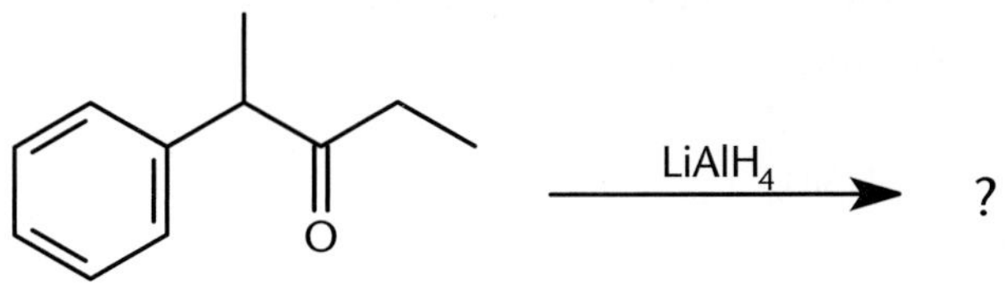


A. 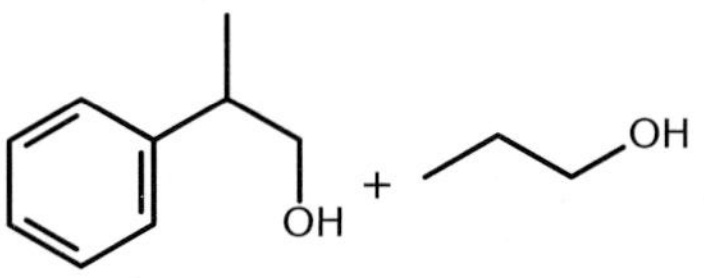


B. 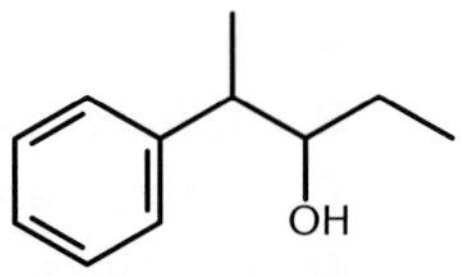


C. 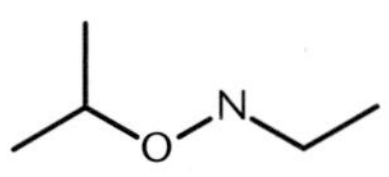


D. 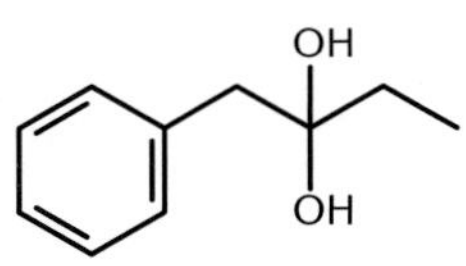


7. What is the product of the reaction between benzaldehyde and an excess of ethanol ($CH_3CH_2OH$) in the presence of anhydrous HCl?

A. 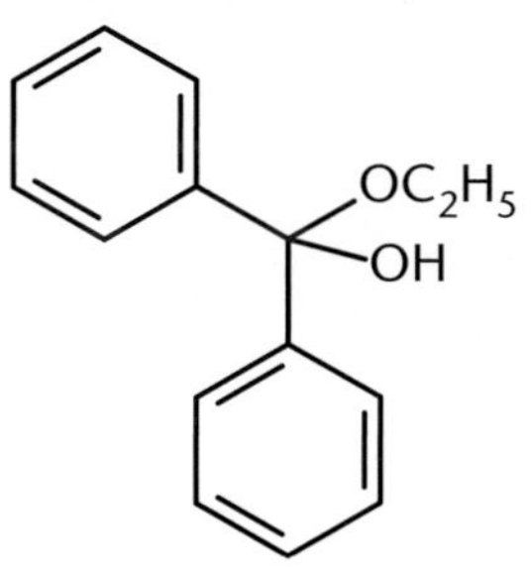


B. 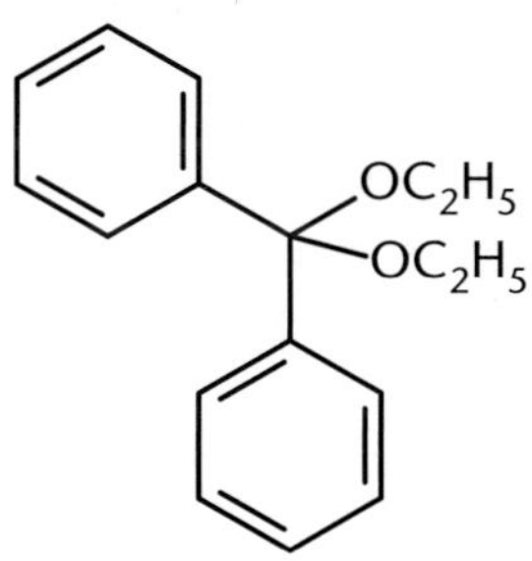


C. 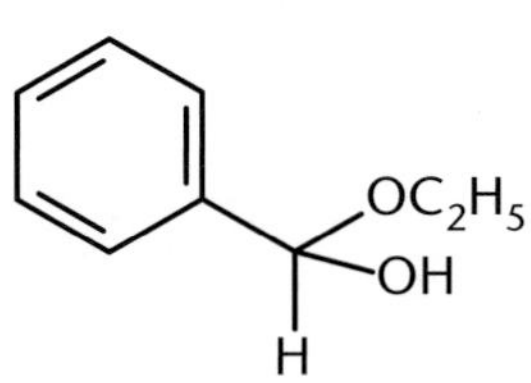


D. 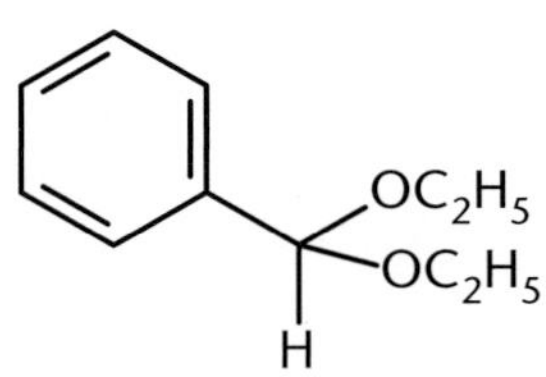


8. Hemiacetals and hemiketals usually keep reacting to form acetals and ketals. Why is it difficult to isolate hemiacetals and hemiketals?
   I. These molecules are unstable.
   II. The hydroxyl group is rapidly protonated and lost as water under acidic conditions, leaving behind a reactive carbocation.
   III. The molecules are extremely basic and react rapidly with one another.

   A. I only
   B. I and II only
   C. II and III only
   D. I, II, and III

9. In a hemiacetal, the central carbon is bonded to:
   A. —OH, —OR, —H and —R.
   B. —H, —OR, —OR, and —R.
   C. —OH, —OR, —R, and —R.
   D. —OR, —OR, —R, and —R.

10. In a reaction between hydrogen cyanide, butyraldehyde, and ethyl methyl ketone, which compounds will come together to form the major product?
   A. Butyraldehyde and hydrogen cyanide
   B. Ethyl methyl ketone and butyraldehyde
   C. Hydrogen cyanide and ethyl methyl ketone
   D. No reaction will occur.

11. Which of the following describe(s) pyridinium chlorochromate (PCC)?
   I. An oxidant that can form aldehydes from primary alcohols
   II. An oxidant that can completely oxidize primary alcohols
   III. An oxidant that can completely oxidize secondary alcohols

   A. I only
   B. I and II only
   C. I and III only
   D. I, II, and III

12. To form a geminal diol, which of the following could attack a carbonyl carbon?
    - **A.** Hydrogen peroxide
    - **B.** Water
    - **C.** Potassium dichromate
    - **D.** Ethanol

13. In a reaction between ammonia and glutaraldehyde, what is the major product?
    - **A.** An imine
    - **B.** A cyanohydrin
    - **C.** A semicarbazone
    - **D.** A hydrazone

14. Which of the following can be used to reduce a ketone to a secondary alcohol?
    - **A.** $CrO_3$
    - **B.** $KMnO_4$
    - **C.** $LiAlH_4$
    - **D.** $Ag_2O$

15. Imines naturally tautomerize to form:
    - **A.** oximes.
    - **B.** hydrazones.
    - **C.** semicarbazones.
    - **D.** enamines.

**Answer Key follows on next page.**

## Answer Key

1. **D** (See section 6.1)
2. **B** (See section 6.1)
3. **C** (See section 6.2)
4. **A** (See section 6.2)
5. **B** (See section 6.1)
6. **B** (See section 6.1)
7. **D** (See section 6.2)
8. **B** (See section 6.2)
9. **A** (See section 6.1)
10. **A** (See section 6.2)
11. **C** (See section 6.1)
12. **B** (See section 6.1)
13. **A** (See section 6.2)
14. **C** (See section 6.1)
15. **D** (See section 6.1)

*The relevant section of the chapter to review for each question is given in parentheses after the correct answer. Detailed explanations can be found at the end of the chapter.*

CHAPTER 6

# ALDEHYDES AND KETONES I: ELECTROPHILICITY AND OXIDATION–REDUCTION

## In This Chapter



## Introduction

This chapter focuses on an important functional group for the MCAT: the carbonyl. Aldehydes and ketones, the two functional groups highlighted here, have a lot in common because they both contain a **carbonyl**—a double bond between a carbon and an oxygen. The only difference between the two is what is attached to the carbonyl carbon.

The carbonyl group is one of the most common functional groups in organic chemistry for two reasons. First, the carbonyl is a component of many different functional groups. In addition to aldehydes and ketones, the carbonyl is found in carboxylic acids, esters, amides, anhydrides, and several other compounds. More importantly, the carbonyl has the unique ability to behave as either a nucleophile (as in condensation reactions) or an electrophile (as in nucleophilic addition reactions). In this chapter, we will investigate the overall properties of aldehydes and ketones, as well as their oxidation–reduction reactions and electrophilic properties. In the following chapter, we will investigate their nucleophilic properties through enolate chemistry.

**CHAPTER PROFILE**

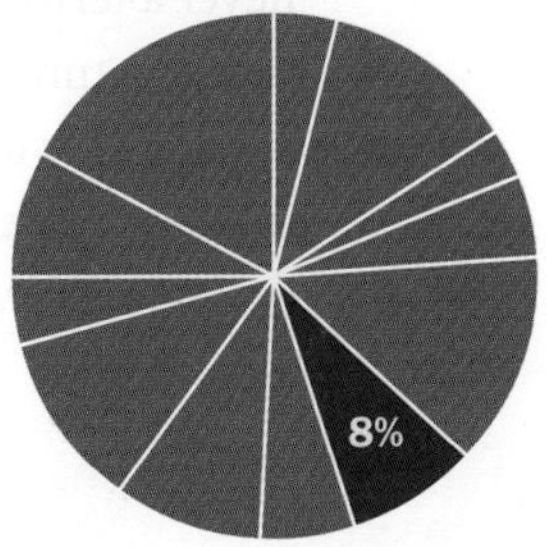


The content in this chapter should be relevant to about 8% of all questions about organic chemistry on the MCAT.

This chapter covers material from the following AAMC content category:

**5D:** Structure, function, and reactivity of biologically-relevant molecules

## 6.1 Description and Properties

**LEARNING OBJECTIVES**

After Chapter 6.1, you will be able to:

- Name aldehydes and ketones using the proper suffixes
- Describe the reactivity of the carbonyl carbon
- Recognize common reactions used to form aldehydes and ketones
- Predict the boiling point of a compound based on its oxidation level

A **ketone** has two alkyl groups bonded to the carbonyl, whereas an **aldehyde** has one alkyl group and one hydrogen. This means that the carbonyl in a ketone is never a terminal group, whereas it always is in an aldehyde. Figure 6.1 compares the structures of aldehydes and ketones. Like many organic compounds, aldehydes and ketones are often strong-smelling compounds. Volatile carbonyls are found in many spices, including cinnamon (*cinnamaldehyde*), vanilla (*vanillin*), cumin (*cuminaldehyde*), dill (*carvenone*), and ginger (*zingerone*).

**KEY CONCEPT**

An aldehyde is a terminal functional group. A ketone, on the other hand, will always be internal and can never be a terminal functional group.

**Figure 6.1** General Structures of Aldehydes and Ketones

## Nomenclature

Aldehydes are named by replacing the –e at the end of the alkane name with the suffix –**al**. Common names for the first five aldehydes, shown in Figure 6.2, are *formaldehyde, acetaldehyde, propionaldehyde, butyraldehyde,* and *valeraldehyde.* When aldehydes are named as substituents, use the prefix **oxo**–.

**MCAT EXPERTISE**

Notice that these common names have a pattern that can help us: form– will also be seen in *formic acid* (a one-carbon carboxylic acid), and acet– is seen in many two-carbon compounds (*acetylene, acetic acid,* and *acetyl-CoA*).

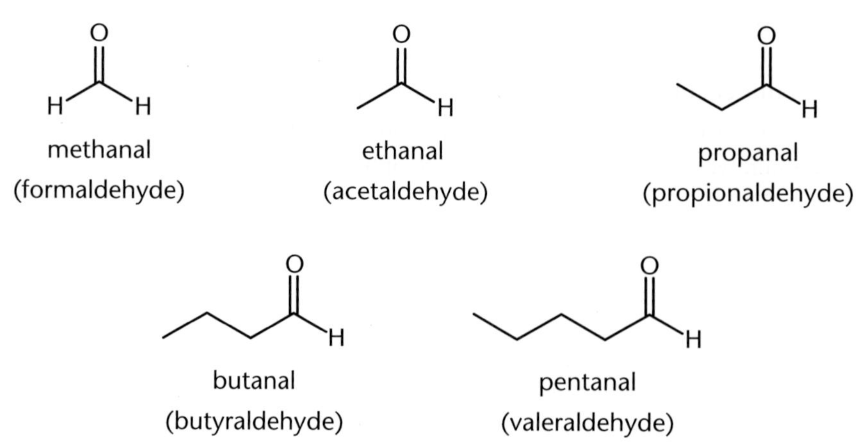


**Figure 6.2** Naming Aldehydes

If the aldehyde is attached to a ring, the suffix –**carbaldehyde** is used instead. This is shown in Figure 6.3.

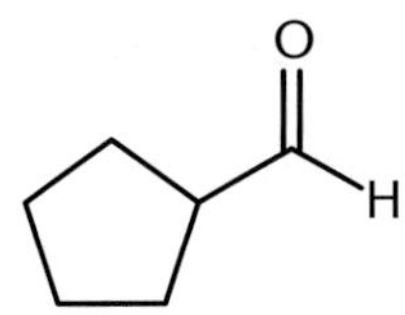

cyclopentanecarbaldehyde

**Figure 6.3** Naming Cyclic Aldehydes

Ketones are named by replacing the –e with the suffix –**one**. When naming ketones by their common names, the two alkyl groups are named alphabetically, followed by **ketone**. When ketones are named as substituents, use either the prefix **oxo**– or **keto**–. Figure 6.4 shows some examples of ketones.

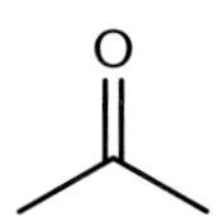

2-propanone
(dimethyl ketone)
(acetone)

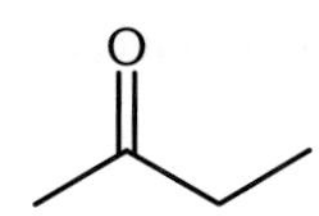

2-butanone
(ethyl methyl ketone)

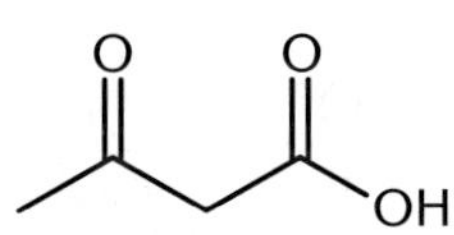

3-oxobutanoic acid

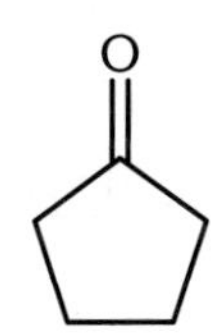

cyclopentanone

**Figure 6.4** Naming Ketones

### KEY CONCEPT

While the dipole moment in the carbonyl group increases the intermolecular forces (and therefore boiling points) of aldehydes and ketones relative to alkanes, this is not as significant as the impact of hydrogen bonding seen in alcohols.

## Physical Properties

The physical properties of aldehydes and ketones are governed by the presence of the carbonyl group. The dipole of the carbonyl is stronger than the dipole of an alcohol because the double-bonded oxygen is more electron-withdrawing than the single bond to oxygen in the hydroxyl group. In solution, the dipole moments associated with these polar carbonyl groups increase intermolecular attractions, causing an elevation in boiling point relative to their parent alkanes. However, even though aldehydes and ketones have dipoles more polar than those of alcohols, the elevation in boiling point is less than that in alcohols because no hydrogen bonding is present. In reactions, aldehydes and ketones both act as electrophiles, making good targets for nucleophiles. This is due to the electron-withdrawing properties of the carbonyl oxygen, which leaves a partial positive charge on the carbon, as shown in Figure 6.5. Generally, aldehydes are more reactive toward nucleophiles than ketones because they have less steric hindrance and fewer electron-donating alkyl groups.

### MCAT EXPERTISE

The carbonyl carbon is the most common electrophile you'll see on Test Day. Remember why this group has a dipole moment: oxygen is more electronegative and pulls electrons away from the carbon, making the carbon electrophilic and a good target for nucleophiles.

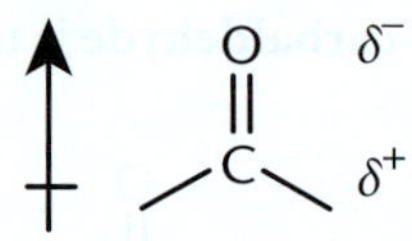


**Figure 6.5** Polarity of the Carbonyl Group

## Formation

Aldehydes and ketones can be produced by several mechanisms. An aldehyde can be obtained from the partial oxidation of a primary alcohol, although only by **pyridinium chlorochromate (PCC; $[C_5H_5NH]^+[CrO_3Cl]^-$)**. With any stronger oxidants, aldehydes will continue to be oxidized to carboxylic acids. A ketone can be obtained from the oxidation of a secondary alcohol. This can be performed using reagents ranging from sodium or potassium dichromate salts ($Na_2Cr_2O_7$ or $K_2Cr_2O_7$) to chromium trioxide ($CrO_3$) to PCC. When oxidizing a secondary alcohol, there is no concern for oxidizing too far because the reaction will stop at the ketone stage, as demonstrated in Figure 6.6.

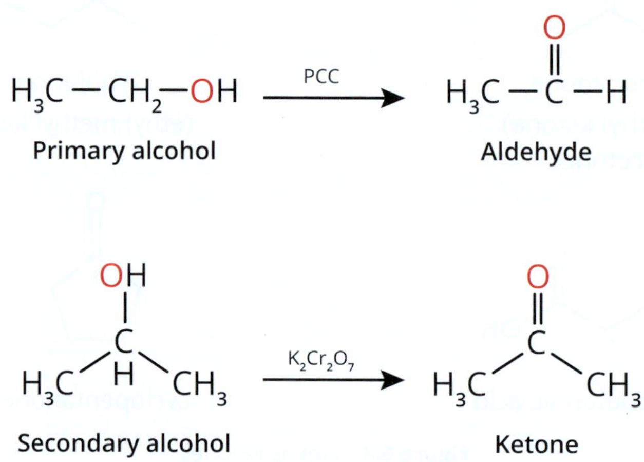


**Figure 6.6** Aldehyde and Ketone Formation

## MCAT CONCEPT CHECK 6.1

Before you move on, assess your understanding of the material with these questions.

1. Name the following two compounds:

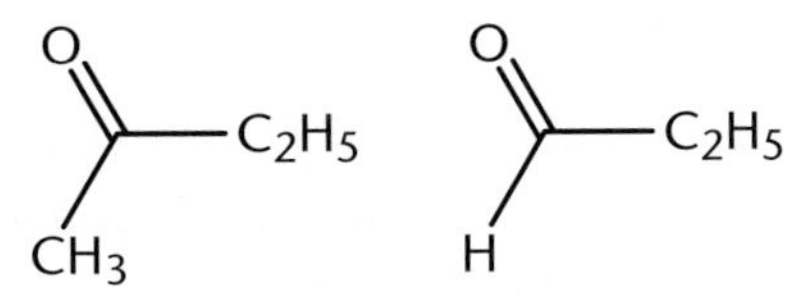


_______________________________________________

2. Given an alkane, an aldehyde, and an alcohol with equal-length carbon chains, which will have the highest boiling point? Why?

_______________________________________________

3. Is the carbon of a carbonyl electrophilic or nucleophilic? Why?

_______________________________________________

4. What is one method for forming an aldehyde? A ketone?
   - Aldehyde:

   _______________________________________________

   - Ketone:

   _______________________________________________

## 6.2 Nucleophilic Addition Reactions

### LEARNING OBJECTIVES

After Chapter 6.2, you will be able to:

- Predict the products of reacting aldehydes or ketones with alcohols, in the presence or absence of acidic conditions
- Recall the functional group formed when nitrogen-containing derivatives react with aldehydes or ketones
- Predict the product of the reaction of HCN with aldehydes or ketones, including the reactivity of the product:

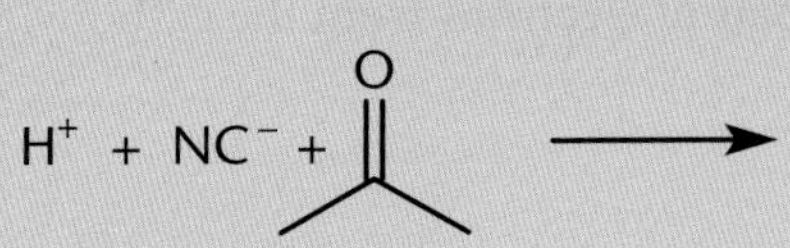

In each of the following reactions, the general reaction mechanism is the same: nucleophilic addition to a carbonyl. This is one of the most important reaction mechanisms on the MCAT, and many of the reactions of aldehydes, ketones, and more complex molecules share this general reaction mechanism. Rather than memorizing each reaction individually, focus on the overall pattern—then learn how a particular reaction exemplifies it.

As we have seen, the C=O bond is polarized, with a partial positive charge on the carbonyl carbon and a partial negative charge on the oxygen. This makes the carbonyl carbon an electrophile, ripe for nucleophilic attack.

When the nucleophile attacks, it forms a covalent bond to the carbon, breaking the $\pi$ bond in the carbonyl. The electrons from the $\pi$ bond are pushed onto the oxygen atom. Oxygen happily accepts extra electrons due to its electronegativity. Breaking the $\pi$ bond forms a tetrahedral intermediate. Any time a carbonyl is opened, one should ask: *Can I reform the carbonyl?* If no good leaving group is present (as is the case with aldehydes and ketones), the carbonyl will not reform. Generally, $O^-$ will accept a proton from the solvent to form a hydroxyl group, resulting in an alcohol. However, if a good leaving group is present (as is the case with carboxylic acids and their derivatives), the carbonyl double bond can reform, pushing off the leaving group. Figure 6.7 shows the reaction mechanism of nucleophilic addition for an aldehyde.

**MCAT EXPERTISE**

Memorizing one reaction may help you to get one question right on the MCAT, but understanding trends and overarching concepts will allow you to answer many more questions correctly. You will see that the carbonyl carbon is a great target for nucleophilic attack in many of the reactions in this chapter.

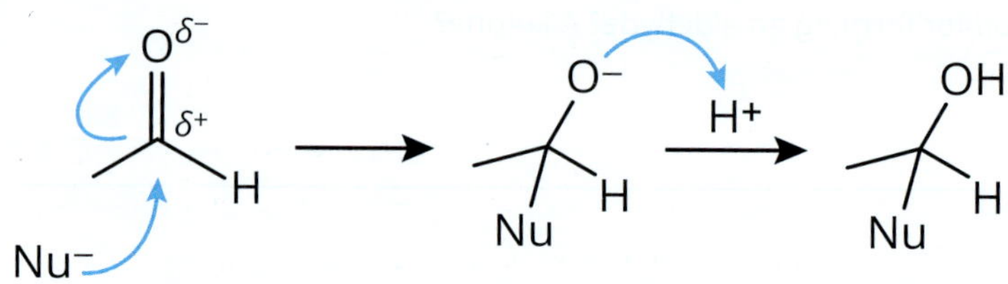


**Figure 6.7** Nucleophilic Addition Reaction Mechanism
*The nucleophile attacks the carbonyl carbon, opening the carbonyl. The carbonyl cannot reform because there is no good leaving group; thus, the $O^-$ is protonated to generate an alcohol.*

## Hydration

In the presence of water, aldehydes and ketones react to form **geminal diols** (1,1-diols), as shown in Figure 6.8. In this case, the nucleophilic oxygen in water attacks the electrophilic carbonyl carbon. This hydration reaction normally proceeds slowly, but we can increase the rate by adding a small amount of catalytic acid or base. In acidic conditions, protonation of the carbonyl oxygen creates an activated electrophilic carbonyl carbon, which allows for the addition of a relatively weak nucleophile like water. By the end of the reaction, the proton is regenerated, making the acid a catalyst. In basic conditions, hydroxide is a relatively strong nucleophile and can directly attack the electrophilic carbonyl carbon without any activation. The resulting negative charge on the oxygen (after gaining a pair of electrons from the carbonyl bond) picks up a proton from water, regenerating a hydroxide.

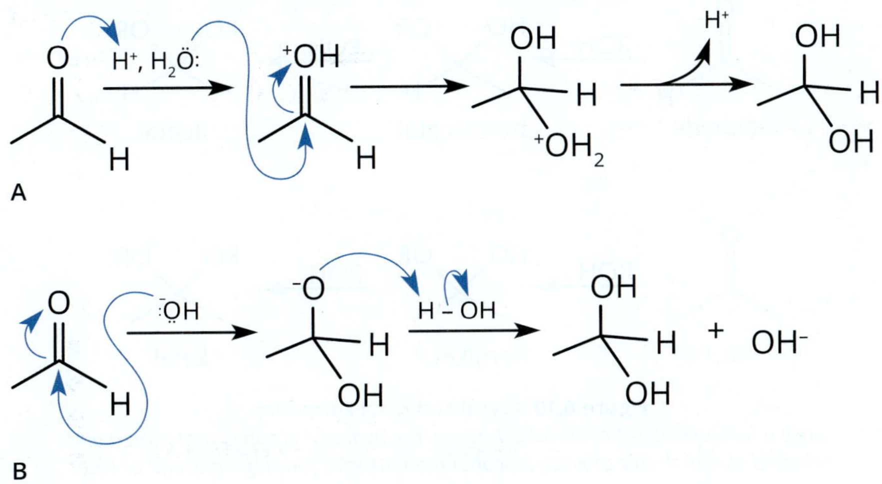


**Figure 6.8** Nucleophilic Addition Reaction Mechanism in Acidic and Basic Conditions

## Acetals and Hemiacetals

A similar reaction occurs when aldehydes and ketones are treated with alcohols. When one equivalent of alcohol (the nucleophile in this reaction) is added to an aldehyde or ketone, the product is a **hemiacetal** or **hemiketal**, respectively, as shown in Figure 6.9. Hemiacetals and hemiketals can be recognized by the retention of the hydroxyl group. This "halfway" step (hence the *hemi–* prefix) is the endpoint in basic conditions.

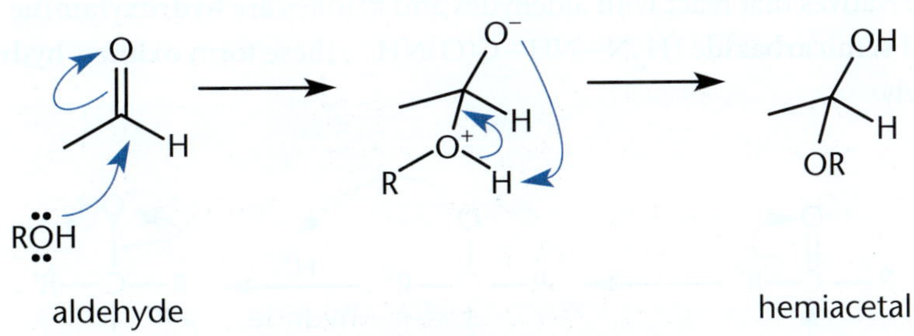


**Figure 6.9** Hemiacetal Formation
*The oxygen in the alcohol functions as the nucleophile, attacking the carbonyl carbon and generating a hemiacetal.*

When two equivalents of alcohol are added, the reaction proceeds to completion, resulting in the formation of an **acetal** or **ketal**, as shown in Figure 6.10. This reaction proceeds by a nucleophilic substitution reaction ($S_N1$) and is catalyzed by anhydrous acid. The hydroxyl group of a hemiacetal or hemiketal is protonated under acidic conditions and lost as a molecule of water. A carbocation is thus formed, and another equivalent of alcohol attacks this carbocation, resulting in the formation of an acetal or ketal. Acetals and ketals, which are comparatively inert, are frequently used as protecting groups for carbonyl functionalities. Molecules with protecting groups can easily be converted back to carbonyls with aqueous acid and heat.

**KEY CONCEPT**

In the formation of hemiacetals and hemiketals, alcohol is the nucleophile and the carbonyl carbon is the electrophile. In the formation of acetals and ketals, alcohol is the nucleophile, and the carbocation carbon (formerly the carbonyl carbon) is the electrophile.

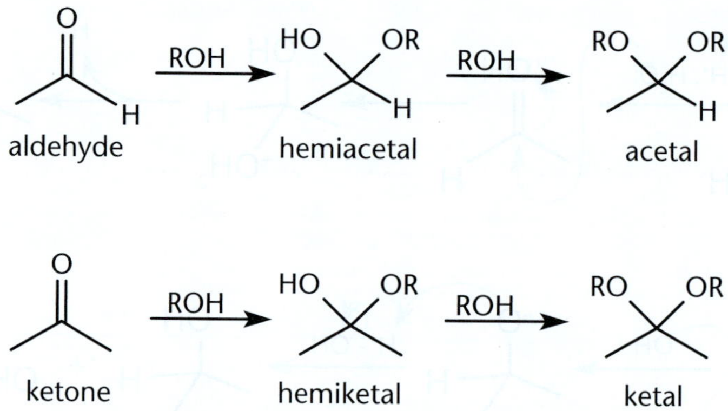


**Figure 6.10** Acetal and Ketal Formation
*Once a hemiacetal or hemiketal is formed, the hydroxyl group is protonated and released as a molecule of water; alcohol then attacks, forming an acetal or ketal.*

## Imines and Enamines

Nitrogen and nitrogen-based functional groups act as good nucleophiles due to the lone pair of electrons on nitrogen, and react readily with the electrophilic carbonyls of aldehydes and ketones. In the simplest case, ammonia adds to the carbon atom and water is lost, producing an **imine**, a compound with a nitrogen atom double-bonded to a carbon atom. This reaction is shown in Figure 6.11. Because a small molecule is lost during the formation of a bond between two molecules, this is an example of a **condensation reaction**. Because nitrogen replaces the carbonyl oxygen, this is also an example of a **nucleophilic substitution**. Some common ammonia derivatives that react with aldehydes and ketones are **hydroxylamine** ($H_2N-OH$), **hydrazine** ($H_2N-NH_2$), and **semicarbazide** ($H_2N-NH-C(O)NH_2$); these form **oximes**, **hydrazones**, and **semicarbazones**, respectively.

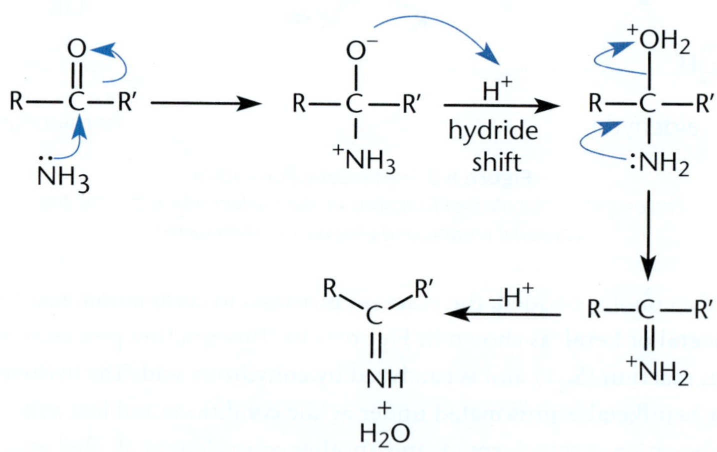


**Figure 6.11** Imine Formation
*Ammonia is added to the carbonyl, resulting in the elimination of water and generation of an imine.*

Imines and related compounds can undergo tautomerization to form **enamines**, which contain both a double bond and a nitrogen-containing group. This is analogous to the keto–enol tautomerization of carbonyl compounds and will be explored in Chapter 7 of *MCAT Organic Chemistry Review*.

## Cyanohydrins

Hydrogen cyanide (HCN) is a classic nucleophile on the MCAT. HCN has both triple bonds and an electronegative nitrogen atom, rendering it relatively acidic with a p$K_a$ of 9.2. After the hydrogen dissociates, the nucleophilic cyanide anion can attack the carbonyl carbon atom, as shown in Figure 6.12. Reactions of hydrogen cyanide with aldehydes and ketones produce stable compounds called **cyanohydrins** once the oxygen has been reprotonated. The cyanohydrin gains its stability from the newly formed C—C bond.

**KEY CONCEPT**

In a reaction with HCN, $^-$:CN is the nucleophile; the carbonyl carbon is the electrophile.

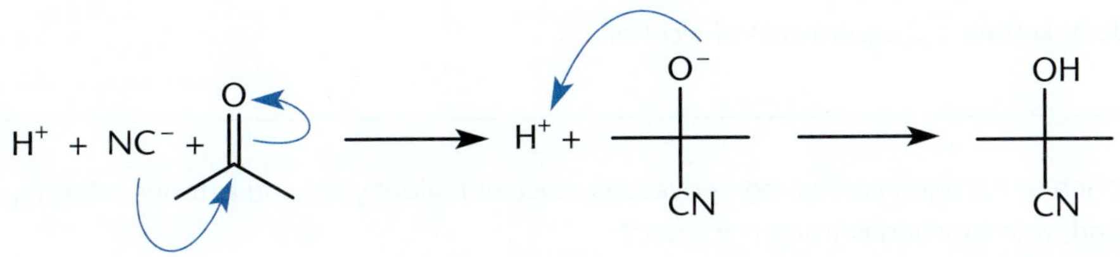


**Figure 6.12** Cyanohydrin Formation
*Cyanide functions as a nucleophile, attacking the carbonyl carbon and generating a cyanohydrin.*

## Grignard Reagents

Organometallic reagents, such as Grignard reagents (R–MgX), are powerful nucleophiles due to a highly polarized carbon-metal bond, which places significant negative charge character on the carbon. These reagents readily attack the electrophilic carbonyl carbon of aldehydes and ketones. The initial product is an alkoxide, which is then protonated in a subsequent acid workup step to yield an alcohol, as shown in Figure 6.13. Addition to formaldehyde gives primary alcohols, addition to other aldehydes gives secondary alcohols, and addition to ketones gives tertiary alcohols.

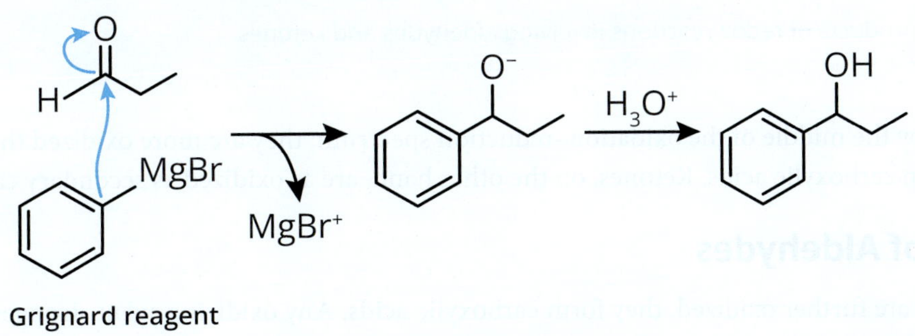


**Figure 6.13** Grignard Reaction

### MCAT CONCEPT CHECK 6.2

Before you move on, assess your understanding of the material with these questions.

1. When an aldehyde or ketone is reacted with one equivalent of an alcohol, what occurs? What would be different if it were reacted with two equivalents in acidic conditions?
   - Aldehyde or ketone + 1 equivalent of alcohol:

   ___

   - Aldehyde or ketone + 2 equivalents of alcohol:

   ___

2. When nitrogen or nitrogen-containing derivatives react with aldehydes and ketones, what type of reaction happens, and what functional group is formed?

   ___

3. When HCN reacts with an aldehyde or ketone, what functional group is produced? Is the product stable?

   ___

## 6.3 Oxidation–Reduction Reactions

### LEARNING OBJECTIVES

After Chapter 6.3, you will be able to:

- Recall common oxidizing and reducing agents used on aldehydes and ketones
- Predict the products of redox reactions involving aldehydes and ketones

Aldehydes occupy the middle of the oxidation–reduction spectrum; they are more oxidized than alcohols but less oxidized than carboxylic acids. Ketones, on the other hand, are as oxidized as secondary carbons can get.

### Oxidation of Aldehydes

When aldehydes are further oxidized, they form carboxylic acids. Any oxidizing agent stronger than PCC can perform this reaction. Some examples include potassium permanganate ($KMnO_4$), chromium trioxide ($CrO_3$), silver(I) oxide ($Ag_2O$), and hydrogen peroxide ($H_2O_2$). This is shown in Figure 6.14.

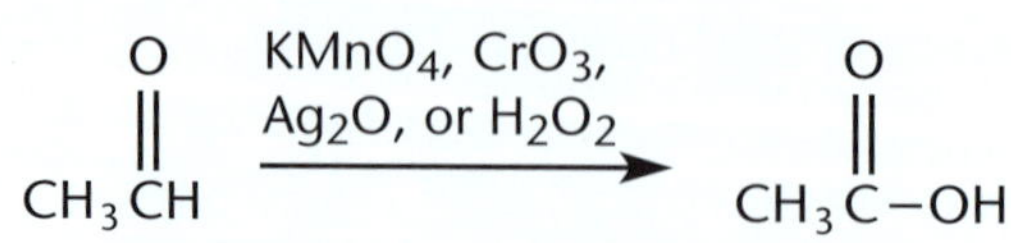


**Figure 6.14** Aldehyde Oxidation
*Most oxidizing agents will turn aldehydes into carboxylic acids; PCC, however, is anhydrous and is not strong enough to oxidize past the point of an aldehyde.*

## Reduction by Hydride Reagents

Aldehydes and ketones can also undergo reduction to form alcohols. This is often performed with **hydride reagents**. The most common of these seen on the MCAT are **lithium aluminum hydride** ($LiAlH_4$) and **sodium borohydride** ($NaBH_4$), which is often used when milder conditions are needed. This reaction is shown in Figure 6.15.

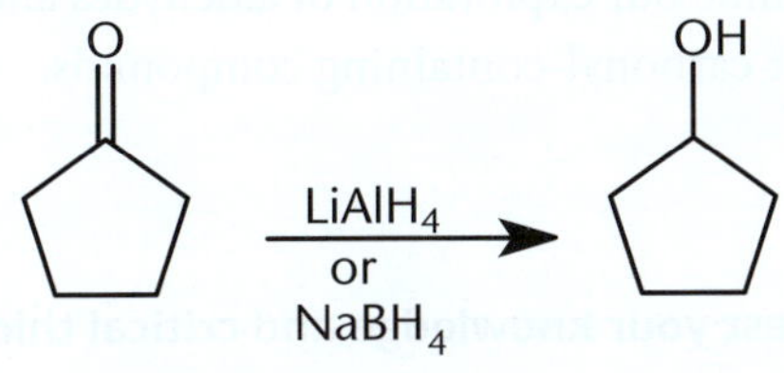


**Figure 6.15** Ketone Reduction
*Ketones are easily reduced to their respective alcohols using hydride reagents.*

### MCAT CONCEPT CHECK 6.3

Before you move on, assess your understanding of the material with these questions.

1. What functional group is formed when an aldehyde is oxidized? What are some common oxidizing agents that assist this reaction?
   - Functional group:

     ______________________________
   - Oxidizing agents:

     ______________________________
2. What functional group is formed when aldehydes and ketones are reduced? What are some common reducing agents that assist this reaction?
   - Functional group:

     ______________________________
   - Reducing agents:

     ______________________________
3. A chemistry student reacts butanone and butanal each with PCC and $KMnO_4$. What are the expected products of each reaction?
   - Butanone:

     ______________________________
   - Butanal:

     ______________________________

## Conclusion

In this chapter, we have examined the properties of aldehydes and ketones. Specifically, we have taken a look at the reactivity of the carbonyl carbon in nucleophilic addition reactions and examined how aldehydes and ketones can be oxidized and reduced. Carbonyls are common reaction sites in many biosynthetic processes, which helps explain their importance on the MCAT.

In the following chapter, we will continue our exploration of aldehydes and ketones by looking at the chemistry of enolates, which are nucleophilic carbonyl-containing compounds.

### GO ONLINE

**You've reviewed the content, now test your knowledge and critical thinking skills by completing a test-like passage set in your online resources!**

# CONCEPT SUMMARY

## Description and Properties

- **Aldehydes** are terminal functional groups containing a carbonyl bonded to at least one hydrogen. In nomenclature, they use the suffix –**al** and the prefix **oxo**–. In rings, they are indicated by the suffix –**carbaldehyde**.
- **Ketones** are internal functional groups containing a carbonyl bonded to two alkyl chains. In nomenclature, they use the suffix –**one** and the prefix **oxo**– or **keto**–.
- The reactivity of a **carbonyl** (C=O) is dictated by the polarity of the double bond. The carbon has a partial positive charge and is therefore electrophilic.
- Carbonyl-containing compounds have higher boiling points than equivalent alkanes because of dipole interactions. Alcohols have higher boiling points than carbonyls because of hydrogen bonding.
- Aldehydes and ketones are commonly produced by oxidation of primary and secondary alcohols, respectively.
  - Weaker, anhydrous oxidizing agents like **pyridinium chlorochromate** (**PCC**) must be used for synthesizing aldehydes, or the reaction will continue oxidizing to the level of the carboxylic acid.
  - Various oxidizing agents can be used for ketones, such as dichromate, chromium trioxide, or PCC because ketones are the most oxidized functional group for secondary carbons.

## Nucleophilic Addition Reactions

- When a nucleophile attacks and forms a bond with a carbonyl carbon, electrons in the $\pi$ bond are pushed to the oxygen atom.
  - If there is no good leaving group (aldehydes and ketones), the carbonyl will remain open and is protonated to form an alcohol.
  - If there is a good leaving group (carboxylic acids and derivatives), the carbonyl will reform and kick off the leaving group.
- In **hydration** reactions, water adds to a carbonyl, forming a **geminal diol**.
- When one equivalent of alcohol reacts with an aldehyde (via nucleophilic addition), a **hemiacetal** is formed. When the same reaction occurs with a ketone, a **hemiketal** is formed.
- When another equivalent of alcohol reacts with a hemiacetal (via nucleophilic substitution), an **acetal** is formed. When the same reaction occurs with a **hemiketal**, a ketal is formed.
- Nitrogen and nitrogen derivatives react with carbonyls to form **imines**, oximes, hydrazones, and semicarbazones. Imines can tautomerize to form **enamines**.
- Hydrogen cyanide reacts with carbonyls to form **cyanohydrins**.

## Oxidation–Reduction Reactions

- Aldehydes can be oxidized to carboxylic acids using an oxidizing agent like $KMnO_4$, $CrO_3$, $Ag_2O$, or $H_2O_2$. They can be reduced to primary alcohols via **hydride reagents** ($LiAlH_4$, $NaBH_4$).
- Ketones cannot be further oxidized, but can be reduced to secondary alcohols using the same hydride reagents.

## ANSWERS TO CONCEPT CHECKS

### 6.1

1. The molecule on the left is butanone. The molecule on the right is propanal.
2. The alkane will have the lowest boiling point, followed by the aldehyde, and then the alcohol. The boiling point of the aldehyde is elevated by its dipole,
but the boiling point of an alcohol is further elevated by hydrogen bonding.
3. The carbon in a carbonyl is electrophilic; it is partially positively charged because oxygen is highly electron-withdrawing.
4. Aldehydes can be formed by the oxidation of primary alcohols, but can only be produced using weaker (and anhydrous) oxidizing agents like PCC—otherwise, they will oxidize fully to carboxylic acids. Ketones can be formed by the oxidation of secondary alcohols. Other methods can be used as well (ozonolysis, Friedel–Crafts acylation), but these are outside the scope of the MCAT.

### 6.2

1. With one equivalent of alcohol, aldehydes and ketones will form hemiacetals and hemiketals, respectively. With two equivalents of alcohol, the reaction will run to completion, forming acetals and ketals, respectively.
2. The reaction that occurs is a condensation reaction because a small molecule is lost, and also a nucleophilic substitution reaction. This reaction results in the formation of an imine (or, for nitrogen-containing derivatives: oximes, hydrazones, or semicarbazones).
3. When HCN reacts with an aldehyde or ketone, a cyanohydrin is produced, which is a stable product.

### 6.3

1. Oxidizing an aldehyde yields a carboxylic acid. Common oxidizing agents include $KMnO_4$, $CrO_3$, $Ag_2O$, and $H_2O_2$.
2. Reducing an aldehyde or ketone yields an alcohol. Under certain conditions not tested on the MCAT, aldehydes and ketones can be reduced all the way to alkanes. Common reducing agents include $LiAlH_4$ and $NaBH_4$.
3. Butanone reacts with neither PCC nor $KMnO_4$ because ketones cannot be oxidized with common oxidizing reagent that cannot break the carbon–carbon bond. Butanal is oxidized by $KMnO_4$ to form butanoic acid, but does not react with PCC, which is not a strong enough oxidant.

# SCIENCE MASTERY ASSESSMENT EXPLANATIONS

**1. D**

The reactivity of the carbonyl can be attributed to the difference in electronegativity between the carbon and oxygen atoms. The more electronegative oxygen atom attracts the bonding electrons and is therefore electron-withdrawing. Thus, the carbonyl carbon is electrophilic. One resonance structure of the carbonyl pushes the $\pi$ electrons onto the oxygen, resulting in a positively charged carbonyl carbon.

2. **B**

Assuming the length of the carbon chain remains the same, the alkane consistently has the lowest boiling point. The boiling point of the ketone is elevated by the dipole in the carbonyl. The boiling point of the alcohol is elevated further by hydrogen bonding.

3. **C**

The reaction between a ketone and one equivalent of alcohol produces a hemiketal. This has an –OR group, an –OH group, and two alkyl groups attached at the same carbon. **(A)** is a ketal, with two –OR groups and two –R groups. **(B)** is a hemiacetal, with an –OH group, an –OR group, one R group, and a hydrogen atom (not drawn). **(D)** is a ketone. Note that a hemiketal is a very unstable compound, and will react rapidly with a second equivalent of alcohol to form a ketal in acidic conditions.

4. **A**

Aldehydes and ketones react with ammonia and nitrogen-based derivatives to form imines—compounds with a double bond between carbon and nitrogen.

5. **B**

Aldehydes are easily oxidized to the corresponding carboxylic acids by $KMnO_4$. In **(A)**, the aldehyde has been reduced to an alcohol. In **(C)**, the molecule has not reacted. In **(D)**, the aldehyde has been oxidized, but a $-CH_2-$ group has been removed.

6. **B**

$LiAlH_4$ reduces aldehydes to primary alcohols and ketones to secondary alcohols. In this reaction, a ketone is converted to a secondary alcohol.

7. **D**

Because an excess of ethanol is present, the product of the reaction between this aldehyde and ethanol will be an acetal. The benzaldehyde will first be converted to a hemiacetal, shown in **(C)**, but will then proceed to completion as an acetal. **(A)** and **(B)** are incorrect because they show the presence of two benzene rings in the final product.

8. **B**

Hemiacetals and hemiketals are usually short-lived because the –OH group will rapidly become protonated in acidic conditions and is lost as water, leaving behind a carbocation that is very susceptible to attack by an alcohol. Once the alcohol has been added, the acetal or ketal becomes more stable because the newly added group is less likely to become protonated and leave as compared to –OH.

9. **A**

A hemiacetal is a molecule in which one equivalent of alcohol has been added to a carbonyl (–OR) and the carbonyl oxygen has been protonated (–OH). Otherwise, there is the same alkyl group (–R) and hydrogen atom (–H) as the parent aldehyde. **(B)** describes an acetal, **(C)** a hemiketal, and **(D)** a ketal.

10. **A**

Although both the aldehyde and ketone listed will be reactive with the strongly nucleophilic hydrogen cyanide, aldehydes are slightly more reactive toward nucleophiles than ketones for steric reasons, so the aldehyde and HCN will form the major product (which will be a cyanohydrin).

11. **C**

PCC is a mild anhydrous oxidant that can oxidize primary alcohols to aldehydes, and secondary alcohols to ketones. It is not strong enough to oxidize alcohols or aldehydes to carboxylic acids.

12. **B**

In a hydration reaction, water adds to a carbonyl, forming a geminal diol—a compound with two hydroxyl groups on the same carbon. Hydrogen peroxide and potassium dichromate are oxidizing agents that can convert an aldehyde to a carboxylic acid. Ethanol will react with a carbonyl compound to form an acetal or a ketal, if excess ethanol is available.

13. **A**

Ammonia, or $NH_3$, will react with an aldehyde like glutaraldehyde to form an imine. This is a condensation and a substitution reaction, as the C=O of the carbonyl will be replaced with a C=N bond.

14. **C**

Hydrides like $LiAlH_4$ and $NaBH_4$ are reducing agents; as such, they will reduce aldehydes and ketones to alcohols. The other reagents listed are oxidizing agents, which will not act on a ketone.

15. **D**

During tautomerization, the double bond between the carbon and nitrogen in an imine is moved to lie between two carbons. This results in an enamine—a compound with a double bond and an amine.

**GO ONLINE**

**Consult your online resources for additional practice.**

## SHARED CONCEPTS

**Biochemistry Chapter 4**
Carbohydrate Structure and Function

**General Chemistry Chapter 11**
Oxidation–Reduction Reactions

**Organic Chemistry Chapter 1**
Nomenclature

**Organic Chemistry Chapter 4**
Analyzing Organic Reactions

**Organic Chemistry Chapter 7**
Aldehydes and Ketones II

**Organic Chemistry Chapter 8**
Carboxylic Acids

CHAPTER 7

# ALDEHYDES AND KETONES II: ENOLATES

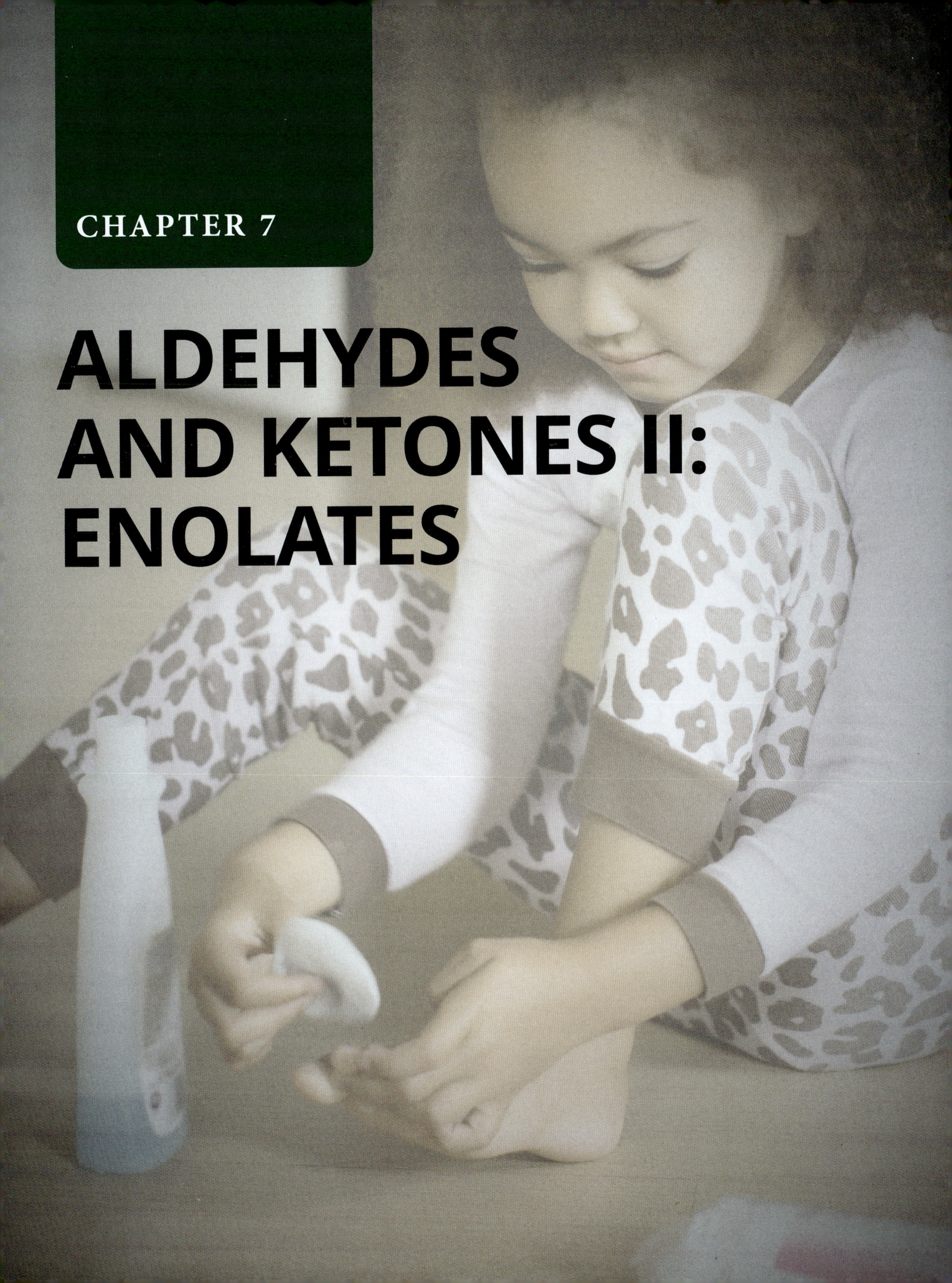

# SCIENCE MASTERY ASSESSMENT

Every pre-med knows this feeling: there is so much content I have to know for the MCAT! How do I know what to do first or what's important?

While the high-yield badges throughout this book will help you identify the most important topics, this Science Mastery Assessment is another tool in your MCAT prep arsenal. This quiz (which can also be taken in your online resources) and the guidance below will help ensure that you are spending the appropriate amount of time on this chapter based on your personal strengths and weaknesses. Don't worry though—skipping something now does not mean you'll never study it. Later on in your prep, as you complete full-length tests, you'll uncover specific pieces of content that you need to review and can come back to these chapters as appropriate.

## How to Use This Assessment

**If you answer 0–7 questions correctly:**

Spend about 1 hour to read this chapter in full and take limited notes throughout. Follow up by reviewing **all** quiz questions to ensure that you now understand how to solve each one.

**If you answer 8–11 questions correctly:**

Spend 20–40 minutes reviewing the quiz questions. Beginning with the questions you missed, read and take notes on the corresponding subchapters. For questions you answered correctly, ensure your thinking matches that of the explanation and you understand why each choice was correct or incorrect.

**If you answer 12–15 questions correctly:**

Spend less than 20 minutes reviewing all questions from the quiz. If you missed any, then include a quick read-through of the corresponding subchapters, or even just the relevant content within a subchapter, as part of your question review. For questions you got correct, ensure your thinking matches that of the explanation and review the Concept Summary at the end of the chapter.

1. What is the product of the reaction below?

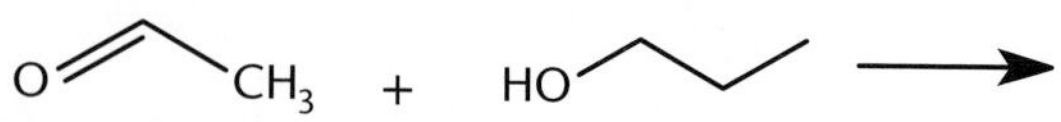

A. 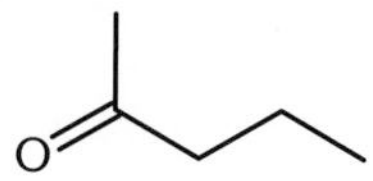

B. 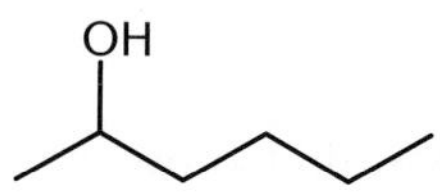

C. 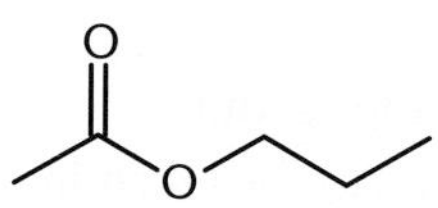

D. 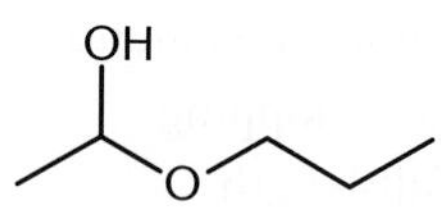

2. The reaction below is an example of:

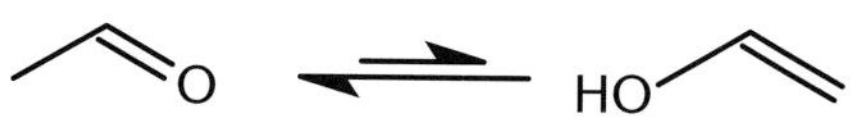

A. esterification.
B. tautomerization.
C. elimination.
D. dehydration.

3. Which of the following reactions would produce the compound below?

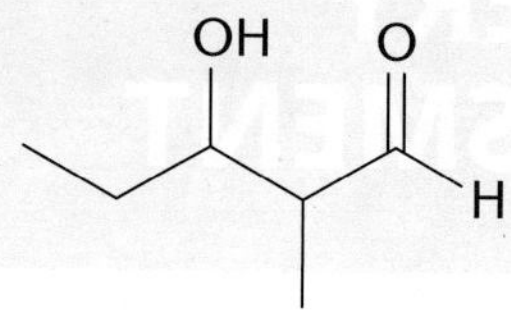

A. $CH_3CHO + CH_3CH_2CH_2CHO \rightarrow$
B. $CH_3COCH_3 + CH_3CH_2CH_2CHO \rightarrow$
C. $CH_3CH_2COCH_3 + CH_3CHO \rightarrow$
D. $CH_3CH_2CHO + CH_3CH_2CHO \rightarrow$

4. Why does the equilibrium between keto and enol tautomers lie far to the keto side?

I. The keto form is more thermodynamically stable.
II. The enol form is lower energy.
III. The enol form is more thermodynamically stable.

A. I only
B. III only
C. I and II only
D. II and III only

5. The aldol condensation is an example of which reaction type(s)?

I. Dehydration
II. Cleavage
III. Nucleophilic addition

A. I only
B. I and III only
C. II and III only
D. I, II, and III

6. Which of the hydrogens in the following molecule is the most acidic?

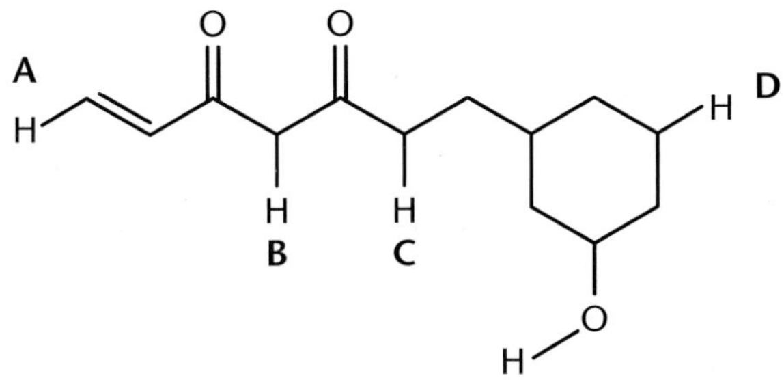


A. A
B. B
C. C
D. D

7. When reacted with ammonia ($NH_3$) at 200°C, which enolate of a carbonyl-containing compound would predominate?
A. Kinetic enolate
B. Thermodynamic enolate
C. Neither enolate; they would be present in roughly equal proportions.
D. Neither enolate; these reaction conditions would not form either enolate.

8. Which of the following compounds would be most reactive toward a nucleophile?
A. Pentanal
B. 3-Pentanone
C. Pentane
D. 2-Nonanone

9. $\alpha$-hydrogens of a ketone are acidic due to:
I. resonance stabilization.
II. the electron-withdrawing properties of the alkyl groups.
III. the electronegative carbonyl oxygen.
A. I only
B. I and III only
C. II and III only
D. I, II, and III

10. Which of the following is considered a tautomer of the imine functional group?
A. Cyanohydrin
B. Hydrazone
C. Enamine
D. Semicarbazone

11. When succinaldehyde is treated with lithium diisopropylamide (LDA), it:
I. becomes more nucleophilic.
II. becomes less nucleophilic.
III. generates a carbanion.
A. I only
B. II only
C. I and III only
D. II and III only

12. Which of the following best describes the final product of an aldol condensation?
A. 1,3-dicarbonyl
B. 1,2-dicarbonyl
C. $\alpha,\beta$-unsaturated carbonyl
D. $\beta,\gamma$-unsaturated carbonyl

13. When benzaldehyde is reacted with acetone, which will act as the nucleophile?
A. Benzaldehyde, after addition of strong acid
B. Benzaldehyde, after reaction with strong base
C. Acetone, after addition of strong acid
D. Acetone, after reaction with strong base

14. 3-Hydroxybutanal can be formed by the reaction of:
A. methanol in diethyl ether.
B. ethanal in base, then in acid.
C. butanal in strong acid.
D. methanal and ethanal in catalytic base.

15. The catalytic production of dihydroxyacetone and glyceraldehyde 3-phosphate (2-hydroxy-3-oxopropyl dihydrogen phosphate) from fructose-1,6-bisphosphate ([(2S,3S,4S,5R)-2,3,4-trihydroxy-5-(phosphonooxymethyl)oxolan-2-yl]methyl dihydrogen phosphate) is what type of reaction?
A. Aldol condensation
B. Retro-aldol reaction
C. Dehydration
D. Nucleophilic attack

## Answer Key

1. **D** (See section 7.2)
2. **B** (See section 7.2)
3. **D** (See section 7.2)
4. **A** (See section 7.1)
5. **B** (See section 7.3)
6. **B** (See section 7.1)
7. **B** (See section 7.2)
8. **A** (See section 7.2)
9. **B** (See section 7.1)
10. **C** (See section 7.1)
11. **C** (See section 7.2)
12. **C** (See section 7.3)
13. **D** (See section 7.2)
14. **B** (See section 7.2)
15. **B** (See section 7.1)

*The relevant section of the chapter to review for each question is given in parentheses after the correct answer. Detailed explanations can be found at the end of the chapter.*

CHAPTER 7

# ALDEHYDES AND KETONES II: ENOLATES

## In This Chapter



**CHAPTER PROFILE**

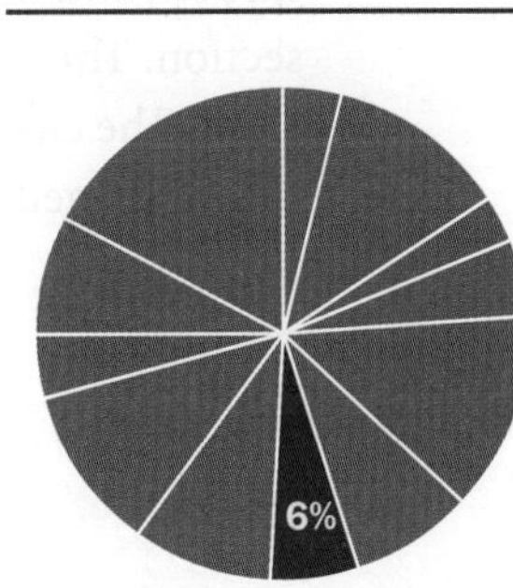


The content in this chapter should be relevant to about 6% of all questions about organic chemistry on the MCAT.

This chapter covers material from the following AAMC content category:

**5D:** Structure, function, and reactivity of biologically-relevant molecules

## Introduction

In the previous chapter, we took a look at a few key properties and reactions of aldehydes and ketones. These molecules have highly predictable chemistry centered on their electrophilic, positively charged carbonyl carbon and will be sure to show up on Test Day. In this chapter, we take a look at several more properties of aldehydes and ketones, and focus on the reactivity of the $\alpha$-hydrogen of carbonyl-containing compounds. The acidity of this $\alpha$-hydrogen allows many aldehydes and ketones to act as both electrophiles and nucleophiles. Sometimes, they can even serve both functions in the same reaction. But don't worry—we'll also review some tips about how to understand when and how aldehydes and ketones will react.

## 7.1 General Principles

**LEARNING OBJECTIVES**

After Chapter 7.1, you will be able to:

- Explain the acidic nature of $\alpha$-hydrogens on aldehydes and ketones
- Compare the acidity of the $\alpha$-hydrogens of aldehydes to those of ketones
- Describe the relationship between steric hindrance and reactivity

In the previous chapter, we focused on how the electronegativity of the oxygen atom in a carbonyl pulls electrons away from the carbonyl carbon, making it partially positively charged. In this chapter, we take the electron-withdrawing characteristics of oxygen one bond further, focusing on the $\alpha$-carbon in an aldehyde or ketone.

## Acidity of $\alpha$-Hydrogens

An **$\alpha$-carbon** is adjacent to the carbonyl carbon, and the hydrogens connected to the $\alpha$-carbon are termed **$\alpha$-hydrogens**. Through induction, oxygen pulls some of the electron density out of these C—H bonds, weakening them. This makes it relatively easy to deprotonate the $\alpha$-carbon of an aldehyde or ketone, as shown in Figure 7.1. The acidity of $\alpha$-hydrogens is augmented by resonance stabilization of the conjugate base. Specifically, when the $\alpha$-hydrogen is removed, the extra electrons that remain can resonate between the $\alpha$-carbon, the carbonyl carbon, and the carbonyl oxygen. This increases the stability of this enolate intermediate, described in the next section. Through this resonance, the negative charge can be distributed to the more electronegative oxygen atom. The electron-withdrawing oxygen atom thereby helps stabilize the **carbanion** (a molecule with a negatively charged carbon atom). When in basic solutions, $\alpha$-hydrogens will easily deprotonate.

**KEY CONCEPT**

Electron-withdrawing groups like oxygen stabilize organic anions. Electron-donating groups like alkyl groups destabilize organic anions.

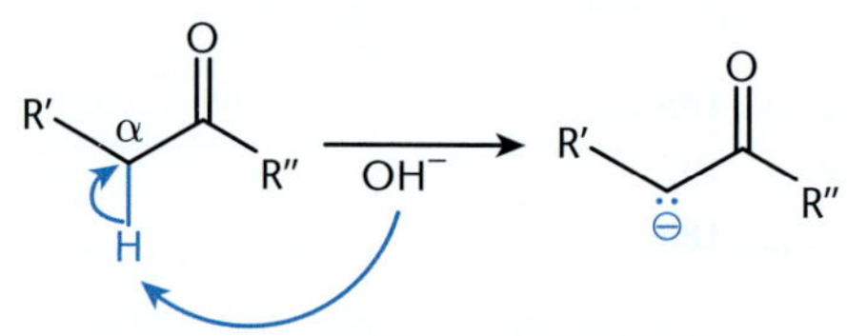


**Figure 7.1** Deprotonation of an $\alpha$-Carbon, Forming a Carbanion

The $\alpha$-hydrogens of ketones tend to be slightly less acidic than those of aldehydes due to the electron-donating properties of the additional alkyl group in a ketone. This property is the same reason that alkyl groups help to stabilize carbocations—but in this case, they destabilize the carbanion.

## Steric Hindrance

In reactions, aldehydes are slightly more reactive to nucleophiles than ketones. This is due in part to steric hindrance in the ketone, which arises from the additional alkyl group that ketones contain. When the nucleophile approaches the ketone or aldehyde in order to react, the additional alkyl groups on the ketone are in the way, more so than the single hydrogen of the aldehyde (see Figure 7.2). This makes for a higher-energy, more crowded intermediate step. Remember, higher-energy intermediates mean that the reaction is less likely to proceed.

**KEY CONCEPT**

Ketones are slightly less likely to react with nucleophiles than aldehydes because the extra alkyl group destabilizes the carbanion and increases steric hindrance.

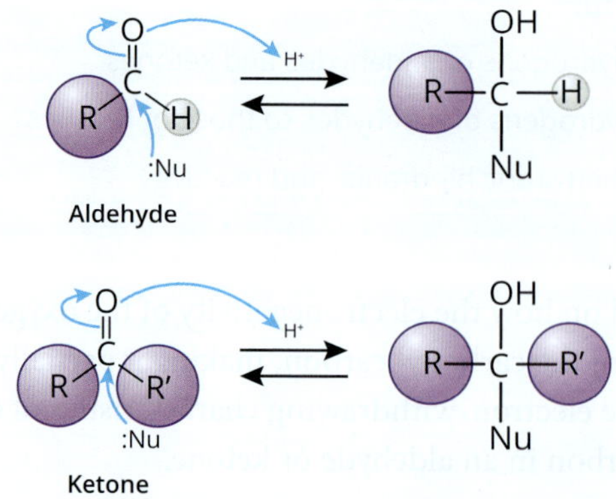


**Figure 7.2** Comparison of Steric Hindrance in Aldehydes and Ketones
*Aldehydes are more prone to nucleophilic attack, as their carbonyl carbon is bonded to a small hydrogen, while ketones are sterically hindered by two bulky alkyl groups.*

### MCAT CONCEPT CHECK 7.1

Before you move on, assess your understanding of the material with these questions.

1. Why are the $\alpha$-hydrogens of aldehydes and ketones acidic?

_______________________________________________

2. Which has a lower p$K_a$: 3-pentanone or pentanal? Why?

_______________________________________________

3. How does steric hindrance affect the relative reactivity of aldehydes and ketones?

_______________________________________________

## 7.2 Enolate Chemistry

### LEARNING OBJECTIVES

After Chapter 7.2, you will be able to:

- Define tautomerization
- Predict the role of an enolate carbanion in a reaction
- Describe the conditions that favor keto and enol forms
- Identify the thermodynamically favored tautomer of an aldehyde or ketone:

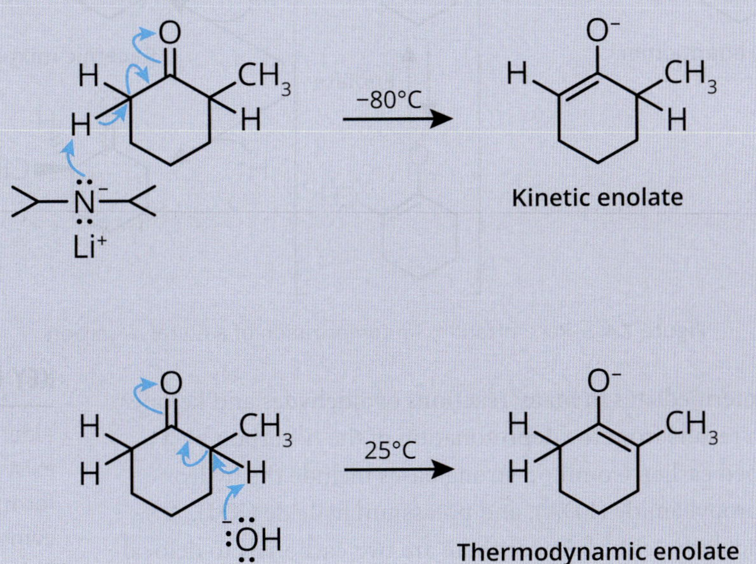


Due to the acidity of the $\alpha$-hydrogen, aldehydes and ketones exist in solution as a mixture of two isomers: the familiar keto form, and the enol form.

## Keto–Enol Tautomerization

The **enol** form gets its name from the presence of a carbon–carbon double bond (the *en–* component) and an alcohol (the *–ol* component). The two isomers, which differ in the placement of a proton and the double bond, are called **tautomers**. The equilibrium between the tautomers lies far to the keto side, so there will be many more keto isomers in solution. The process of interconverting from the keto to the enol tautomer, shown in Figure 7.3, is called **enolization**, or, more generally, **tautomerization**.

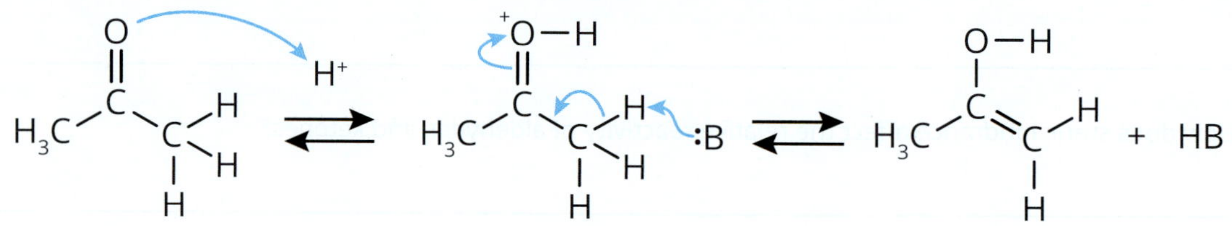


**Figure 7.3** Enolization (Tautomerization)
*On the left is the keto form, which is thermodynamically favored over the enol form on the right.*

By extension, any aldehyde or ketone with a chiral $\alpha$-carbon will rapidly become a racemic mixture as the keto and enol forms interconvert, a phenomenon known as **$\alpha$-racemization**, as shown in Figure 7.4.

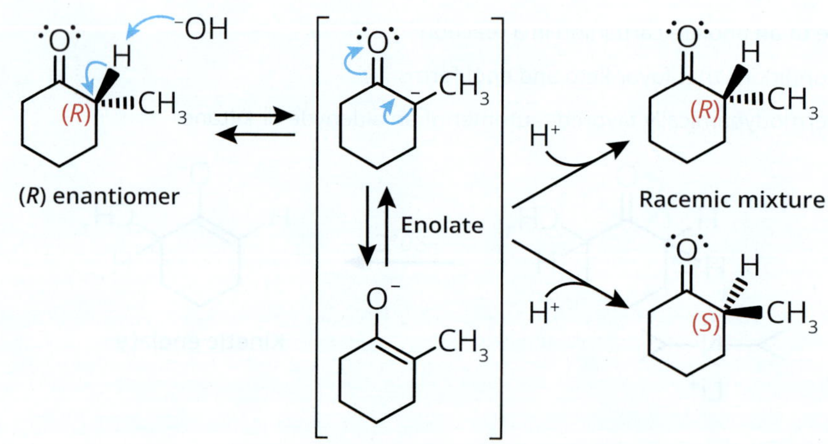


**Figure 7.4** $\alpha$-Racemization: Tautomerization of a Chiral $\alpha$-Carbon

Enols are important intermediates in many reactions of aldehydes and ketones. The enolate carbanion results from the deprotonation of the $\alpha$-carbon by a strong base, as described earlier. Common strong bases include the hydroxide ion, lithium diisopropyl amide (LDA), and potassium hydride (KH). A 1,3-dicarbonyl is particularly acidic because there are two carbonyls to delocalize negative charge and, as such, is often used to form enolate carbanions. Once formed, the nucleophilic carbanion reacts readily with electrophiles. We will see one example of this shortly in the aldol condensation. Another example of this type of reaction is a **Michael addition**, shown in Figure 7.5, in which the carbanion attacks an $\alpha,\beta$-unsaturated carbonyl compound—a molecule with a multiple bond between the $\alpha$- and $\beta$-carbons next to a carbonyl.

**KEY CONCEPT**

Aldehydes and ketones exist in the traditional keto form (C=O) and as the less common enol tautomer (enol = ene + ol). The deprotonated enolate form can act as a nucleophile. Note that tautomers are *not* resonance structures because they differ in their connectivity of atoms.

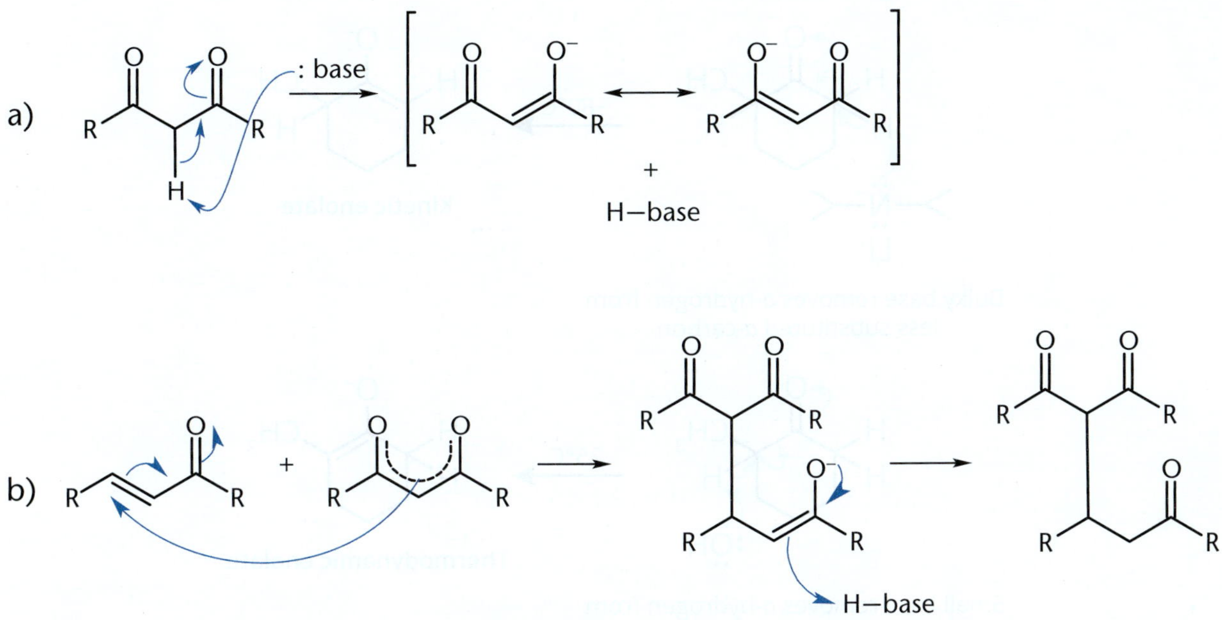


**Figure 7.5** Michael Addition
*(a) The base deprotonates the α-carbon, making it a good nucleophile;*
*(b) The carbanion attacks the double bond, resulting in a Michael addition.*

This reaction proceeds as shown due to the resonance stabilization of the intermediates. The better you understand the resonance forms of molecules, the more you will be able to predict the specific location on a molecule where a reaction will occur.

## Kinetic and Thermodynamic Enolates

Given a ketone that has two different alkyl groups, each of which may have $\alpha$-hydrogens, two forms of the enolate can form, with the carbon–carbon double bond between the carbonyl carbon and either the more or less substituted carbon, as shown in Figure 7.6. The equilibrium between these forms is dictated by the kinetic and thermodynamic control of the reaction. The kinetically controlled product is formed more rapidly but is less stable. This form has the double bond to the less substituted $\alpha$-carbon. As expected, this product is formed by the removal of the $\alpha$-hydrogen from the less substituted $\alpha$-carbon because it offers less steric hindrance. The thermodynamically controlled product is formed more slowly, but is more stable and features the double bond being formed with the more substituted $\alpha$-carbon. Accordingly, this is formed by the removal of the $\alpha$-hydrogen from the more substituted $\alpha$-carbon.

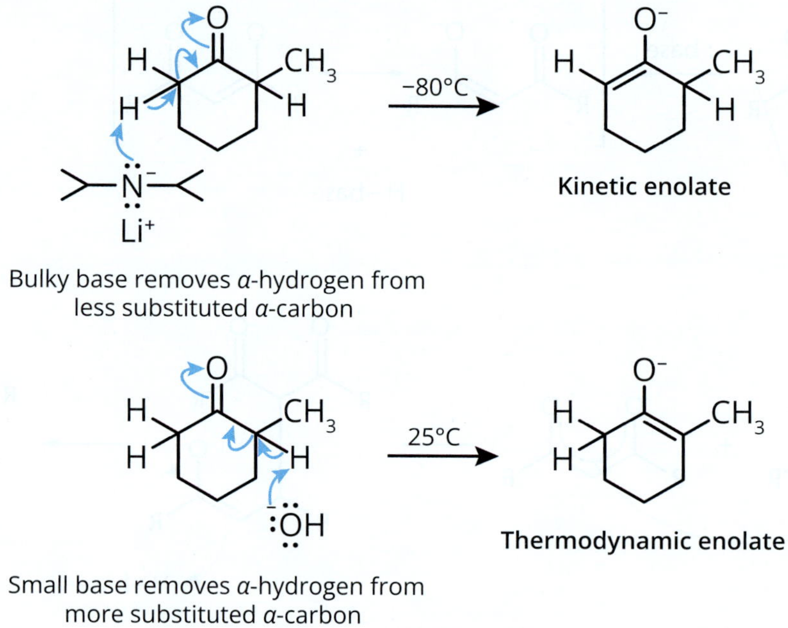


**Figure 7.6** Kinetic and Thermodynamic Enolates
*The kinetic enolate forms more quickly, but is less stable than the thermodynamic enolate.*

Each of these two products is favored by different conditions. The kinetic product is favored in reactions that are rapid, irreversible, at lower temperatures, and with a strong, sterically hindered base. If the reaction is reversible, the kinetic product can revert to the original reactant and react again to form the thermodynamic product. The thermodynamic product is favored with higher temperatures; slow, reversible reactions; and weaker, smaller bases.

## Enamines

Just as enols are tautomers of carbonyls, enamines are tautomers of imines. An imine is a compound that contains a C=N bond. The nitrogen in the imine may or may not be bonded to an alkyl group or other substituent. Through tautomerization (movement of a hydrogen and a double bond), imines can be converted into enamines, as shown in Figure 7.7.

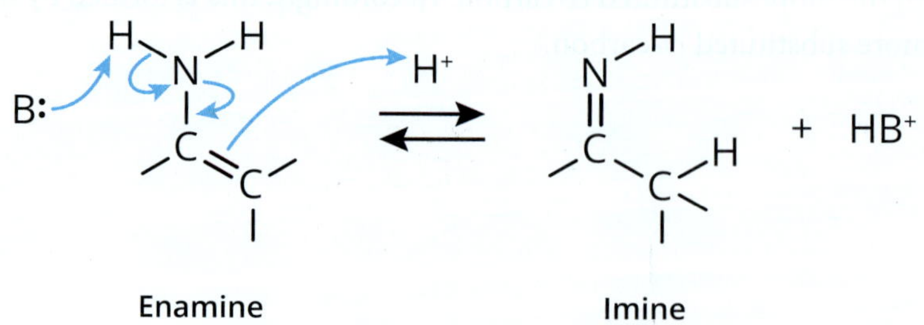


**Figure 7.7** Enamination (Tautomerization)
*On the right is the imine form, which is thermodynamically favored over the enamine form on the left.*

## MCAT CONCEPT CHECK 7.2

Before you move on, assess your understanding of the material with these questions.

1. What are tautomers?

_______________________________________________

2. Which tautomer of aldehydes and ketones is thermodynamically favored: keto or enol?

_______________________________________________

3. Which role does the enolate carbanion play in organic reactions: nucleophile, electrophile, oxidizing agent, or reducing agent?

_______________________________________________

4. In the following reaction, which product is the kinetic enolate? The thermodynamic? What conditions favor the formation of each?

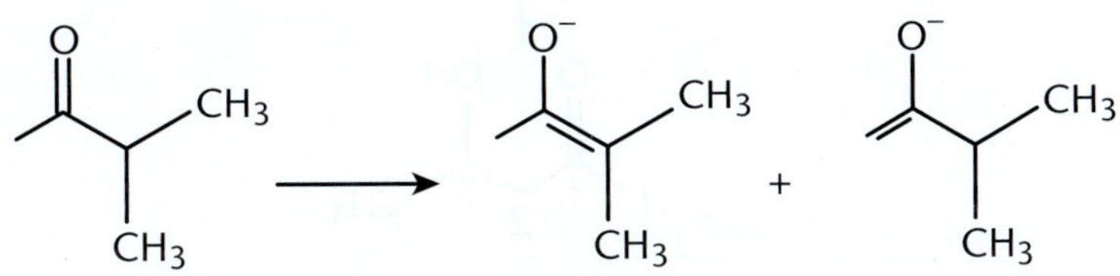


- Kinetic enolate:

_______________________________________________

- Thermodynamic enolate:

_______________________________________________

# 7.3 Aldol Condensation

## LEARNING OBJECTIVES

After Chapter 7.3, you will be able to:

- Identify the species that act as nucleophiles and electrophiles in aldol condensations
- Describe the conditions, reactants, and products involved in a retro-aldol reaction
- List the reaction types associated with aldol condensation

The **aldol condensation** is another vital reaction for the MCAT. This reaction follows the same general mechanism of nucleophilic addition to a carbonyl as previously described. In this case, however, an aldehyde or ketone acts both as an electrophile (in its keto form) and a nucleophile (in its enolate form), and the end result is the formation of a carbon–carbon bond.

As shown in Figure 7.8, when acetaldehyde (ethanal) is treated with a catalytic amount of base, an enolate ion is produced. The enolate is more nucleophilic than the enol because it is negatively charged.

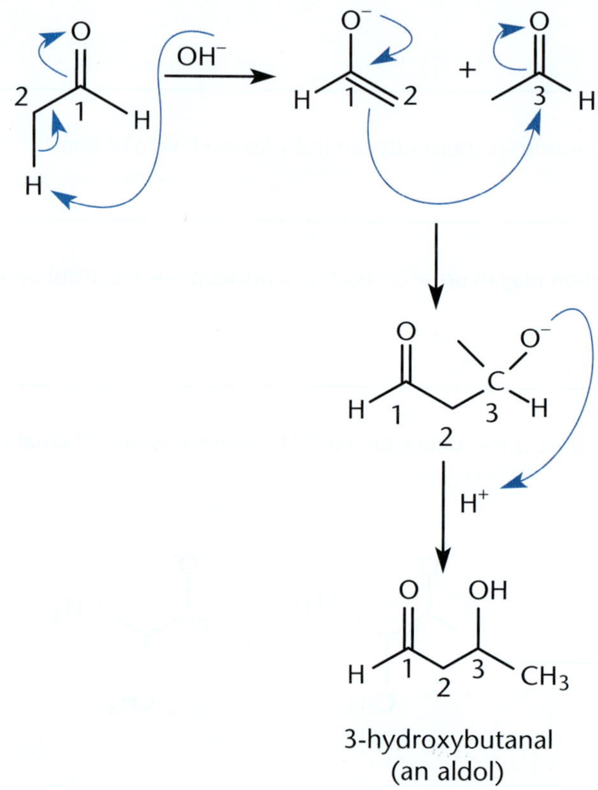


**Figure 7.8** Aldol Condensation, Step 1: Forming the Aldol
*An enolate ion is formed, which then attacks the carbonyl carbon, forming an aldol.*

**KEY CONCEPT**

In aldol condensations, it's the same nucleophilic addition reaction that we have seen before with carbonyl compounds—just with the carbonyl-containing compound acting as both a nucleophile and an electrophile.

This nucleophilic enolate ion can react with the electrophilic carbonyl group of another acetaldehyde molecule. The key to this reaction is that both species are in the same flask. The product is 3-hydroxybutanal, which is an example of an **aldol** (a molecule that contains both **ald**ehyde and alco**hol** functional groups). Note that the mechanism is still called an aldol reaction even when the reactants are ketones.

With a strong base and high temperatures, dehydration occurs by an E1 or E2 mechanism: we kick off a water molecule and form a double bond, producing an $\alpha$, $\beta$-unsaturated carbonyl, as shown in Figure 7.9.

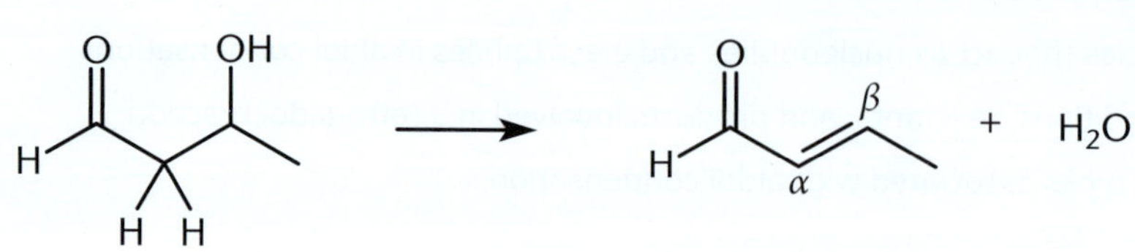

**Figure 7.9** Aldol Condensation, Step 2: Dehydration of the Aldol
*The –OH is removed as water (dehydration), forming a double bond.*

Aldol condensations are most useful if we only use one type of aldehyde or ketone. If there are multiple aldehydes or ketones, we cannot easily control which will act as the nucleophile and which will act as the electrophile, and a mixture of products will result. This can be prevented if one of the molecules has no $\alpha$-hydrogens because the $\alpha$-carbons are quaternary (like benzaldehyde).

This reaction is referred to as a **condensation reaction** because two molecules are joined with the loss of a small molecule. This type of reaction is also a **dehydration reaction** because the small molecule that is lost is water.

## The Retro-Aldol Reaction

The reverse of this reaction is called a **retro-aldol reaction**. To push the reaction in a retro-aldol direction, aqueous base is added and heat is applied. The retro-aldol reaction is useful for breaking bonds between the $\alpha$-and $\beta$-carbons of a carbonyl, as shown in Figure 7.10. This reaction is facilitated if the intermediate can be stabilized in the enolate form, just as in the forward reaction.

**KEY CONCEPT**

In a retro-aldol reaction, a bond is broken between the $\alpha$-and $\beta$-carbons of a carbonyl, forming two aldehydes, two ketones, or one aldehyde and one ketone.

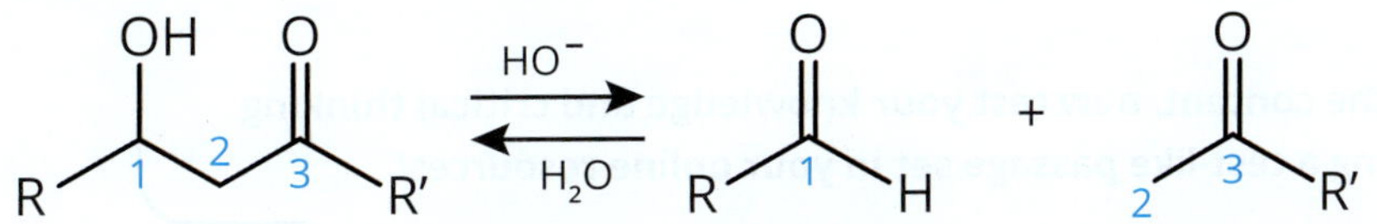


**Figure 7.10** Retro-Aldol Reaction
*The bond between the α- and β-carbons of a carbonyl is broken.*

### MCAT CONCEPT CHECK 7.3

Before you move on, assess your understanding of the material with these questions.

1. In the following reaction, an aldehyde is treated with a catalytic amount of base and an enolate ion is formed. The enolate then reacts with another aldehyde molecule leading to an aldol condensation. Identify the nucleophile and electrophile in the aldol condensation.

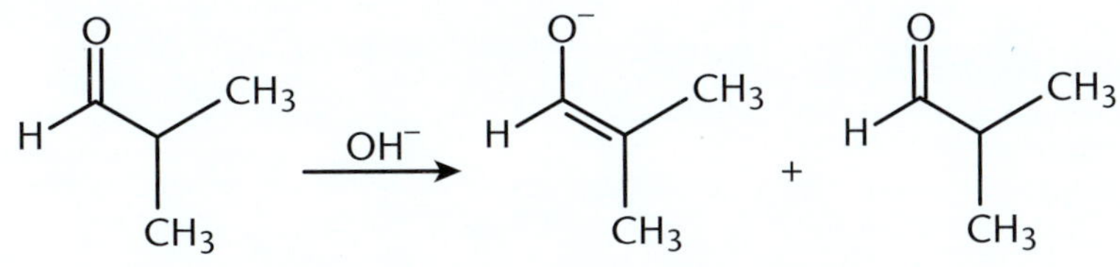


______________________________

2. What is a retro-aldol reaction? What conditions favor retro-aldol reactions?

______________________________

3. The aldol condensation can be classified under many categories of reactions. List some of these reaction types, and provide a short description of each.

______________________________

## Conclusion

In this second chapter on aldehydes and ketones, we've taken a look at the important resonance structures that the carbonyl of aldehydes and ketones allows. The high electronegativity of the oxygen atom in a carbonyl not only makes the carbonyl carbon electrophilic, but also weakens the C–H bonds on $\alpha$-carbons. Deprotonation of this $\alpha$-carbon results in an enolate, a nucleophilic version of carbonyl-containing compounds. Thus, while the carbonyl carbon dictates the electrophilic chemistry of carbonyls, it is the $\alpha$-carbon, along with its acidic hydrogens, that dictates the nucleophilic chemistry of carbonyls.

Aldehydes and ketones are not the only carbonyl-containing compounds, of course. Carboxylic acids and their derivatives, including esters, anhydrides, and amides, also have chemistry controlled by a carbonyl. But there is one critical difference between aldehydes and ketones, and carboxylic acids and their derivatives: the absence or presence of a leaving group. While aldehydes and ketones lack leaving groups, carboxylic acids and carboxylic acid derivatives have leaving groups with varying degrees of stability. Over the next two chapters, we'll explore the chemistry of these interesting groups of compounds.

**GO ONLINE**

**You've reviewed the content, now test your knowledge and critical thinking skills by completing a test-like passage set in your online resources!**

# CONCEPT SUMMARY

## General Principles

- The carbon adjacent to the carbonyl carbon is termed an **$\alpha$-carbon**; the hydrogens attached to the $\alpha$-carbon are called **$\alpha$-hydrogens**.
- $\alpha$-hydrogens are relatively acidic and can be removed by a strong base.
  - The electron-withdrawing oxygen of the carbonyl weakens the C—H bonds on $\alpha$-carbons.
  - The **enolate** resulting from deprotonation can be stabilized by resonance with the carbonyl.
- Ketones are less reactive toward nucleophiles because of steric hindrance and $\alpha$-carbanion destabilization.
  - The presence of an additional alkyl group crowds the transition step and increases its energy.
  - The alkyl group also donates electron density to the carbanion, making it less stable.

## Enolate Chemistry

- Aldehydes and ketones exist in the traditional **keto form** (C=O) and in the less common **enol form** (ene + ol = double bond + hydroxyl group).
  - **Tautomers** are isomers that can be interconverted by moving a hydrogen and a double bond. The keto and enol forms are tautomers of each other.
  - The enol form can be deprotonated to form an **enolate**. Enolates are good nucleophiles.
- In the **Michael addition**, an enolate attacks an $\alpha,\beta$-unsaturated carbonyl, creating a bond.
- The **kinetic enolate** is favored by fast, irreversible reactions at lower temperatures with strong, sterically hindered bases. The **thermodynamic enolate** is favored by slower, reversible reactions at higher temperatures with weaker, smaller bases.
- **Enamines** are tautomers of imines. Like enols, enamines are the less common tautomer.

## Aldol Condensation

- In the **aldol condensation**, the aldehyde or ketone acts as both nucleophile and electrophile, resulting in the formation of a carbon–carbon bond in a new molecule called an aldol.
  - An **aldol** contains both aldehyde and alcohol functional groups.
  - The nucleophile is the enolate formed from the deprotonation of the $\alpha$-carbon.
  - The electrophile is the aldehyde or ketone in the form of the keto tautomer.
  - First, a **condensation reaction** occurs in which the two molecules come together.
  - After the aldol is formed, a **dehydration reaction** (loss of a water molecule) occurs. This results in an $\alpha$, $\beta$-unsaturated carbonyl.
- **Retro-aldol reactions** are the reverse of aldol condensations.
  - Retro-aldol reactions are catalyzed by heat and base.
  - In these reactions, the bond between an $\alpha$- and $\beta$-carbon is cleaved.

# ANSWERS TO CONCEPT CHECKS

## 7.1

1. The $\alpha$-hydrogens of aldehydes and ketones are acidic, or deprotonate easily, due to both inductive effects and resonance effects. The electronegative oxygen atom pulls electron density from the C—H bond, weakening it. Once deprotonated, the resonance stabilization of the negative charge between the $\alpha$-carbon, carbonyl carbon, and electron-withdrawing carbonyl oxygen increases the stability of this form.
2. The $\alpha$-hydrogens of aldehydes are slightly more acidic than those of ketones due to the electron-donating characteristics of the second alkyl group in ketones. This extra alkyl group destabilizes the carbanion, which slightly disfavors the loss of the $\alpha$-hydrogens in ketones as compared to aldehydes. Therefore, pentanal is a stronger acid than 3-pentanone and will have a lower p$K_a$.
3. Steric hindrance is one of the two reasons that aldehydes are slightly more reactive than ketones. The additional alkyl group gets in the way and makes for a higher-energy, crowded intermediate.

## 7.2

1. Tautomers are isomers that can be interconverted by the movement of a hydrogen and a double bond.
2. The keto form is thermodynamically favored.
3. Enolate carbanions act as nucleophiles.
4. The product with the double bond to the less substituted $\alpha$-carbon is the kinetically controlled product (the product shown on the right). The thermodynamically controlled product has the double bond formed with the more substituted $\alpha$-carbon (the product on the left). Because the kinetic enolate forms rapidly and can interconvert with the thermodynamic form if given time, the kinetic form is favored by fast, irreversible reactions, such as with a strong, sterically hindered base, and lower temperatures. The thermodynamic form, on the other hand, is favored by slower, reversible reactions, with weaker or smaller bases, and higher temperatures.

## 7.3

1. In the aldol condensation reaction, the enolate carbanion (the deprotonated aldehyde or ketone) acts as the nucleophile and the keto form of the aldehyde or ketone acts as the electrophile.
2. A retro-aldol reaction is the reverse of an aldol reaction where instead a bond between the $\alpha$-and $\beta$-carbons of a carbonyl is broken. This can be favored by the addition of base and heat. In this reaction, a bond between the $\alpha$-and $\beta$-carbons of a carbonyl is broken.
3. An aldol condensation is a condensation reaction, in which two molecules are joined to form a single molecule with the loss of a small molecule; a dehydration reaction, in which a molecule of water is lost; and a nucleophile–electrophile reaction, in which a nucleophile pushes an electron pair to form a bond with an electrophile.

## SCIENCE MASTERY ASSESSMENT EXPLANATIONS

1. **D**

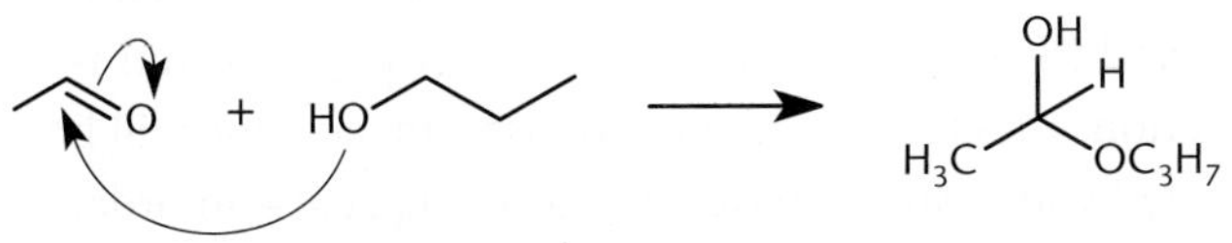


One mole of aldehyde reacts with one mole of alcohol via a nucleophilic addition reaction to form a product called a hemiacetal. In a hemiacetal, an —OH group, an —OR group, a hydrogen atom, and an —R group are attached to the same carbon atom.

2. **B**

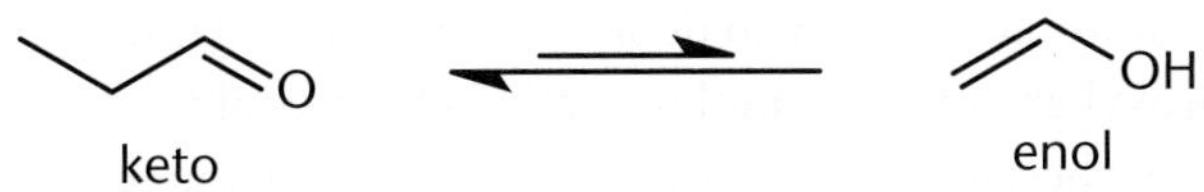


Tautomerization is the interconversion of two isomers in which a hydrogen and a double bond are moved. The keto and enol tautomers of aldehydes and ketones are common examples of tautomers seen on Test Day. Note that the equilibrium lies to the left because the keto form is more stable. Esterification, **(A)**, is the formation of esters from carboxylic acids and alcohols. Elimination, **(C)**, is a reaction in which a part of a reactant is removed and a new multiple bond is introduced. Dehydration, **(D)**, is a reaction in which a molecule of water is eliminated.

3. **D**

The reactions listed in the answer choices are examples of aldol condensations. In the presence of a base, the $\alpha$-hydrogen is abstracted from an aldehyde, forming an enolate ion, $[CH_3CHCHO]^-$. This enolate ion then attacks the carbonyl group of the other aldehyde molecule, $CH_3CH_2CHO$, forming the pictured aldol.

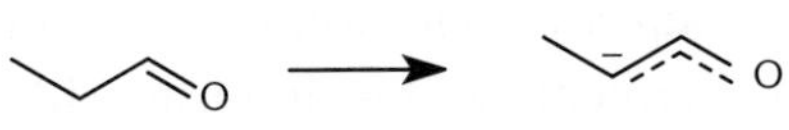


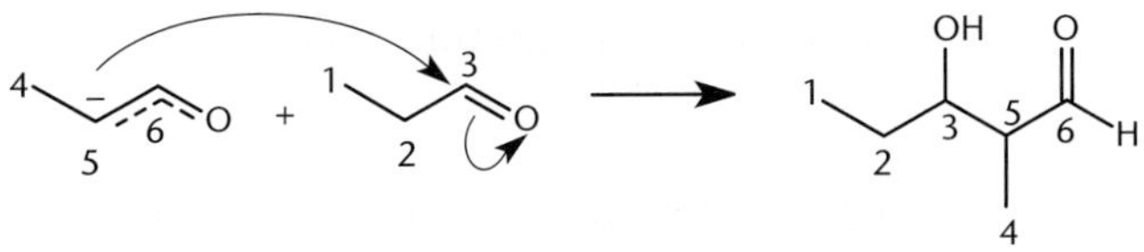


4. **A**

The keto–enol equilibrium lies far to the keto side because the keto form is significantly more thermodynamically stable than the enol form. This thermodynamic stability stems from the fact that the oxygen is more electronegative than the carbon, and the keto tautomer puts more electron density around the oxygen than the enol tautomer. If the enol tautomer is less thermodynamically stable, it is also higher energy than the keto tautomer.

5. **B**

The aldol condensation is both a dehydration reaction because a molecule of water is lost, and a nucleophilic addition reaction because the nucleophilic enolate attacks and bonds to the carbonyl carbon.

6. **B**

This hydrogen is on the carbon between two carbonyls, which means that it is particularly acidic. This is due to both the inductive effects of the two oxygen atoms in the carbonyls and the resonance stabilization of the anion between the carbonyl groups.

7. **B**

At high temperatures and with a weak base like $NH_3$, the thermodynamic enolate will be favored. The reaction proceeds slowly with the weak base, giving the kinetic enolate time to interconvert to the more stable thermodynamic enolate.

8. **A**

Aldehydes are generally more reactive than ketones because the additional alkyl group of a ketone is sterically hindering; this alkyl group is also electron-donating, destabilizing the carbanion intermediate. This eliminates **(B)** and **(D)**. The carbonyl carbon is highly electrophilic; alkanes lack any significant electrophilicity, eliminating **(C)**.

9. **B**

When $\alpha$-carbons are deprotonated, the negative charge is resonance stabilized in part by the electronegative carbonyl oxygen, which is electron-withdrawing. Alkyl groups are actually electron-donating, which destabilizes carbanion intermediates; this invalidates statement II.

10. **C**

All of the answer choices are nitrogen-containing functional groups, but only enamines are tautomers of imines. Imines contain a double bond between a carbon and a nitrogen; enamines contain a double bond between two carbons as well as an amine.

11. **C**

When succinaldehyde (or any aldehyde or ketone with $\alpha$-hydrogens) is treated with a strong base like lithium diisopropylamide (LDA), it forms the more nucleophilic enolate carbanion.

12. **C**

Aldol condensations contain two main steps. In the first step, the $\alpha$-carbon of an aldehyde or ketone is deprotonated, generating the enolate carbanion. This carbanion can then attack another aldehyde or ketone, generating the aldol. In the second step, the aldol is dehydrated, forming a double bond. This double bond is between the $\alpha$- and $\beta$-carbons, so the molecule is an $\alpha,\beta$-unsaturated carbonyl.

13. **D**

Because benzaldehyde lacks an $\alpha$-proton, it cannot be reacted with base to form the nucleophilic enolate carbanion. Therefore, acetone will act as our nucleophile, and both **(A)** and **(B)** can be eliminated. In order to perform this reaction, which is an aldol condensation, acetone will be reacted with a strong base—not a strong acid—in order to extract the $\alpha$-hydrogen and form the enolate anion, which will act as a nucleophile.

14. **B**

This is an example of an aldol condensation, but stopped after aldol formation (before dehydration). After the aldol is formed using strong base, the reaction may be halted by the addition of acid. Butanal in strong acid, described in **(C)**, would be likely to deprotonate without gaining the hydroxyl group. Methanol in diethyl ether would not be reactive because diethyl ether is not a strong enough base to abstract the $\alpha$-hydrogen, eliminating **(A)**. Reaction of the two aldehydes methanal and ethanal in catalytic base would form 3-hydroxypropanal (which would dehydrate to form propenal), not 3-hydroxybutanal.

15. **B**

The nomenclature in this question is well above what one needs to be able to draw on the MCAT; however, we can discern that we are forming a ketone and an aldehyde from a single molecule. The hallmark of a reverse aldol reaction is the breakage of a carbon–carbon bond, forming two aldehydes, two ketones, or one of each. In an aldol condensation, **(A)**, we would expect to form a single product by combining two aldehydes, two ketones, or one of each. A dehydration reaction, **(C)**, should release a water molecule, rather than breaking apart a large organic molecule into two smaller molecules. A nucleophilic attack, **(D)**, should feature the formation of a bond between a nucleophile and an electrophile; again, we would not expect to break apart a large organic molecule into two smaller molecules. Note that simply noting how many reactants and products are present in the reaction is sufficient to determine the answer.

**GO ONLINE**

**Consult your online resources for additional practice.**

## SHARED CONCEPTS

**General Chemistry Chapter 5**
Chemical Kinetics

**Organic Chemistry Chapter 4**
Analyzing Organic Reactions

**Organic Chemistry Chapter 6**
Aldehydes and Ketones I

**Organic Chemistry Chapter 8**
Carboxylic Acids

**Organic Chemistry Chapter 9**
Carboxylic Acid Derivatives

**Organic Chemistry Chapter 10**
Nitrogen- and Phosphorus-Containing Compounds

CHAPTER 8

# CARBOXYLIC ACIDS

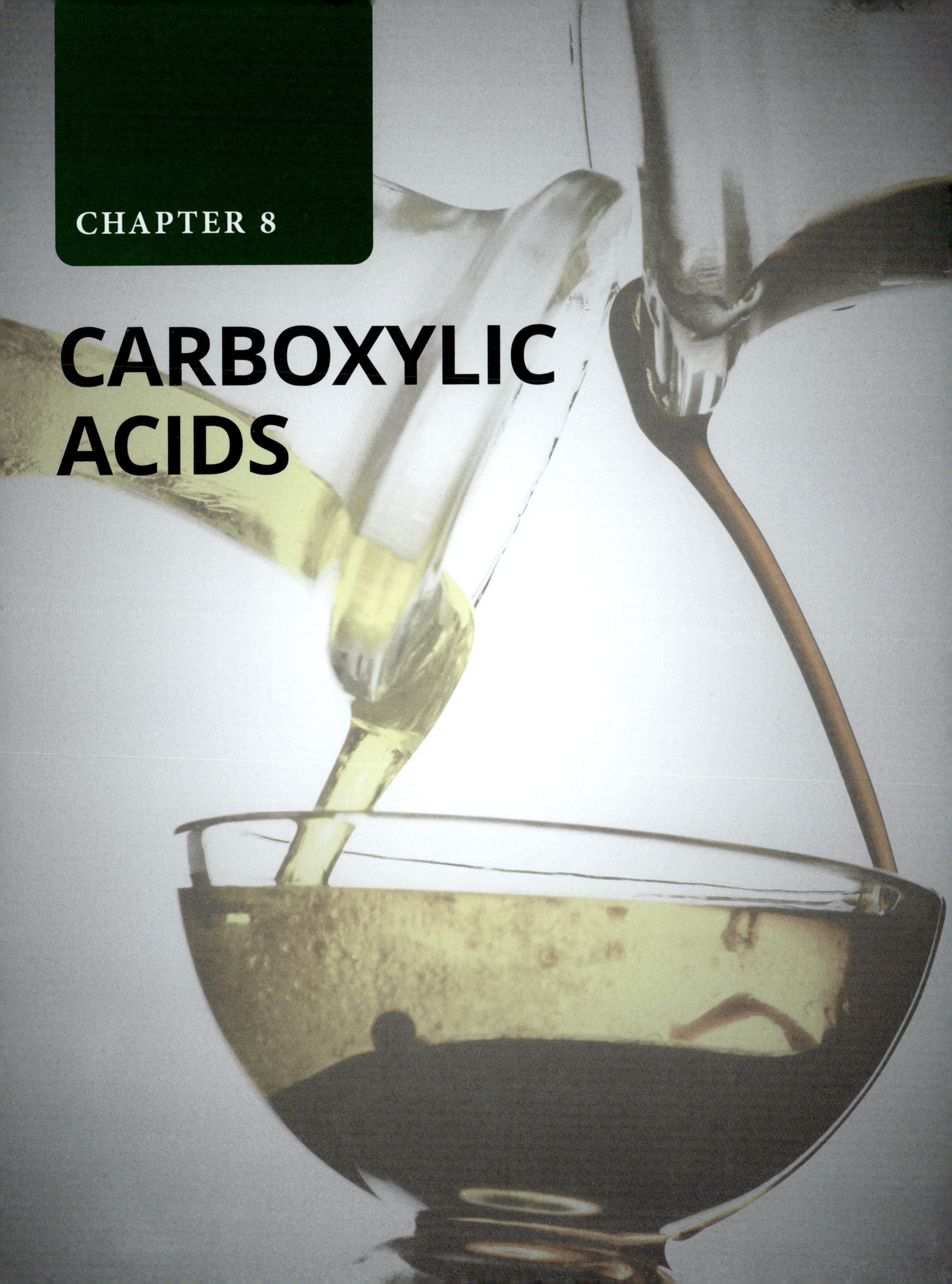

# SCIENCE MASTERY ASSESSMENT

Every pre-med knows this feeling: there is so much content I have to know for the MCAT! How do I know what to do first or what's important?

While the high-yield badges throughout this book will help you identify the most important topics, this Science Mastery Assessment is another tool in your MCAT prep arsenal. This quiz (which can also be taken in your online resources) and the guidance below will help ensure that you are spending the appropriate amount of time on this chapter based on your personal strengths and weaknesses. Don't worry though—skipping something now does not mean you'll never study it. Later on in your prep, as you complete full-length tests, you'll uncover specific pieces of content that you need to review and can come back to these chapters as appropriate.

## How to Use This Assessment

### If you answer 0–7 questions correctly:

Spend about 1 hour to read this chapter in full and take limited notes throughout. Follow up by reviewing **all** quiz questions to ensure that you now understand how to solve each one.

### If you answer 8–11 questions correctly:

Spend 20–40 minutes reviewing the quiz questions. Beginning with the questions you missed, read and take notes on the corresponding subchapters. For questions you answered correctly, ensure your thinking matches that of the explanation and you understand why each choice was correct or incorrect.

### If you answer 12–15 questions correctly:

Spend less than 20 minutes reviewing all questions from the quiz. If you missed any, then include a quick read-through of the corresponding subchapters, or even just the relevant content within a subchapter, as part of your question review. For questions you got correct, ensure your thinking matches that of the explanation and review the Concept Summary at the end of the chapter.

1. Which of these compounds would be expected to decarboxylate when heated?

A. 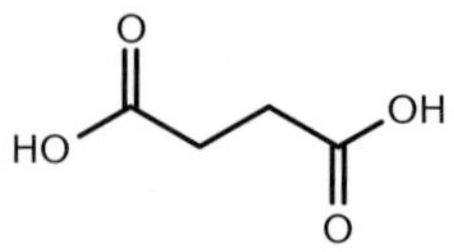

B. 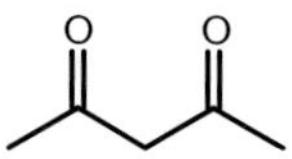

C. 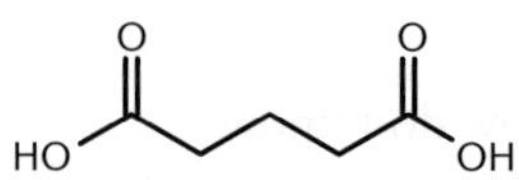

D. 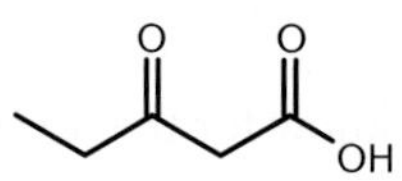

2. Carboxylic acids have higher boiling points than their corresponding alcohols primarily because:
   - **A.** molecular weight is increased by the additional carboxyl group.
   - **B.** the pH of the compound is lower.
   - **C.** acid salts are soluble in water.
   - **D.** hydrogen bonding is much stronger than in alcohols.

3. Which of the following carboxylic acids will be the most acidic?
   - **A.** $CH_3CHClCH_2COOH$
   - **B.** $CH_3CH_2CCl_2COOH$
   - **C.** $CH_3CH_2CHClCOOH$
   - **D.** $CH_3CH_2CH_2COOH$

4. Which of the following molecules could be classified as a soap?
   - **A.** $CH_3(CH_2)_{19}COOH$
   - **B.** $CH_3COOH$
   - **C.** $CH_3(CH_2)_{19}COO^-Na^+$
   - **D.** $CH_3COO^-Na^+$

5. What is the final product of the following reaction?

$$CH_3(CH_2)_4CH_2OH \xrightarrow[\text{acetone}]{CrO_3,\ H_2SO_4}$$

   - **A.** $CH_3(CH_2)_4CHO$
   - **B.** $CH_3(CH_2)_4COOH$
   - **C.** $CH_3(CH_2)_4CH_3$
   - **D.** $HOOC(CH_2)_4COOH$

6. Carboxylic acids can be reacted with one reagent (in addition to acid) to form all of the following compounds EXCEPT:
   - **A.** esters.
   - **B.** amides.
   - **C.** alkenes.
   - **D.** alcohols.

7. The reduction of a carboxylic acid using lithium aluminum hydride will yield what final product?
   - **A.** An aldehyde
   - **B.** An ester
   - **C.** A ketone
   - **D.** An alcohol

8. Which of the following is true with respect to a micelle in a hydrophilic environment?
   - **A.** The interior is hydrophilic.
   - **B.** The structure, as a whole, is hydrophobic.
   - **C.** It is composed of short-chain fatty acids with polar heads.
   - **D.** It can dissolve nonpolar molecules deep in its core.

9. In the presence of an acid catalyst, the major product of butanoic acid and 1-pentanol is:
   - **A.** 1-butoxy-1-pentanol.
   - **B.** butyl pentanoate.
   - **C.** 1-pentoxy-1-butanol.
   - **D.** pentyl butanoate.

10. The $\alpha$-hydrogen of a carboxylic acid is:
    - **I.** more acidic than the hydroxyl hydrogen.
    - **II.** less acidic than the hydroxyl hydrogen.
    - **III.** relatively acidic, as organic compounds go.
    - **A.** I only
    - **B.** II only
    - **C.** I and III only
    - **D.** II and III only

11. The reaction of formic acid with sodium borohydride will yield what final product?
    - **A.** An aldehyde
    - **B.** A carboxylic acid
    - **C.** A ketone
    - **D.** An alcohol

12. The intramolecular reaction of 5-aminopentanoic acid through nucleophilic acyl substitution would result in a(n):
    - **A.** anhydride.
    - **B.** lactone.
    - **C.** lactam.
    - **D.** carboxylic acid.

13. Butanoic anhydride can be produced by the reaction of butanoic acid with which of the following compounds?
    - **A.** Butanoic acid
    - **B.** Ethanoic acid
    - **C.** Butanol
    - **D.** Methanal

14. Nucleophilic acyl substitution is favored by:
    - **I.** basic solution.
    - **II.** acidic solution.
    - **III.** leaving groups that are strong bases.
    - **A.** I only
    - **B.** II only
    - **C.** I and II only
    - **D.** I, II, and III

15. The reaction of ammonia with caprylic acid, found in coconuts, would produce a(n):
    - **A.** ester.
    - **B.** anhydride.
    - **C.** alcohol.
    - **D.** water molecule.

## Answer Key

1. **D** (See section 8.2)
2. **D** (See section 8.1)
3. **B** (See section 8.1)
4. **C** (See section 8.1)
5. **B** (See section 8.2)
6. **C** (See section 8.2)
7. **D** (See section 8.2)
8. **D** (See section 8.1)
9. **D** (See section 8.2)
10. **D** (See section 8.1)
11. **B** (See section 8.2)
12. **C** (See section 8.2)
13. **A** (See section 8.2)
14. **C** (See section 8.2)
15. **D** (See section 8.2)

*The relevant section of the chapter to review for each question is given in parentheses after the correct answer. Detailed explanations can be found at the end of the chapter.*

CHAPTER 8

# CARBOXYLIC ACIDS

## In This Chapter



**CHAPTER PROFILE**

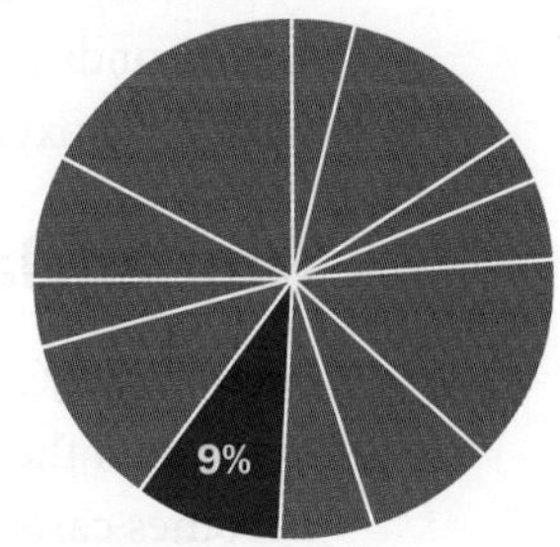


The content in this chapter should be relevant to about 9% of all questions about organic chemistry on the MCAT.

This chapter covers material from the following AAMC content category:

**5D:** Structure, function, and reactivity of biologically-relevant molecules

## Introduction

Carboxylic acids, with both carbonyl and hydroxyl groups, are some of the most reactive organic molecules you'll encounter on Test Day. As we will see in this chapter, these molecules can react as acids (as their name suggests), nucleophiles, and electrophiles and are integral to many biological processes. Carboxylic acids are found in soaps, oils, preservatives, skin care products, clothing, and—most importantly for the MCAT—amino acids. Carboxylic acids often have strong, unpleasant odors. For example, acetic acid (ethanoic acid) is the main ingredient in vinegar; propionic acid (propanoic acid) gives Swiss cheese its smell; butyric acid (butanoic acid) is found in rancid butter and body odor.

So what makes carboxylic acids so interesting and versatile? First, they're acids, so they like to give away protons—particularly because when they do so, the remaining negative charge resonates between two oxygen atoms, making the anion very stable. This makes carboxylic acids some of the most acidic compounds encountered in organic chemistry, with p$K_a$ values between 3 and 6. Compare this with alcohols, which have an average p$K_a$ around 17. Carboxylic acids are also excellent at hydrogen bonding, which results in large intermolecular forces and high boiling points. Finally, carboxylic acids are ubiquitous in nature and are synthesized by all living organisms.

## 8.1 Description and Properties

### LEARNING OBJECTIVES

After Chapter 8.1, you will be able to:

- Explain the underlying cause of the relatively high acidity of carboxylic acids
- Predict the effects of additional substituents on the acidity of a carboxylic acid
- Rank the acidity of comparable carboxylic acids based on their structure

A **carboxylic acid** contains both a carbonyl group and a hydroxyl group, bonded to the same carbon. With three bonds to oxygen atoms, this is one of the most oxidized functional groups encountered in organic chemistry. Carboxylic acids are always terminal groups.

### Nomenclature

In the IUPAC system of nomenclature, carboxylic acids are named by adding the suffix **–oic acid** to the parent root when the carboxylic acid is the highest-priority functional group. When this is true, the carbonyl carbon becomes carbon number 1. Figure 8.1 shows two examples.

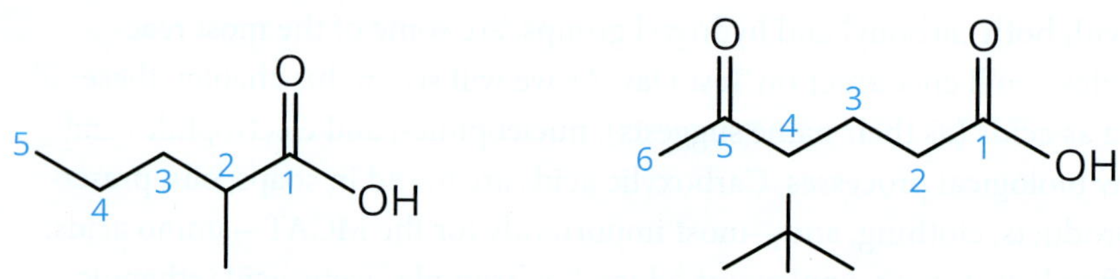

2-methylpentanoic acid

4-isopropyl-5-oxohexanoic acid

**Figure 8.1** IUPAC Names of Carboxylic Acids

Like the other functional groups, many carboxylic acids are also named by their common names. Make note of the common prefixes used in the examples in Figure 8.2.

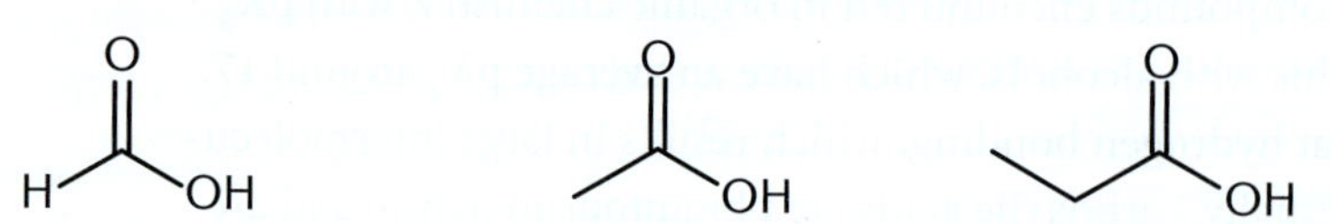

methanoic acid
(formic acid)

ethanoic acid
(acetic acid)

propanoic acid
(propionic acid)

**Figure 8.2** IUPAC and Common Names of Carboxylic Acids
*Common names are in parentheses.*

#### MCAT EXPERTISE

The same common-name prefixes are used for both aldehydes and carboxylic acids: form– for one carbon, acet– for two, and propion– for three.

Cyclic carboxylic acids are named by listing the cycloalkane with the suffix **carboxylic acid**. Salts of carboxylic acids are named beginning with the cation, followed by the name of the acid with the ending **–oate** replacing **–oic acid**. Typical examples are shown in Figure 8.3.

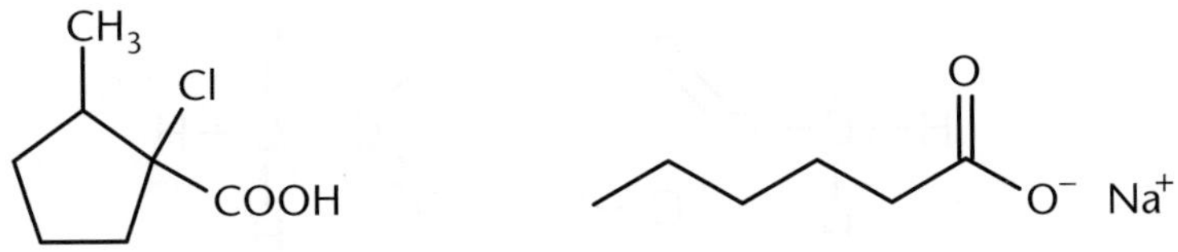


1-chloro-2-methylcyclo-pentane carboxylic acid

sodium hexanoate

**Figure 8.3** Cyclic Carboxylic Acid and Carboxylic Acid Salt

Finally, **dicarboxylic acids**, which have a carboxylic acid group on each end of the molecule, are common in biological systems. The smallest dicarboxylic acid is *oxalic acid*, with two carbons. The next five straight-chain dicarboxylic acids are *malonic*, *succinic*, *glutaric*, *adipic*, and *pimelic* acids. Their IUPAC names have the suffix **–dioic acid**: ethanedioic acid, propanedioic acid, butanedioic acid, pentanedioic acid, hexanedioic acid, and heptanedioic acid. Figure 8.4 shows several examples.

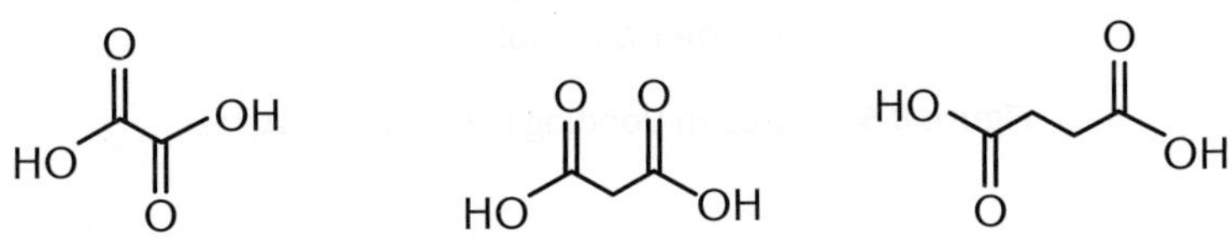


ethanedioic acid (oxalic acid)

propanedioic acid (malonic acid)

butanedioic acid (succinic acid)

**Figure 8.4** IUPAC and Common Names of Dicarboxylic Acids

## Physical Properties

Many of the physical properties of carboxylic acids are similar to those of aldehydes and ketones because they both contain carbonyl groups. However, the additional hydroxyl group permits carboxylic acids to hydrogen bond and provides another acidic hydrogen that can participate in reactions.

### Hydrogen Bonding

Carboxylic acids are polar because they contain a carbonyl group and can also form hydrogen bonds because they contain a hydrogen bonded to a very electronegative atom (in this case, the hydroxyl oxygen). Carboxylic acids display particularly strong intermolecular attractions because both the hydroxyl oxygen and carbonyl oxygen can participate in hydrogen bonding. As a result, carboxylic acids tend to form **dimers**: pairs of molecules connected by two hydrogen bonds. An example of a carboxylic acid that forms dimers is oxalic acid, seen in Figure 8.5. Multiple hydrogen bonds elevate the boiling and melting points of carboxylic acids past those of corresponding alcohols. Boiling points also increase with increasing molecular weight.

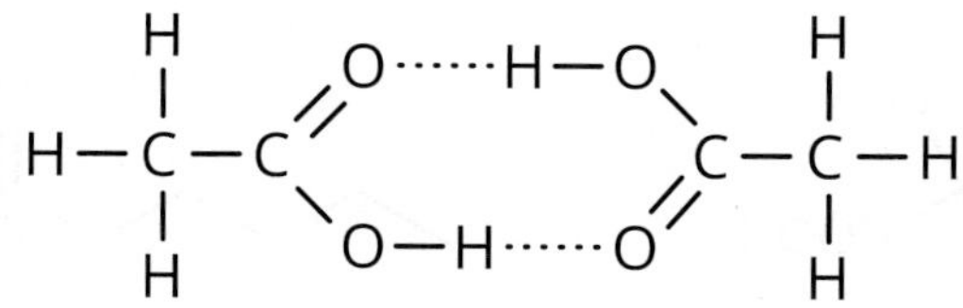

**Acetic acid**
Boiling point 118 °C

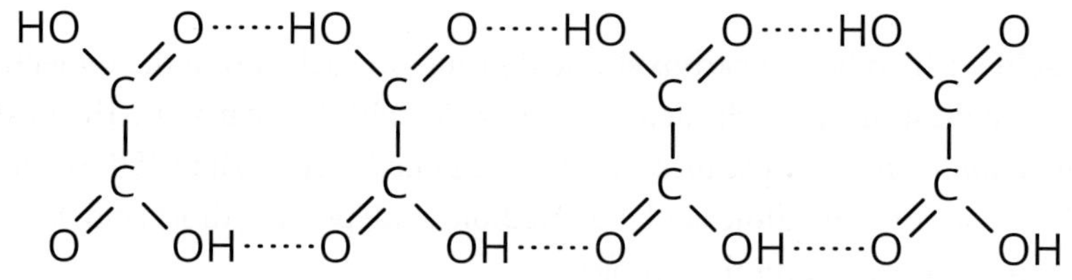

**Oxalic acid**
Boiling point 365 °C

**Figure 8.5** Hydrogen Bonding in Carboxylic Acids

### Acidity

The hydroxyl hydrogen of a carboxylic acid is quite acidic. This results in a negative charge that remains after the hydrogen is removed and resonance stabilization occurs between both of the electronegative oxygen atoms. Delocalization of the negative charge results in a very stable carboxylate anion, which is demonstrated in Figure 8.6.

**KEY CONCEPT**

Carboxylic acids are polar and can form hydrogen bonds. Their acidity is due to resonance stabilization and can be enhanced by the addition of electronegative groups or a greater ability to delocalize charge.

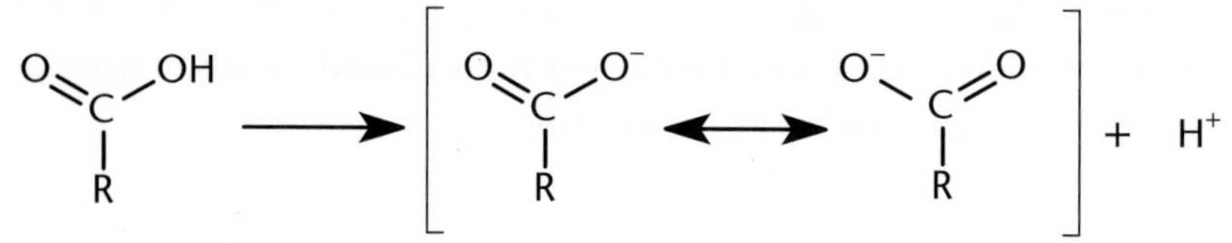

**Figure 8.6** Carboxylate Anion Stability
*The negative charge from deprotonation is stabilized through resonance.*

The more stable the conjugate base is, the easier it is for the proton to leave, and thus, the stronger the acid. Carboxylic acids are relatively acidic, with p$K_a$ values on the order of 4.8 for ethanoic acid and 4.9 for propanoic acid. However, keep in mind that although these are quite acidic for organic compounds, they do not compare to strong acids like HCl (p$K_a$ = −8.0) or even $HSO_4^-$ (p$K_a$ = 1.99). Remember, lower p$K_a$ values indicate stronger acids.

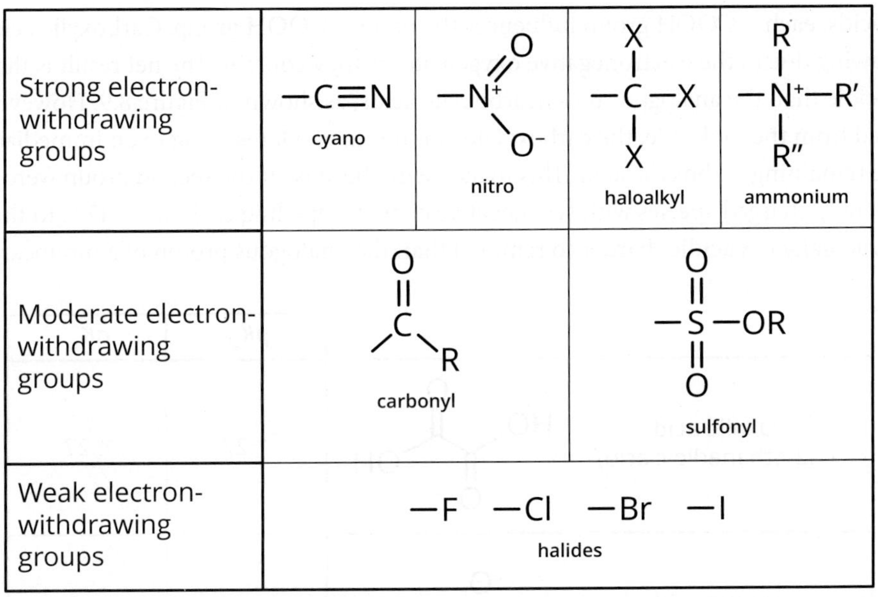


**Figure 8.7** Electron-Withdrawing Groups

Substituents on carbon atoms near a carboxyl group influence anion stability and therefore affect acidity. Groups like $-NO_2$ or halides are electron-withdrawing (Figure 8.7) and increase acidity. In contrast, $-NH_2$ or $-OCH_3$ are electron-donating groups (Figure 8.8) that destabilize the negative charge, decreasing the acidity of the compound. The closer the substituent groups are to the carboxyl group, the greater the effect will be.

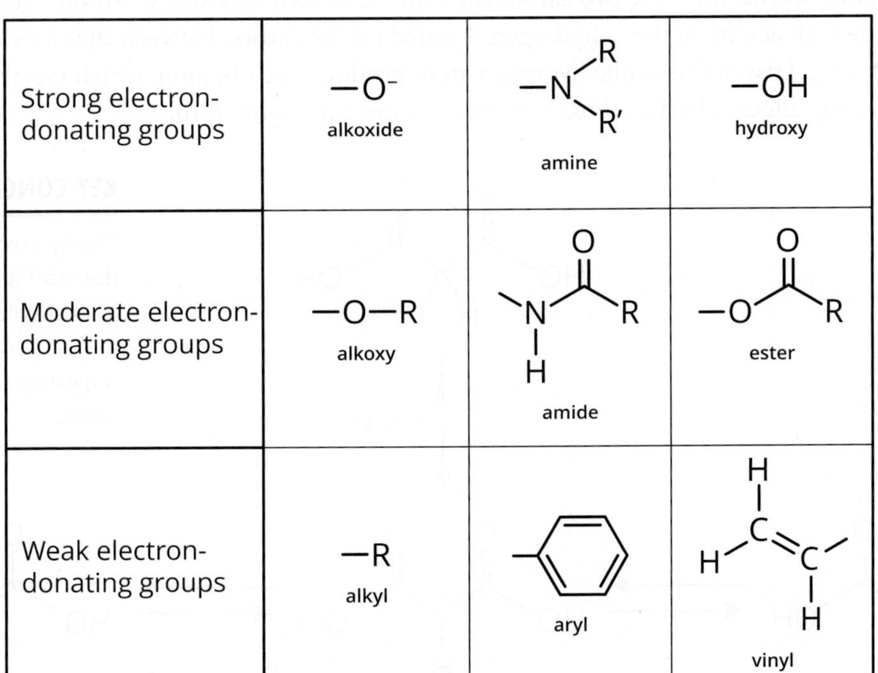


**Figure 8.8** Electron-Donating Groups

In dicarboxylic acids, each $-COOH$ group influences the other $-COOH$ group. Carboxylic acids are electron-withdrawing due to the electronegative oxygen atoms they contain. The net result is that dicarboxylic acids are more acidic than the analogous monocarboxylic acids, as shown in Figure 8.9. However, when one proton is removed from the molecule, the carboxylate anion is formed, resulting in an immediate decrease in the acidity of the remaining carboxylic acid. This makes sense because if the second group were deprotonated, it would create a doubly charged species with two negative charges repelling each other. Due to this instability, the second proton is actually *less* acidic (harder to remove) than the analogous proton of a monocarboxylic acid.

| | | $pK_{a1}$ | $pK_{a2}$ |
|---|---|---|---|
| **Oxalic acid** (1,2-ethanedioic acid) | 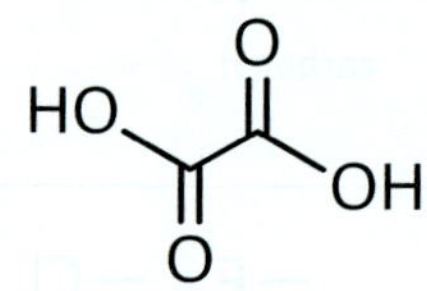 | 1.27 | 4.27 |
| **Acetic acid** (ethanoic acid) | 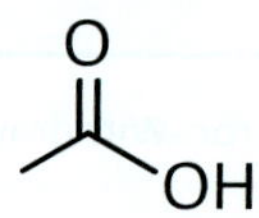 | 4.7 | |

**Figure 8.9** Acidity Comparison: Monocarboxylic vs. Dicarboxylic Acids

**$\beta$-dicarboxylic acids** are dicarboxylic acids in which each carboxylic acid is positioned on the $\beta$-carbon of the other; in other words, there are two carboxylic acids separated by a single carbon. These compounds are notable for the high acidity of the $\alpha$-hydrogens located on the carbon between the two carboxyl groups ($pK_a \approx 9-14$). Loss of this acidic hydrogen atom produces a carbanion, which is stabilized by the electron-withdrawing effect of both carboxyl groups, as shown in Figure 8.10.

**KEY CONCEPT**

The hydroxyl hydrogen is the most acidic proton on a carboxylic acid. However, in 1,3-dicarbonyls, the $\alpha$-hydrogen is also quite acidic.

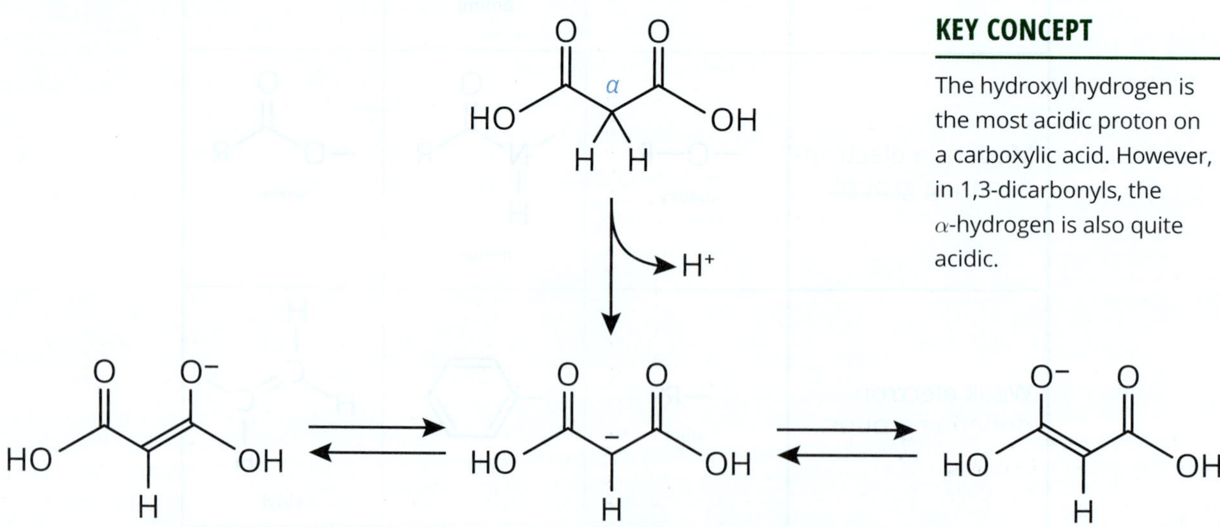

**Figure 8.10** Acidity of the $\alpha$-Hydrogen in $\beta$-Dicarboxylic Acids
*Note that the $\alpha$-hydrogen is less acidic than the hydroxyl hydrogens; the hydroxyl groups are left protonated in this example for demonstration purposes only.*

Note that this also applies to the $\alpha$-hydrogens in a $\beta$-diketone, $\beta$-ketoacids, $\beta$-dialdehydes, and other molecules that share the 1,3-dicarbonyl structure shown in Figure 8.11.

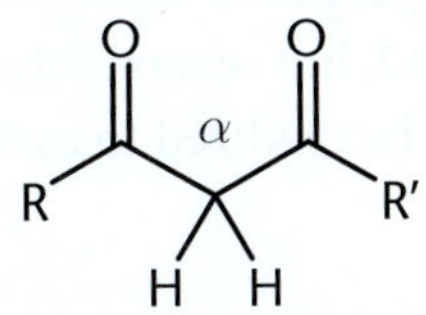


**Figure 8.11** General Structure of 1,3-Dicarbonyl Compounds

### MCAT CONCEPT CHECK 8.1

Before you move on, assess your understanding of the material with these questions.

1. What causes the relatively high acidity of carboxylic acids?

   ______________________________

2. Among a monocarboxylic acid, a dicarboxylic acid, and a dicarboxylic acid that has been deprotonated once, which will be the most acidic? Why?

   ______________________________

3. What effects do additional substituents have on the acidity of carboxylic acids?

   ______________________________

## 8.2 Reactions of Carboxylic Acids

High Yield

### LEARNING OBJECTIVES

After Chapter 8.2, you will be able to:

- Recall the reactant types used in acyl substitution reactions to form the major carboxylic acid derivatives, such as amides and esters
- Describe the mechanism of nucleophilic acyl substitution reactions
- Identify the conditions that would lead to spontaneous decarboxylation of a carboxylic acid
- Predict the products of an acyl substitution reaction:

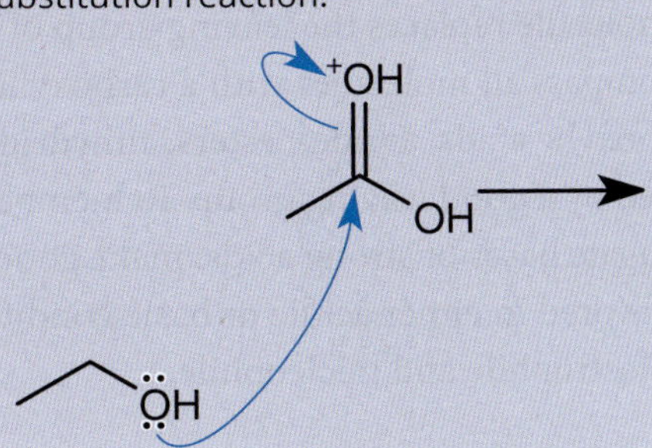


The properties of carboxylic acids make them highly reactive in a number of different categories. Several of the most important reactions are described here.

## Synthesis of Carboxylic Acids

As described in earlier chapters, carboxylic acids can be prepared via oxidation of aldehydes and primary alcohols. The oxidant is often a dichromate salt ($Na_2Cr_2O_7$ or $K_2Cr_2O_7$), chromium trioxide ($CrO_3$), or potassium permanganate ($KMnO_4$), as shown in Figure 8.12, but several other oxidizing agents can also work. Remember that secondary and tertiary alcohols cannot be oxidized to carboxylic acids because they already have at least two bonds to other carbons.

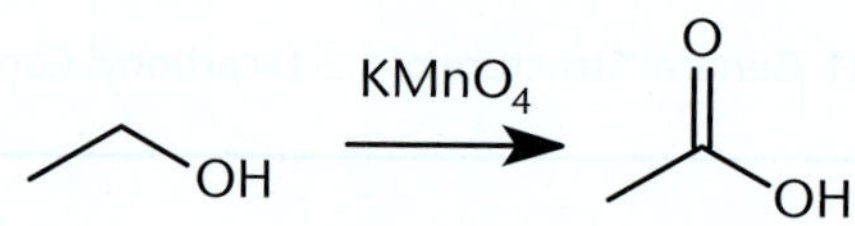


**Figure 8.12** Synthesis of a Carboxylic Acid via Oxidation of a Primary Alcohol

There are many other methods of generating carboxylic acids, including hydrolysis of nitriles (–C≡N), but these are outside the scope of the MCAT.

## Nucleophilic Acyl Substitution

Many of the reactions in which carboxylic acids (and their derivatives) participate proceed via a single mechanism: nucleophilic acyl substitution. This mechanism is similar to nucleophilic addition to an aldehyde or ketone, which was discussed in Chapters 6 and 7 of *MCAT Organic Chemistry Review*. The key difference, however, focuses on the existence of a leaving group in carboxylic acids and their derivatives. In this case, after opening the carbonyl via nucleophilic attack and forming a tetrahedral intermediate, the carbonyl can reform, thereby kicking off the leaving group. This reaction is shown in Figure 8.13.

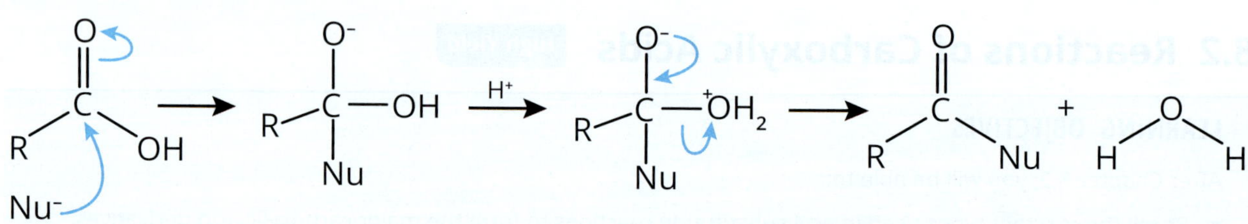


**Figure 8.13** Nucleophilic Acyl Substitution
*Step 1: Nucleophilic addition; Step 2: Elimination of the leaving group and reformation of the carbonyl.*

In these reactions, the nucleophilic molecule replaces the leaving group of an acyl derivative. **Acyl derivatives** encompass all molecules with a carboxylic acid-derived carbonyl, including carboxylic acids, amides, esters, anhydrides, and others. These reactions are favored by a good leaving group. Remember, weak bases, which are often the conjugate bases of strong acids, make good leaving groups. These reactions are also favored in either acidic or basic conditions, which can alter the reactivity of the electrophile and nucleophile.

**MCAT EXPERTISE**

While you may have learned about other acyl derivatives in your organic chemistry classes, such as acyl halides and nitriles, the official content list for the MCAT restricts its focus to carboxylic acids, amides, esters, and anhydrides.

## Amides

Carboxylic acids can be converted into amides if the incoming nucleophile is ammonia ($NH_3$) or an amine, as shown in Figure 8.14. This can be carried out in either an acidic or basic solution to drive the reaction forward.

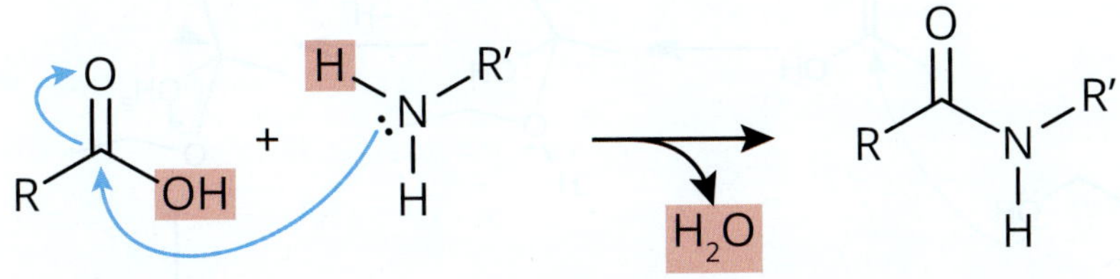


**Figure 8.14** Formation of an Amide by Nucleophilic Acyl Substitution

Amides are named by replacing the –**oic acid** suffix with –**amide** in the name of the parent carboxylic acid. Any alkyl groups on the nitrogen are placed at the beginning of the name with the prefix ***N***–. Amides exist in a resonance state where delocalization of electrons occurs between the oxygen and nitrogen atoms, as shown in Figure 8.15.

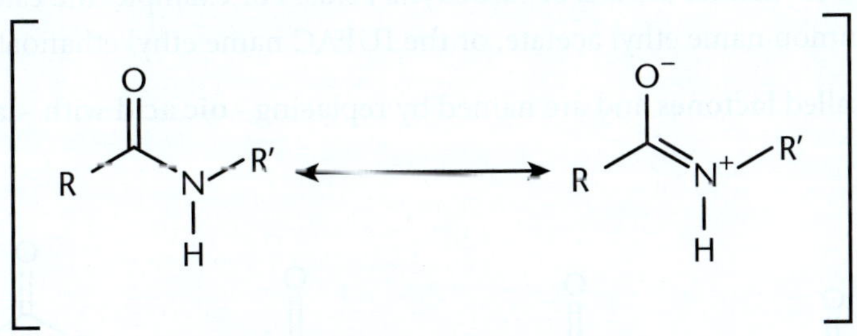


**Figure 8.15** Resonance of Amides
*Resonance between the carbonyl and lone pair on the nitrogen stabilizes this bond and restricts its motion.*

Amides that are cyclic are called **lactams** and are named by replacing –**oic acid** with –**lactam**. They may also be named by indicating the specific carbon that is bonded during cyclization of the compound. Several examples are shown in Figure 8.16.

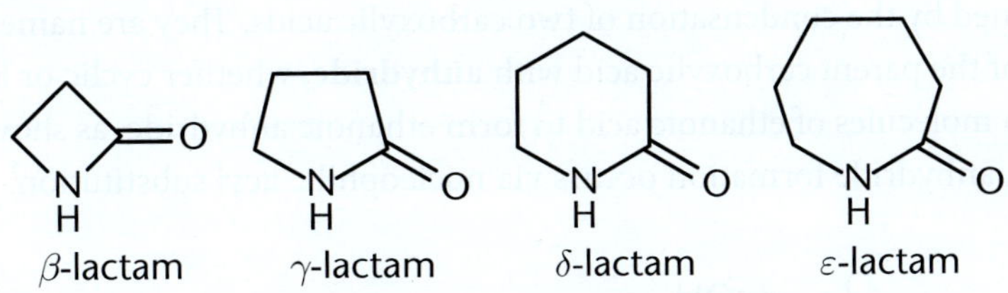


**Figure 8.16** Examples of Lactams

## Esters

**Esters** are a hybrid between a carboxylic acid and an ether (ROR′), which can be made by reacting carboxylic acids with alcohols under acidic conditions, as shown in Figure 8.17. **Esterification** is a **condensation** reaction with water as a side product. In acidic solutions, the carbonyl oxygen can be protonated,

### KEY CONCEPT

Protonating the C=O makes the electrophilic carbon even more ripe for nucleophilic attack.

which enhances the polarity of the bond, thereby placing additional positive charge on the carbonyl carbon and increasing its susceptibility to nucleophilic attack. This condensation reaction occurs most rapidly with primary alcohols.

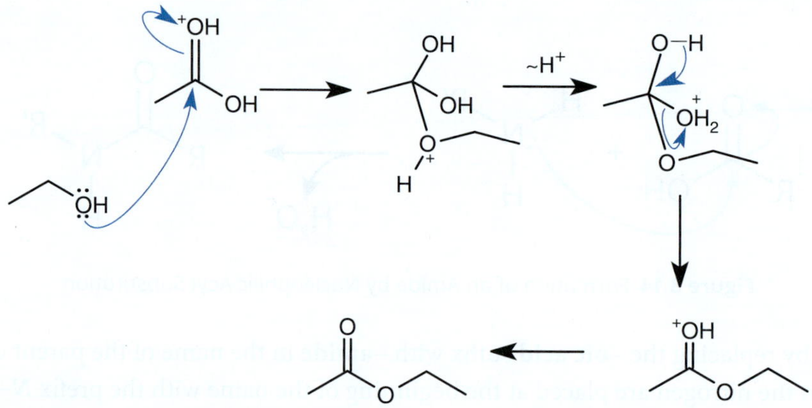


**Figure 8.17** Esterification: Reaction of a Carboxylic Acid with an Alcohol

Esters are named in the same manner as salts of carboxylic acids. For example, the ester shown in the reaction in Figure 8.17 has the common name ethyl acetate, or the IUPAC name ethyl ethanoate.

Esters that are cyclic are called **lactones** and are named by replacing –**oic acid** with –**lactone**. Several examples are shown in Figure 8.18.

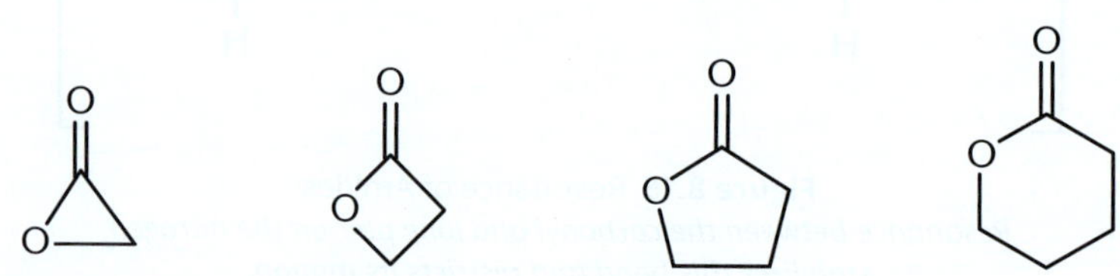

α-acetolactone β-propiolactone γ-butyrolactone δ-valerolactone

**Figure 8.18** Examples of Lactones

## Anhydrides

**Anhydrides** can be formed by the condensation of two carboxylic acids. They are named by replacing the **acid** at the end of the name of the parent carboxylic acid with **anhydride**, whether cyclic or linear. One example is the condensation of two molecules of ethanoic acid to form ethanoic anhydride, as shown in Figure 8.19. Just like the above reactions, anhydride formation occurs via nucleophilic acyl substitution.

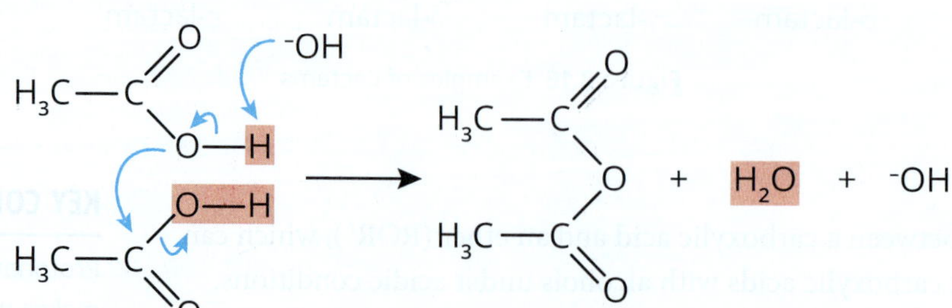


Ethanoic anhydride

**Figure 8.19** Synthesis of an Anhydride via Carboxylic Acid Condensation

## Reduction

Carboxylic acids can be reduced to primary alcohols by the use of lithium aluminum hydride ($LiAlH_4$). Aldehyde intermediates may be formed in the course of this reaction, but they, too, will be reduced to the alcohol. The reaction occurs by nucleophilic addition of hydride to the carbonyl group. The reaction mechanism is shown in Figure 8.20.

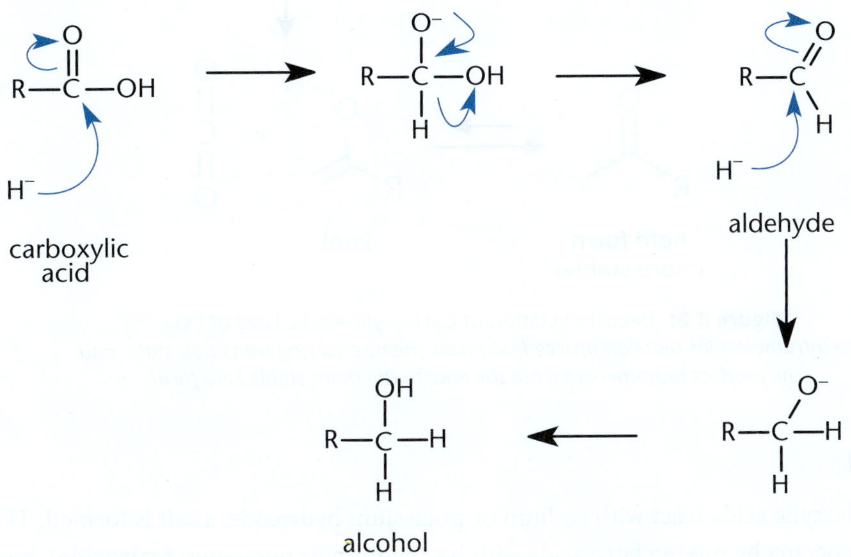


**Figure 8.20** Reduction of a Carboxylic Acid to a Primary Alcohol
*Reaction occurs by nucleophilic addition of hydride and proceeds through an aldehyde intermediate.*

**BRIDGE**

See Chapter 4 of *MCAT Organic Chemistry Review* for more information on redox reagents.

Lithium aluminum hydride is a strong reducing agent that can successfully reduce a carboxylic acid; a gentler reducing agent like sodium borohydride ($NaBH_4$) is not strong enough to reduce carboxylic acids.

**KEY CONCEPT**

Carboxylic acids can be reduced by $LiAlH_4$, but not the less reactive $NaBH_4$.

## Decarboxylation

Decarboxylation describes the complete loss of the carboxyl group as carbon dioxide. This is a common way of getting rid of a carbon from the parent chain. 1,3-Dicarboxylic acids and other *β*-keto acids may spontaneously decarboxylate when heated. Under these conditions, the carboxyl group is lost and replaced with hydrogen. Because both the electrophile and nucleophile are in the same molecule, the reaction proceeds through a six-membered ring in its transition state, as shown in Figure 8.21. The enol that is initially formed from the destruction of the ring tautomerizes to the more stable keto form.

**BRIDGE**

Decarboxylation is common in biochemical pathways in the body. *Pyruvate dehydrogenase complex*, described in Chapter 10 of *MCAT Biochemistry Review*, carries out the decarboxylation of pyruvate to help form acetyl-CoA, which can feed into the citric acid cycle.

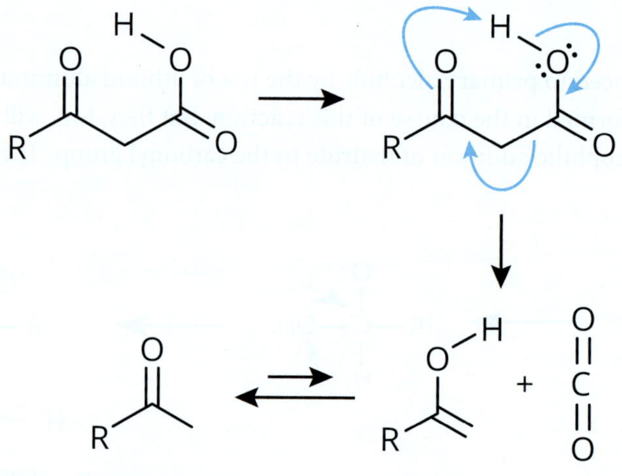


**Figure 8.21** Decarboxylation of Carboxylic Acids: Loss of $CO_2$
*The intramolecular reaction proceeds via a six-membered ring transition state, and the product tautomerizes from the enol to the more stable keto form.*

## Saponification

When long-chain carboxylic acids react with sodium or potassium hydroxide, a salt is formed. This process, called **saponification**, occurs by mixing fatty acids with lye (sodium or potassium hydroxide), resulting in the formation of a salt that we know as **soap**. Soaps can solvate nonpolar organic compounds in aqueous solutions because they contain both a nonpolar tail and a polar carboxylate head, as shown in Figure 8.22.

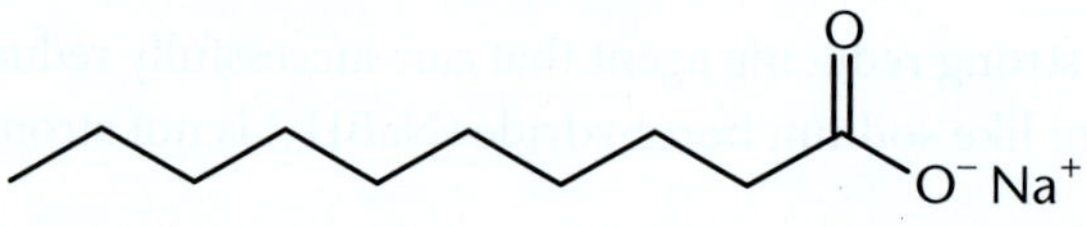


**Figure 8.22** Carboxylic Acid Salt (Soap)

When placed in aqueous solution, soap molecules arrange themselves into spherical structures called **micelles**, as shown in Figure 8.23. The polar heads face outward, where they can be solvated by water, and the nonpolar hydrocarbon chains are oriented toward the inside of the sphere, protected from the solvent. Nonpolar molecules, such as grease, dissolve in the hydrocarbon interior of the spherical micelle; the micelle as a whole then dissolves in water due to the polarity of its exterior surface.

**BRIDGE**

The formation of the phospholipid bilayer, micelles, and liposomes are all contingent on the bipolar nature of carboxylic acids with long hydrocarbon chains. These structures are discussed in Chapter 5 of *MCAT Biochemistry Review*.

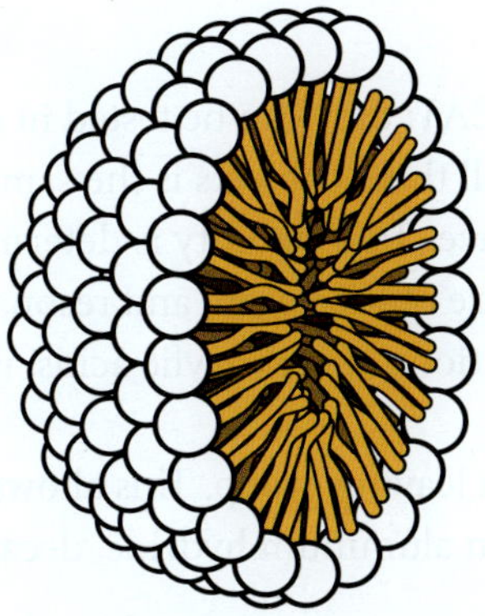

**Figure 8.23** Soap Micelle
*The polar heads interact with the hydrophilic environment; the nonpolar tails are oriented toward the interior of the micelle.*

## MCAT CONCEPT CHECK 8.2

Before you move on, assess your understanding of the material with these questions.

1. For each of the derivatives below, list the nucleophile used to form the derivative in an acyl substitution reaction and the name of the cyclic form of that functional group.

| Carboxylic Acid Derivative | Formed by Reaction with: | Name of Cyclic Form: |
|---|---|---|
| Amide | | |
| Ester | | |
| Anhydride | | |

2. Briefly describe the mechanism of nucleophilic acyl substitution reactions.

______________________________

3. What is the result when butanoic acid is reacted with sodium borohydride? With lithium aluminum hydride?

   - Sodium borohydride:

   ______________________________

   - Lithium aluminum hydride:

   ______________________________

4. Under what conditions will a carboxylic acid spontaneously decarboxylate?

______________________________

## Conclusion

Acids are an important concept on the MCAT: they can be tested in general chemistry, organic chemistry, and biochemistry. The underlying concept in all three subjects is the same: the more stable the conjugate base is, the more likely it is that the proton will leave. This stability is determined by three factors: periodic trends (electronegativity and, thus, induction), size of the anion, and resonance. Understanding these effects is a major key to success on Test Day. The reactions of carboxylic acids, in particular, are dictated by the polarity of the carbonyl group in conjunction with
the ability of the hydroxyl group to act as a leaving group. This allows a diversity of reactions through nucleophilic acyl substitution, reduction by lithium aluminum hydride, decarboxylation, and saponification.

**GO ONLINE**

**You've reviewed the content, now test your knowledge and critical thinking skills by completing a test-like passage set in your online resources!**

# CONCEPT SUMMARY

## Description and Properties

- **Carboxylic acids** contain a carbonyl and a hydroxyl group connected to the same carbon. They are always terminal groups.
- Carboxylic acids are indicated with the suffix –**oic acid**. Salts are named with the suffix –**oate**, and **dicarboxylic acids** are –**dioic acids**.
- Physical Properties
  - Carboxylic acids are polar and hydrogen bond very well, resulting in high boiling points. They often exist as **dimers** in solution.
  - The acidity of a carboxylic acid is enhanced by the resonance between its oxygen atoms.
  - Acidity can be further enhanced by substituents that are electron-withdrawing, and decreased by substituents that are electron-donating.
  - **$\beta$-dicarboxylic acids**, like other 1,3-dicarbonyl compounds, have an $\alpha$-hydrogen that is also highly acidic.

## Reactions of Carboxylic Acids

- Carboxylic acids can be made by the oxidation of primary alcohols or aldehydes using an oxidizing agent like potassium permanganate ($KMnO_4$), dichromate salts ($Na_2Cr_2O_7$ or $K_2Cr_2O_7$), or chromium trioxide ($CrO_3$).
- **Nucleophilic acyl substitution** is a common reaction in carboxylic acids.
  - A nucleophile attacks the electrophilic carbonyl carbon, opening the carbonyl and forming a tetrahedral intermediate.
  - The carbonyl reforms, kicking off the leaving group.
  - If the nucleophile is ammonia or an amine, an **amide** is formed. Amides are given the suffix –**amide**. Cyclic amides are called **lactams**.
  - If the nucleophile is an alcohol, an **ester** is formed. Esters are given the suffix –**oate**. Cyclic esters are called **lactones**.
  - If the nucleophile is another carboxylic acid, an **anhydride** is formed. Both linear and cyclic anhydrides are given the suffix **anhydride**.
- Carboxylic acids can be reduced to a primary alcohol with a strong reducing agent like lithium aluminum hydride ($LiAlH_4$).
  - Aldehyde intermediates are formed, but are also reduced to primary alcohols.
  - Sodium borohydride ($NaBH_4$) is a common reducing agent for other organic reactions, but is not strong enough to reduce a carboxylic acid.

- $\beta$-dicarboxylic acids and other $\beta$-keto acids can undergo spontaneous **decarboxylation** when heated, losing a carbon as carbon dioxide. This reaction proceeds via a six-membered cyclic intermediate.
- Mixing long-chain carboxylic acids (fatty acids) with a strong base results in the formation of a salt we call **soap**. This process is called **saponification**.
  - Soaps contain hydrophilic carboxylate heads and hydrophobic alkyl chain tails.
  - Soaps organize in hydrophilic environments to form **micelles**. A micelle dissolves nonpolar organic molecules in its interior, and can be solvated with water due to its exterior shell of hydrophilic groups.

## ANSWERS TO CONCEPT CHECKS

### 8.1

1. Carboxylic acids are particularly acidic due to the electron-withdrawing oxygen atoms in the functional group and the high stability of the carboxylate anion, which is resonance stabilized by delocalization with two electronegative oxygen atoms.
2. A dicarboxylic acid would be the most acidic, as the second carboxyl group is electron-withdrawing and therefore contributes to even higher stability of the anion after loss of the first hydrogen. However, a monocarboxylic acid is more acidic than a deprotonated dicarboxylic acid because the carboxylate anion is electron-donating and destabilizes the product of the second deprotonation step, resulting in decreased acidity.
3. Electron-withdrawing substituents make the anion more stable and therefore increase acidity. Electron-donating substituents, on the other hand, destabilize the anion, causing the carboxylic acid to be less acidic. The closer the substituent is to the carboxylic acid on the molecule, the stronger the effect will be.

### 8.2

1.

| Carboxylic Acid Derivative | Formed by Reaction with: | Name of Cyclic Form: |
|---|---|---|
| **Amide** | Ammonia ($NH_3$) or an amine | Lactam |
| **Ester** | Alcohol | Lactone |
| **Anhydride** | Another carboxylic acid | Anhydride |

2. Nucleophilic acyl substitution is the substitution of an attacking nucleophile for the leaving group of an acyl compound, which includes carboxylic acids, amides, esters, and anhydrides. The nucleophile attacks, opening the carbonyl and forming a tetrahedral intermediate. The carbonyl then reforms, kicking off the leaving group. This reaction is favored by acidic or basic conditions.
3. Sodium borohydride is not strong enough to reduce carboxylic acids so there will be no reaction. Lithium aluminum hydride, however, is strong enough to reduce carboxylic acids to primary alcohols—producing 1-butanol.
4. 1,3-Dicarboxylic acids will spontaneously decarboxylate when heated, due to the stable cyclic intermediate step.

# SCIENCE MASTERY ASSESSMENT EXPLANATIONS

1. **D**

This compound is a $\beta$-keto acid: a carbonyl functional group at the $\beta$-position from a carboxyl group. Decarboxylation occurs with $\beta$-keto acids and $\beta$-dicarboxylic acids because they can form a cyclic transition state that permits simultaneous hydrogen transfer and loss of carbon dioxide. **(B)** is a diketone and does not have a single carboxyl group. **(A)** and **(C)** are $\gamma$- and $\delta$-dicarboxylic acids, respectively, and can decarboxylate but with more difficulty.

2. **D**

The boiling points of compounds depend on the strength of the attractive forces between molecules. In both alcohols and carboxylic acids, the major form of intermolecular attraction is hydrogen bonding. However, hydrogen bonding is much stronger in carboxylic acids as compared to alcohols because carboxylic acids are more polar, and the carbonyl also contributes to hydrogen bonding in addition to the hydroxyl group. The stronger hydrogen bonds elevate the boiling points of carboxylic acids compared to alcohols. Boiling points also depend on molecular weight, **(A)**, but in this case, the difference in molecular weight is insignificant compared to the effect of hydrogen bonding. **(B)** and **(C)** are both true but do not explain the difference in boiling points.

3. **B**

The acidity of carboxylic acids is significantly increased by the presence of highly electronegative functional groups. Their electron-withdrawing effect increases the stability of the carboxylate anion, favoring proton dissociation. This effect increases as the number of electronegative groups on the chain increases, and it also increases as the distance between the acid functionality and electronegative group decreases. This answer has two halogens bonded to it at a smaller distance from the carboxyl group compared to the other answers.

4. **C**

Soap is a salt of a carboxylate anion with a long hydrocarbon tail. **(A)** and **(B)** are not salts of anionic compounds. **(D)** is sodium acetate, which is a salt but does not contain the long hydrocarbon tail needed to be considered a soap.

5. **B**

Jones reagent (chromium trioxide in aqueous sulfuric acid) is an oxidizing agent. As such, it oxidizes primary alcohols directly to carboxylic acids. This reagent is too strong an oxidant to give an aldehyde, so **(A)** is incorrect; remember that pyridinium chlorochromate (PCC) is a common oxidizing agent used to convert alcohols to aldehydes without progressing to a carboxylic acid. **(D)**, a dicarboxylic acid, cannot form because there is no functional group on the other end of the molecule for the reagent to attack, and it cannot attack an inert alkane. **(C)** represents reduction, not oxidation.

6. **C**

Carboxylic acids cannot be converted into alkenes with just one reagent. Esters, **(A)**, are formed in nucleophilic acyl substitution reactions with alcohols. Amides, **(B)**, are formed by nucleophilic acyl substitution reactions with ammonia. Alcohols, **(D)**, may be formed using a variety of reducing agents, most notably lithium aluminum hydride. To form alkenes, carboxylic acids may be reduced to alcohols, which can then be transformed into alkenes by elimination in a second step with addition of another reagent.

7. **D**

Lithium aluminum hydride ($LiAlH_4$ or LAH) is a strong reducing agent. LAH can completely reduce carboxylic acids to primary alcohols. Aldehydes are intermediate products of this reaction; therefore, **(A)** is incorrect. The other compounds are not created through the reduction of a carboxylic acid.

8. **D**

Micelles are self-assembled aggregates of soap in which the interior is composed of long hydrocarbon (fatty) tails, which can dissolve nonpolar molecules. The outer surface is covered with carboxylate groups, which makes the overall structure water-soluble. Soaps, in general, are salts of long-chain hydrocarbons with carboxylate head groups.

9. **D**

The reaction described is esterification, in which the nucleophilic oxygen atom of 1-pentanol attacks the electrophilic carbonyl carbon of butanoic acid, ultimately displacing water to form pentyl butanoate. The acid catalyst is regenerated from 1-pentanol's released proton. **(A)** reverses the carbon chains, considering the butyl tail to be the esterifying group. Ethers do not form under these conditions, so **(B)** and **(C)** are also incorrect.

10. **D**

The $\alpha$-hydrogen of a carboxylic acid is relatively acidic as far as organic compounds go, due to resonance stabilization. However, the hydroxyl hydrogen is significantly more acidic because it is able to share the negative charge resulting from deprotonation between both electronegative oxygen atoms in the functional group.

11. **B**

The reaction of formic acid, which is a simple carboxylic acid, with sodium borohydride, which is a mild reducing agent, will result in no reaction, and therefore will result in maintenance of the carboxylic acid. Sodium borohydride is too mild to reduce carboxylic acids, and therefore cannot produce the primary alcohols that lithium aluminum hydride, a strong reducing agent, would.

12. **C**

5-aminopentanoic acid contains a carboxylic acid and an amine. If this molecule undergoes intramolecular nucleophilic acyl substitution, it will form a cyclic amide. These molecules are called lactams. Lactones, **(B)**, are cyclic esters, not amides.

13. **A**

Butanoic anhydride is an anhydride with two butane R groups. Anhydrides are produced by the reaction of two carboxylic acids with the loss of a water molecule. Therefore, butanoic anhydride would be produced by the reaction of two molecules of butanoic acid.

14. **C**

Nucleophilic acyl substitutions are favored in basic solution, which makes the nucleophile more nucleophilic; in acidic solution, which makes the electrophile more electrophilic; and by good leaving groups. However, strong bases do not make good leaving groups; weak bases do.

15. **D**

Based on its name, caprylic acid must be a carboxylic acid. The reaction between a carboxylic acid and ammonia ($NH_3$) would produce an amide—which is not one of the options listed. Instead, we should take a look at the type of reaction occurring. The production of an amide from a carboxylic acid and ammonia occurs through a condensation reaction in which a molecule of water is removed as a leaving group.

**GO ONLINE**
**Consult your online resources for additional practice.**

## SHARED CONCEPTS

**Biochemistry Chapter 1**
Amino Acids, Peptides, and Proteins

**Biochemistry Chapter 5**
Lipid Structure and Function

**Organic Chemistry Chapter 1**
Nomenclature

**Organic Chemistry Chapter 4**
Analyzing Organic Reactions

**Organic Chemistry Chapter 6**
Aldehydes and Ketones I

**Organic Chemistry Chapter 9**
Carboxylic Acid Derivatives

CHAPTER 9

# CARBOXYLIC ACID DERIVATIVES

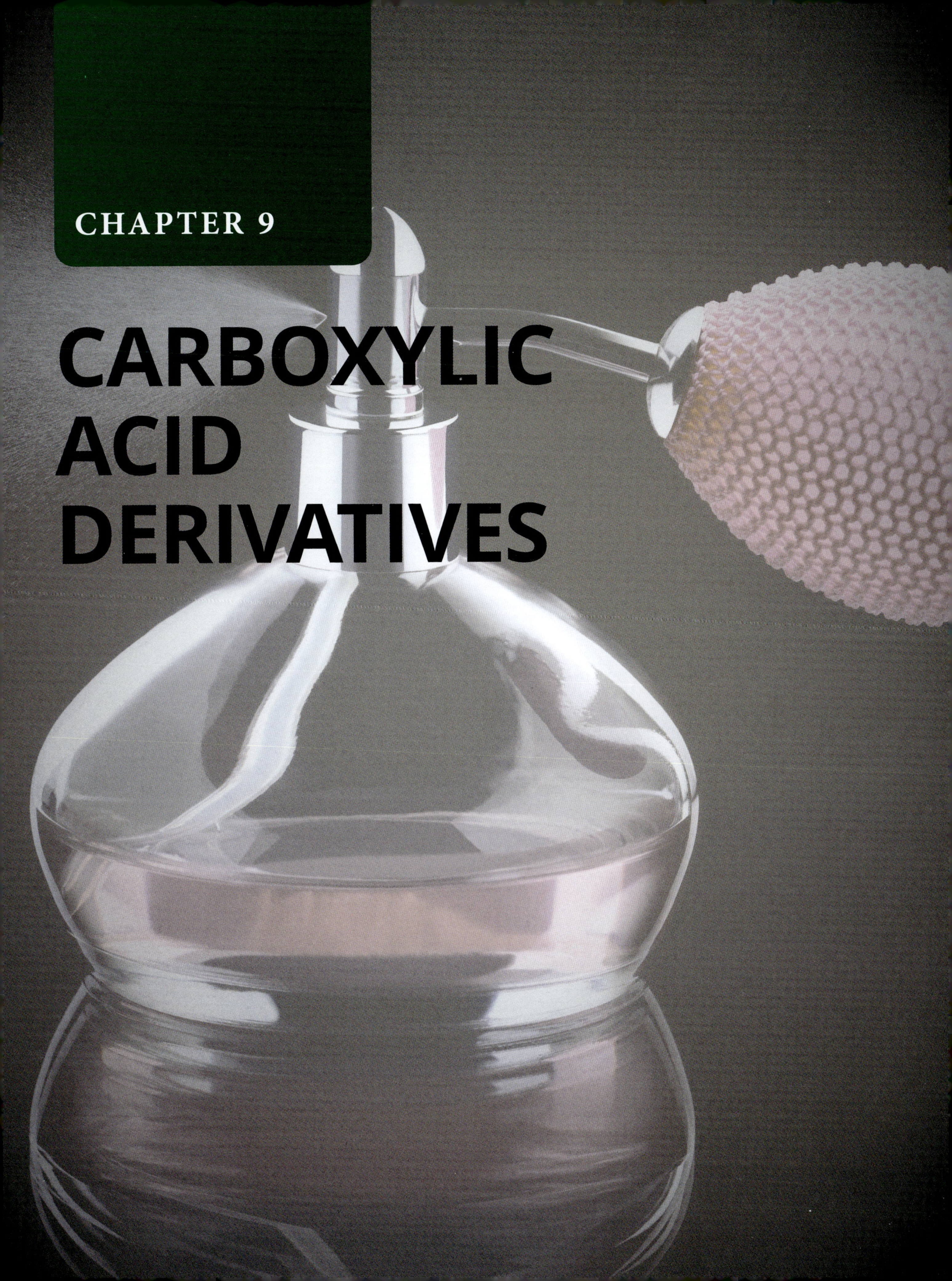

# SCIENCE MASTERY ASSESSMENT

Every pre-med knows this feeling: there is so much content I have to know for the MCAT! How do I know what to do first or what's important?

While the high-yield badges throughout this book will help you identify the most important topics, this Science Mastery Assessment is another tool in your MCAT prep arsenal. This quiz (which can also be taken in your online resources) and the guidance below will help ensure that you are spending the appropriate amount of time on this chapter based on your personal strengths and weaknesses. Don't worry though—skipping something now does not mean you'll never study it. Later on in your prep, as you complete full-length tests, you'll uncover specific pieces of content that you need to review and can come back to these chapters as appropriate.

## How to Use This Assessment

### If you answer 0–7 questions correctly:

Spend about 1 hour to read this chapter in full and take limited notes throughout. Follow up by reviewing **all** quiz questions to ensure that you now understand how to solve each one.

### If you answer 8–11 questions correctly:

Spend 20–40 minutes reviewing the quiz questions. Beginning with the questions you missed, read and take notes on the corresponding subchapters. For questions you answered correctly, ensure your thinking matches that of the explanation and you understand why each choice was correct or incorrect.

### If you answer 12–15 questions correctly:

Spend less than 20 minutes reviewing all questions from the quiz. If you missed any, then include a quick read-through of the corresponding subchapters, or even just the relevant content within a subchapter, as part of your question review. For questions you got correct, ensure your thinking matches that of the explanation and review the Concept Summary at the end of the chapter.

1. Which of the following would be the best method of producing methyl propanoate?
   - **A.** Reacting propanoic acid and methanol in the presence of a mineral acid
   - **B.** Reacting methanoic acid and propanol in the presence of a mineral acid
   - **C.** Reacting propanoic anhydride with an aqueous base
   - **D.** Reacting propanoic acid with an aqueous base

2. What would be the product(s) of the reaction below?

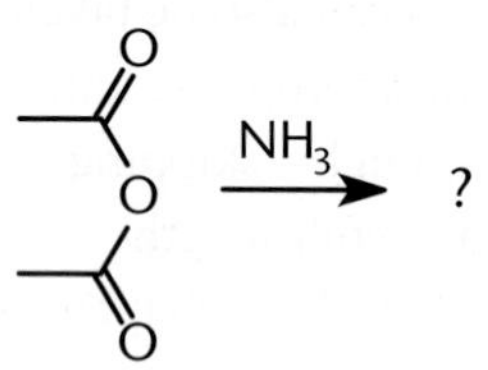


**A.**
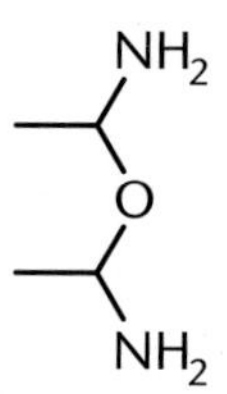

**B.** 2
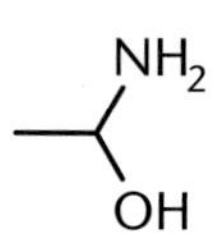

**C.**
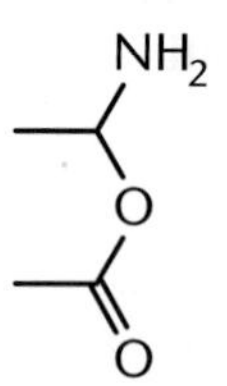

**D.**
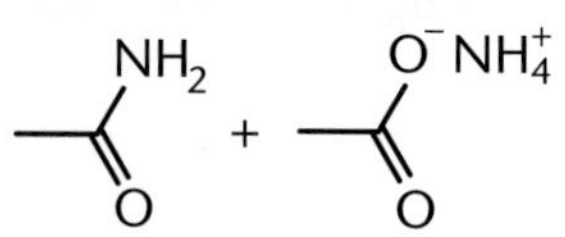

3. Which of the following undergoes a Fischer esterification most rapidly?

**A.**
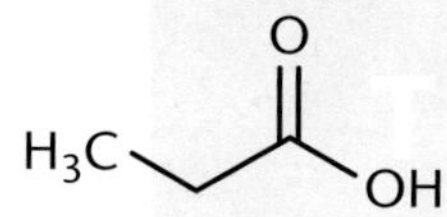

**B.**
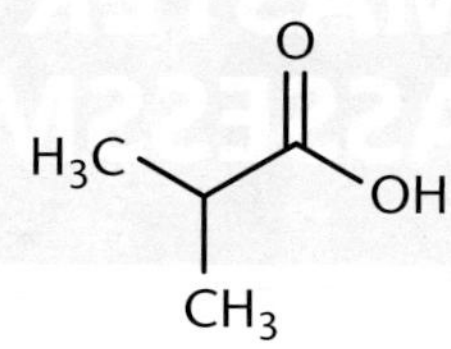

**C.**
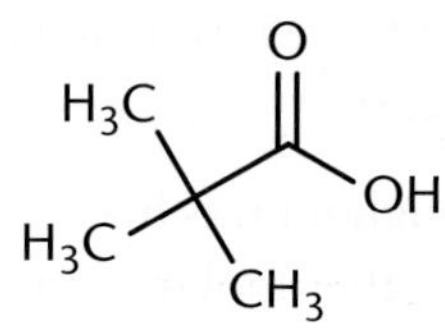

**D.**
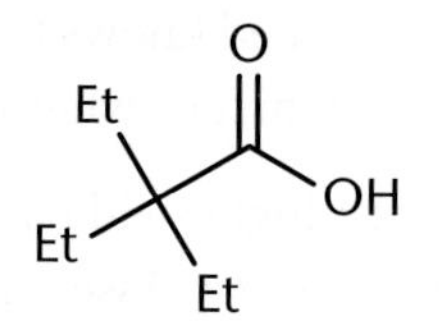

4. Each of the acyl compounds listed below contains a six-membered ring EXCEPT:
   - **A.** $\delta$-lactam.
   - **B.** cyclohexane carboxylic acid.
   - **C.** $\gamma$-butyrolactone.
   - **D.** the anhydride formed from intramolecular ring closure of pentanedioic acid.

5. Which of the following would be most reactive toward nucleophiles?
   - **A.** Propyl ethanoate
   - **B.** Propanoic acid
   - **C.** Propanamide
   - **D.** Propanoic anhydride

**6.** How might succinic anhydride, shown below, be formed from succinic acid (butanedioic acid)?

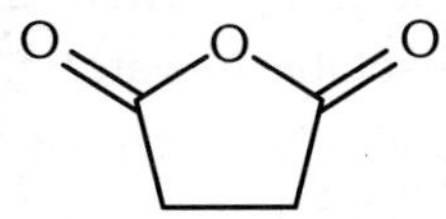

**A.** Catalytic acid
**B.** Catalytic base
**C.** Heat
**D.** Oxidation

**7.** Which of the following would react most readily with a carboxylic acid to form an amide?
**A.** Methylamine
**B.** Triethylamine
**C.** Diphenylamine
**D.** Ethylmethylamine

**8.** If propanamide were treated with water, what product(s) would be observed?
**A.** Propanamide
**B.** Propanoic acid
**C.** Equal concentrations of propanamide and propanoic acid
**D.** Propyl propanoate

**9.** $\beta$-lactams are:
**I.** cyclic forms of the least reactive type of carboxylic acid derivative.
**II.** more reactive than their straight-chain counterparts.
**III.** molecules with high levels of ring strain.
**A.** I only
**B.** II only
**C.** II and III only
**D.** I, II, and III

**10.** The acid-catalyzed conversion of propyl ethanoate to benzyl ethanoate is likely:
**A.** reduction.
**B.** hydrolysis.
**C.** transesterification.
**D.** oxidation.

**11.** The reaction shown, which is important for the breakdown of polypeptides, would be favored under what conditions?

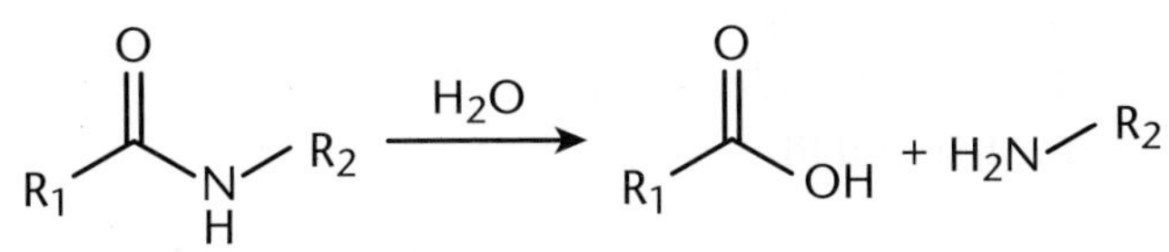


**A.** Mild heat
**B.** Acid environment
**C.** Anhydrous environment
**D.** Nonpolar solvent

**12.** A positive charge on the molecule shown would have greater stability than a positive charge on a straight-chain alkane version of the same molecule. What property most explains this effect?

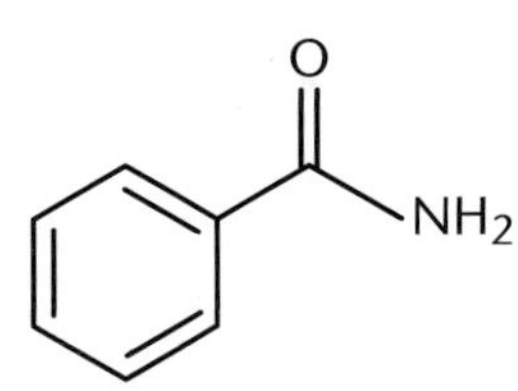

**A.** Steric hindrance
**B.** Nitrogen electronegativity
**C.** Induction
**D.** Conjugation

13. The molecule shown is:

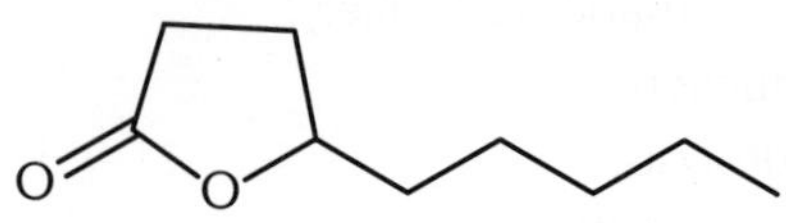


I. synthesizable from a γ-hydroxycarboxylic acid.

II. a lactone.

III. a form of an ester.

A. I only
B. I and II only
C. II and III only
D. I, II, and III

14. Which reactant could be combined with butanol to form butyl acetate?

A. $(CH_3CO)_2O$ and catalytic acid
B. $(CH_3CH_2CO)_2O$ and catalytic acid
C. $CH_3CH_2CONH_2$ and catalytic acid
D. $CH_3CONH_2$ and catalytic acid

15. Why should esterification reactions NOT be carried out in water?

A. Carboxylic acids, from which esters are made, are generally insoluble in water.
B. The polar nature of water overshadows the polar nature of the leaving group.
C. The extensive hydrogen bonding of water interferes with the nucleophilic addition mechanism.
D. Water molecules would hydrolyze the desired products back into the parent carboxylic acid.

**Answer Key follows on next page.**

## Answer Key

1. **A** (See section 9.1)
2. **D** (See section 9.1)
3. **A** (See section 9.1)
4. **C** (See section 9.3)
5. **D** (See section 9.2)
6. **C** (See section 9.1)
7. **A** (See section 9.1)
8. **A** (See section 9.2)
9. **D** (See section 9.1)
10. **C** (See section 9.1)
11. **B** (See section 9.2)
12. **D** (See section 9.2)
13. **D** (See section 9.1)
14. **A** (See section 9.3)
15. **D** (See section 9.2)

*The relevant section of the chapter to review for each question is given in parentheses after the correct answer. Detailed explanations can be found at the end of the chapter.*

CHAPTER 9

# CARBOXYLIC ACID DERIVATIVES

## In This Chapter



**CHAPTER PROFILE**

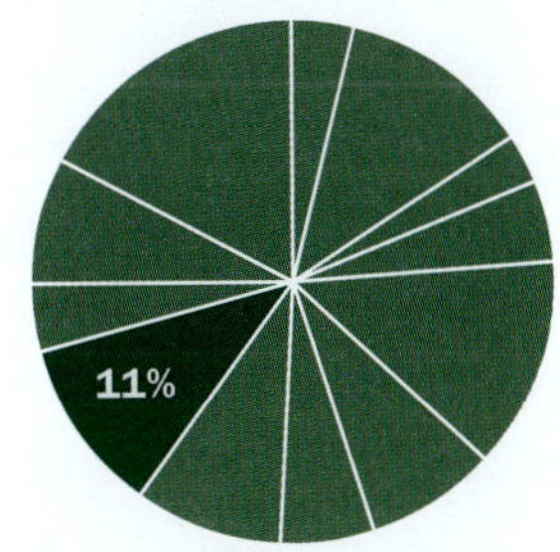


The content in this chapter should be relevant to about 11% of all questions about organic chemistry on the MCAT.

This chapter covers material from the following AAMC content categories:

**1A:** Structure and function of proteins and their constituent amino acids

**5D:** Structure, function, and reactivity of biologically-relevant molecules

## Introduction

We saw in the previous three chapters that carbonyls are susceptible to attack by everything from water to amines to other carbonyl-containing compounds (in the enol or enolate form). These reactions often result in the formation of carboxylic acid derivatives. Our focus in this chapter will be on describing the carboxylic acid derivatives that appear on the MCAT: amides, esters, and anhydrides. Each of these molecules replaces the $-OH$ on the carboxyl group with another leaving group ($-NR_2$, $-OR$, and $-OCOR$, respectively). These each react in similar ways to carboxylic acids. Many of these functional groups are also critical for biochemical processes.

## 9.1 Amides, Esters, and Anhydrides

**LEARNING OBJECTIVES**

After Chapter 9.1, you will be able to:

- Apply the rules for naming carboxylic acid derivatives, including the nomenclature for the cyclic version of the molecule
- Describe a condensation reaction

Amides, esters, and anhydrides are all carboxylic acid derivatives. Each of these is formed by a **condensation** reaction with a carboxylic acid—a reaction that combines two molecules into one, while losing a small molecule. In this case, the small molecule is water, which is created from the hydroxyl group of the carboxylic acid and a hydrogen associated with the incoming nucleophile.

**KEY CONCEPT**

In a condensation reaction, two molecules are combined to form one, with the loss of a small molecule—water, in our case. Carboxylic acid derivatives are formed by this mechanism.

## Descriptions

For each of the carboxylic acid derivatives described in this section, focus on the relevant nucleophile that forms the derivative and the nomenclature of the functional group. In the next section, we'll focus more directly on the relative reactivity of these compounds.

### Amides

**Amides** are compounds with the general formula $RCONR_2$. They are named by replacing the –**oic acid** suffix with –**amide**. Alkyl substituents on the nitrogen atom are listed as prefixes, and their location is specified with the letter ***N***–. Figure 9.1 shows a few examples.

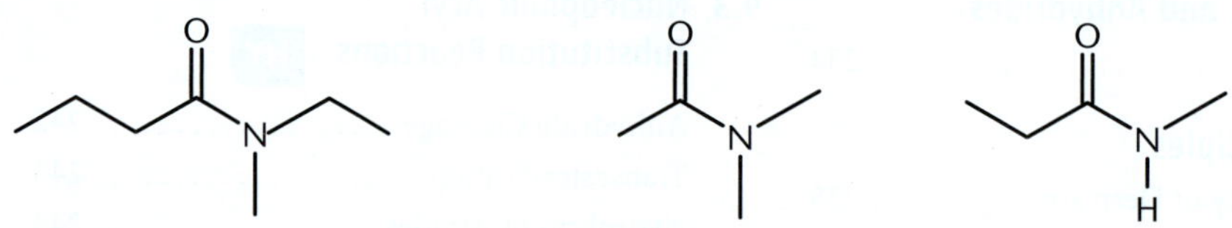


*N*-ethyl-*N*-methylbutanamide *N,N*-dimethylethanamide *N*-methylpropanamide

**Figure 9.1** Naming Amides

Amides are generally synthesized by the reaction of other carboxylic acid derivatives with either ammonia or an amine. Note that loss of hydrogen from the nucleophile is required for this reaction to take place. Thus, only primary and secondary amines will undergo this reaction.

**KEY CONCEPT**

Amides are formed by the condensation reaction of other carboxylic acid derivatives and ammonia or an amine.

Cyclic amides are called **lactams**. These are named according to the carbon atom bonded to the nitrogen: $\beta$-lactams contain a bond between the $\beta$-carbon and the nitrogen, $\gamma$-lactams contain a bond between the $\gamma$-carbon and the nitrogen, and so forth. Structures of lactams are shown in Figure 9.2.

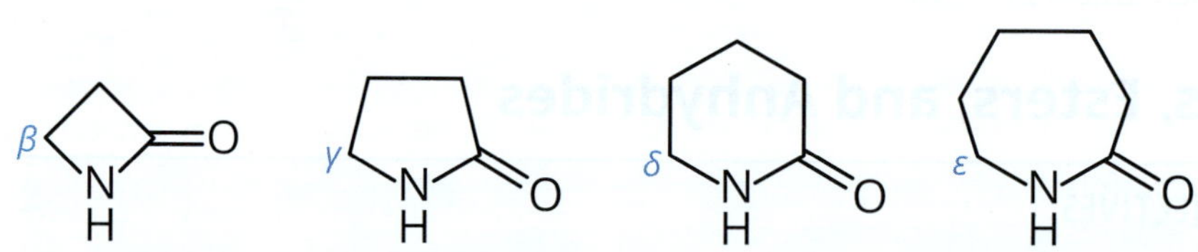


β-lactam γ-lactam δ-lactam ε-lactam

**Figure 9.2** Examples of Lactams

Amides may or may not participate in hydrogen bonding depending on the number of alkyl groups they have bonded, and therefore their boiling points may be lower or on the same level as the boiling points of carboxylic acids.

## Esters

**Esters** are the dehydration synthesis products of other carboxylic acid derivatives and alcohols. They are named by placing the **esterifying group** (the substituent bonded to the oxygen) as a prefix; the suffix –**oate** replaces –**oic acid**. Two examples are shown in Figure 9.3. As mentioned in the last chapter, ethyl acetate, derived from the condensation of acetic acid and ethanol, is called ethyl ethanoate according to IUPAC nomenclature.

**KEY CONCEPT**

Esters are formed by the condensation reaction of carboxylic acids or anhydrides with alcohols.

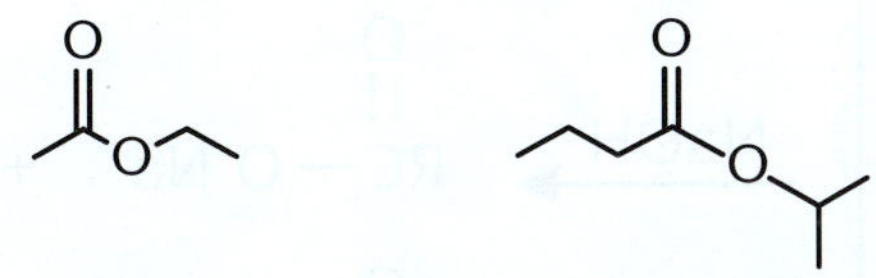


**Figure 9.3** Naming Esters

Under acidic conditions, mixtures of carboxylic acids and alcohols will condense into esters. This reaction, called a **Fischer esterification**, is shown in Figure 9.4. Esters can also be obtained from the reaction of anhydrides with alcohols.

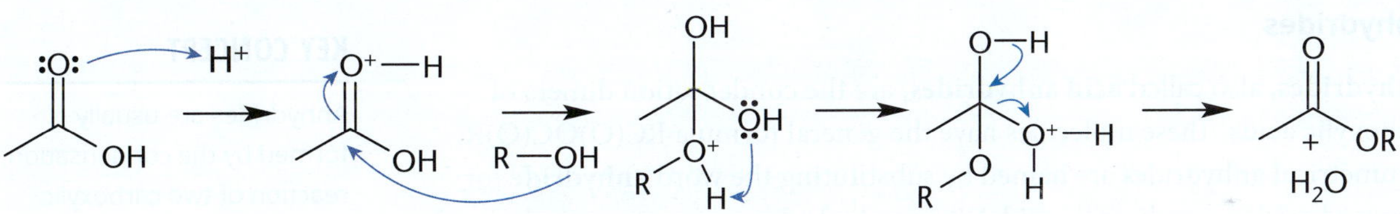


**Figure 9.4** Fischer Esterification

Cyclic esters are called **lactones** and are named in the same manner as lactams, with the name of the precursor acid molecule also included. Examples are shown in Figure 9.5.

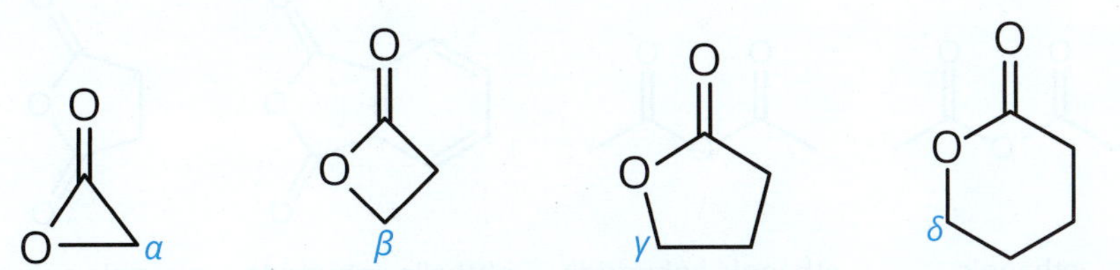


**Figure 9.5** Examples of Lactones

Because they lack hydrogen bonding, esters usually have lower boiling points than their related carboxylic acids.

**Triacylglycerols**, the storage form of fats in the body, are esters of long-chain carboxylic acids (fatty acids) and **glycerol** (1,2,3-propanetriol). **Saponification** is the process by which fats are hydrolyzed under basic conditions to produce soap; saponification of a triacylglycerol is shown in Figure 9.6. Subsequent acidification of the soap regenerates the fatty acids.

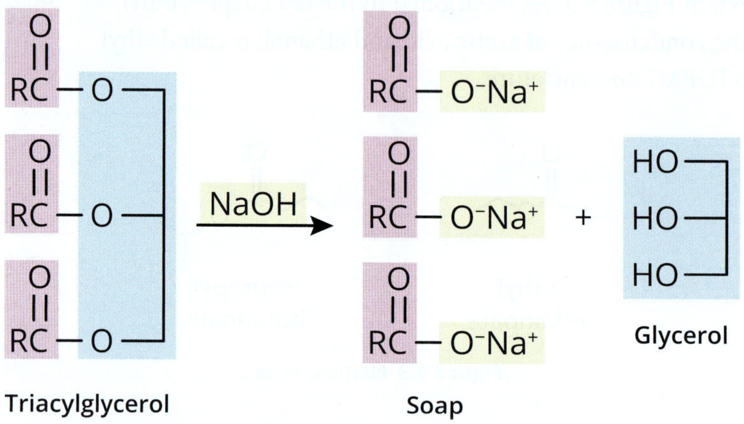


**Figure 9.6** Saponification of a Triacylglycerol
*Treating triacylglycerols with NaOH will produce fatty acid salts (soap) as well as glycerol.*

## Anhydrides

**Anhydrides**, also called **acid anhydrides**, are the condensation dimers of carboxylic acids. These molecules have the general formula RC(O)OC(O)R. Symmetrical anhydrides are named by substituting the word **anhydride** for the word **acid** in a carboxylic acid. When anhydrides are asymmetrical, simply name the two chains alphabetically, followed by **anhydride**, as shown in Figure 9.7. Phthalic and succinic anhydrides are cyclic anhydrides arising from intramolecular condensation or dehydration of diacids; their structures need not be memorized, but recognize them as cyclic anhydrides.

**KEY CONCEPT**

Anhydrides are usually formed by the condensation reaction of two carboxylic acids.

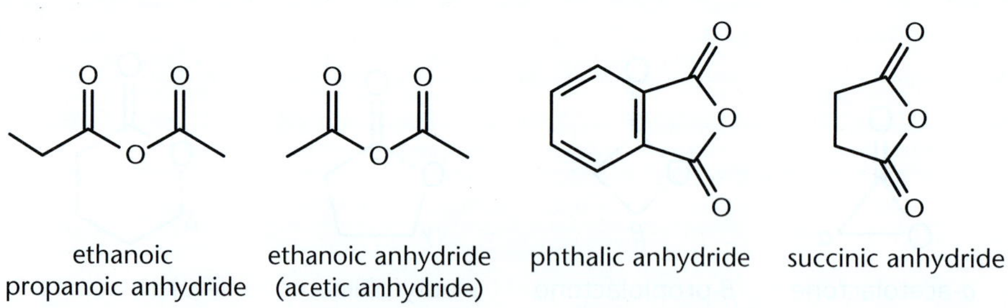


**Figure 9.7** Naming Anhydrides

Acid anhydrides are synthesized, as mentioned previously, by a condensation reaction between two carboxylic acids, with one molecule of water lost in the condensation, as shown in Figure 9.8.

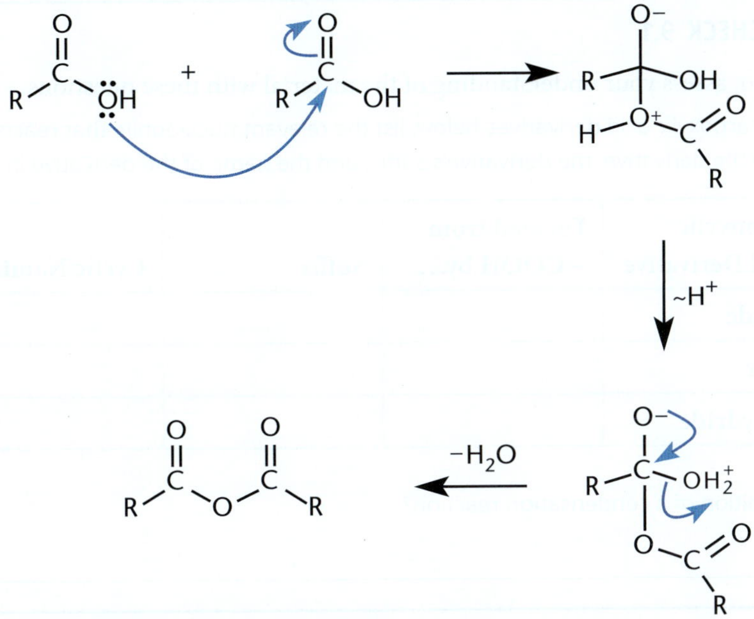


**Figure 9.8** Synthesis of an Anhydride via Carboxylic Acid Condensation
*Two molecules of carboxylic acid come together and lose a molecule of water in the formation of an anhydride.*

Certain cyclic anhydrides can be formed simply by heating carboxylic acids, as shown in Figure 9.9. The reaction is driven forward by the increased stability of the newly formed ring; as such, only anhydrides with five- or six-membered rings are easily made. Just as with all anhydride formations, the hydroxyl group of one –COOH acts as the nucleophile, attacking the carbonyl on the other –COOH.

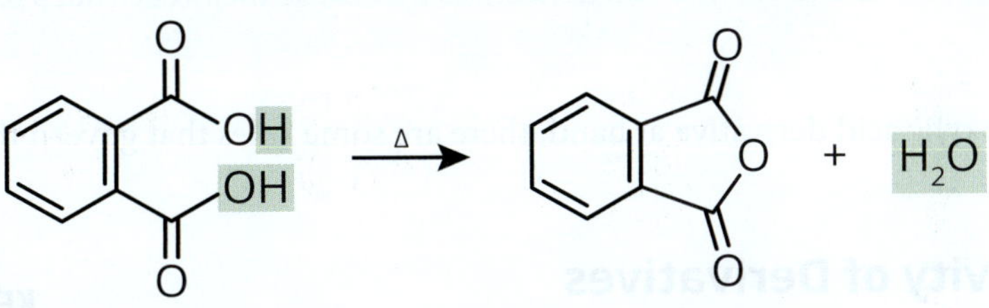


**Figure 9.9** Intramolecular Anhydride Formation
*Heat and the increased stability of the newly formed ring drive this intramolecular ring formation reaction forward.*

Anhydrides often have higher boiling points than their related carboxylic acids, based solely on their much greater weight.

**MCAT CONCEPT CHECK 9.1**

Before you move on, assess your understanding of the material with these questions.

1. For each of the carboxylic acid derivatives below, list the relevant nucleophile that reacts with a carboxylic acid to generate the derivative, the derivative's suffix, and the name of the derivative in cyclic form.

| Carboxylic Acid Derivative | Formed from –COOH by... | Suffix | Cyclic Naming |
|---|---|---|---|
| Amide | | | |
| Ester | | | |
| Anhydride | | | |

2. What is the definition of a condensation reaction?

______________________________

## 9.2 Reactivity Principles

**LEARNING OBJECTIVES**

After Chapter 9.2, you will be able to:

- Order carboxylic acid derivatives, including anhydrides, esters, and amides, based on their reactivity
- Explain the relatively high rate of hydrolysis in $\beta$-lactams
- Identify the properties of the carboxylic acid derivatives that cause their reactivities to differ

Regardless of the carboxylic acid derivative at hand, there are some rules that govern the reactivity of these molecules.

### Relative Reactivity of Derivatives

In a nucleophilic substitution reaction, the reactivity of the carbonyl is determined by its substituents, as seen in Figure 9.10. Anhydrides are most reactive, followed by esters (which are essentially tied with carboxylic acids), then finally amides. This can be explained by the structure of these molecules. Anhydrides, with their resonance stabilization and three electron-withdrawing oxygen atoms, are the most electrophilic. Esters, by comparison, lack one electron-withdrawing carbonyl oxygen and are slightly less reactive. Finally, amides, with an electron-donating amino group, are the least reactive toward nucleophiles.

**KEY CONCEPT**

When considering the reactivity of carboxylic acid derivatives toward nucleophilic attack, anhydrides are the most reactive, followed by esters and carboxylic acids, and then amides.

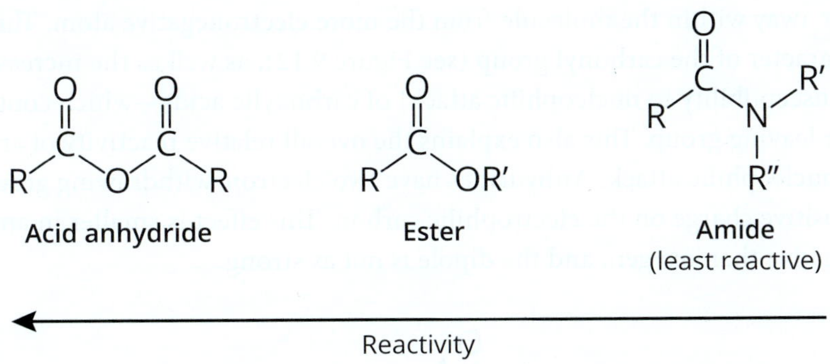


**Figure 9.10** Reactivity of Carboxylic Acid Derivatives

## Steric Effects

Steric hindrance is always worth keeping in mind when considering reactivity. **Steric hindrance** describes when a reaction does not proceed due to the size of the substituents. As seen in Figure 9.11, tertiary carbons exhibit the most steric hindrance, while primary carbons are the least affected. A good example of this is in $S_N2$ reactions, which will not occur at tertiary carbons. This effect, which might sound detrimental, can be used to our advantage—for example, if we want to push a reaction in an $S_N1$ direction, rather than $S_N2$, we can use a tertiary substrate. Another way that this is used synthetically is in the creation of protecting groups. As we saw in Chapter 6 of *MCAT Organic Chemistry Review*, aldehydes and ketones will readily react with strong reducing agents like $LiAlH_4$—but this can be prevented by first reacting the aldehyde or ketone with two equivalents of alcohol, producing a nonreactive acetal or ketal. After we complete the rest of the desired reactions, we can then regenerate the carbonyl with aqueous acid. In the context of carboxylic acid derivatives, the size and substitution of the leaving group can affect the ability of a nucleophile to access the carbonyl carbon, thus affecting the reactivity of the derivative to nucleophilic acyl substitution.

**KEY CONCEPT**

Steric hindrance can be used to control where a reaction occurs in a molecule. Protecting groups may make it too hard for a nucleophile, oxidizing agent, or reducing agent to access or react with a part of the molecule.

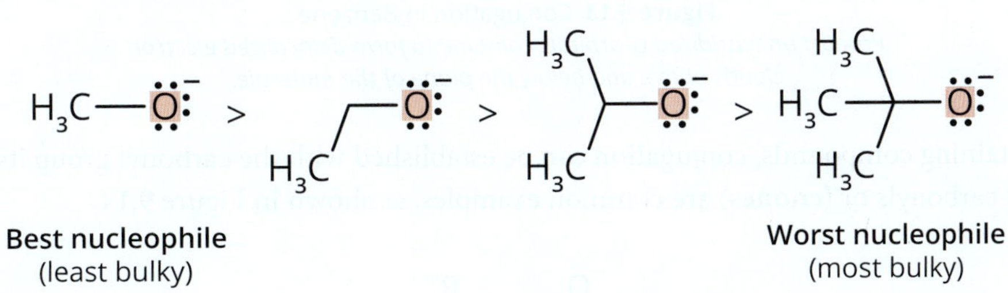


**Figure 9.11** Steric Hindrance of Nucleophiles

## Electronic Effects

There are several electronic effects that must be considered in organic chemistry on the MCAT, and all of them come into play when considering carboxylic acid derivatives. **Induction** refers to the distribution of charge across $\sigma$ bonds. Electrons are attracted to atoms that are more electronegative, generating a dipole across the $\sigma$ bond. The less electronegative atom acquires a slightly positive charge, and the more electronegative atom acquires a slightly negative charge. This effect is relatively weak and gets increasingly weaker as one moves further away within the molecule from the more electronegative atom. This effect is responsible for the dipole character of the carbonyl group (see Figure 9.12), as well as the increased dipole character (and, therefore, susceptibility to nucleophilic attack) of carboxylic acids—which contain an additional oxygen atom in their leaving group. This also explains the overall relative reactivity of anhydrides, esters, and amides toward nucleophilic attack. Anhydrides have two electron-withdrawing groups, which leave a significant partial positive charge on the electrophilic carbon. This effect is smaller in amides because nitrogen is less electronegative than oxygen, and the dipole is not as strong.

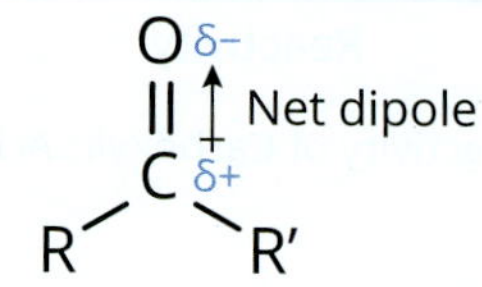


**Figure 9.12** Carbonyl Dipole

Resonance and conjugation also affect the reactivity of a molecule. **Conjugation** refers to the presence of alternating single and multiple bonds. This setup implies that all of the atoms involved in these bonds are either $sp^2$- or $sp$-hybridized—and therefore have unhybridized *p*-orbitals. When these *p*-orbitals align, they can delocalize $\pi$ electrons through resonance, forming clouds of electron density above and below the plane of the molecule. This type of electron sharing is most commonly demonstrated using benzene, as shown in Figure 9.13.

**KEY CONCEPT**

Induction is the distribution of charge across $\sigma$ bonds. Conjugation and resonance are much more powerful effects and occur in systems with alternating single and multiple bonds.

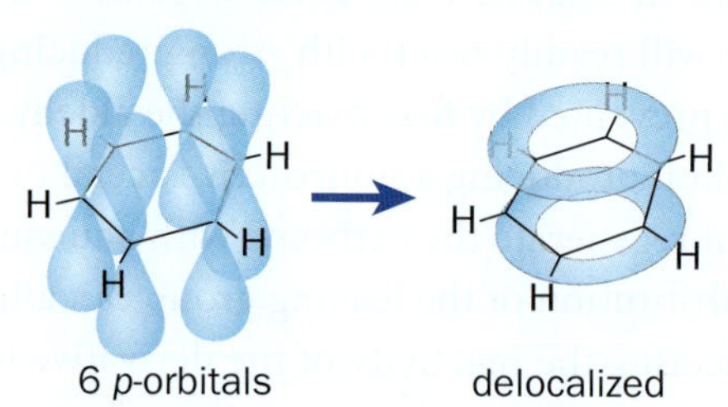


**Figure 9.13** Conjugation in Benzene
*Parallel unhybridized* p*-orbitals combine to form delocalized electron clouds above and below the plane of the molecule.*

In carbonyl-containing compounds, conjugation can be established with the carbonyl group itself. $\alpha,\beta$-unsaturated carbonyls or (**enones**) are common examples, as shown in Figure 9.14.

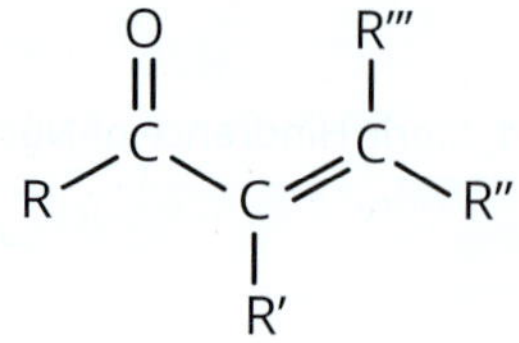


**Figure 9.14** Conjugation in a Carbonyl-Containing Compound

This type of electron sharing makes for very stable compounds because these compounds have multiple resonance structures. This characteristic allows for the stabilization of a positive charge once the nucleophile has bonded, making these compounds more susceptible to nucleophilic attack.

## Strain in Cyclic Derivatives

Lactams and lactones are cyclic amides and esters, respectively. Certain lactams and lactones are more reactive to hydrolysis because they contain more strain. $\beta$-lactams, for example, are four-membered cyclic amides and are highly reactive due to significant ring strain; four-membered rings have both torsional strain from eclipsing interactions and angle strain from compressing the normal $sp^3$ angle of 109.5°. These molecules are part of the core structure of several antibiotic families, as shown in Figure 9.15. The ring strain, and therefore the reactivity, is increased by fusion to a second ring. The four-membered structure of a $\beta$-lactam also forces a trigonal pyramidal bond geometry on the nitrogen atom in the ring, which reduces resonance, making hydrolysis more likely.

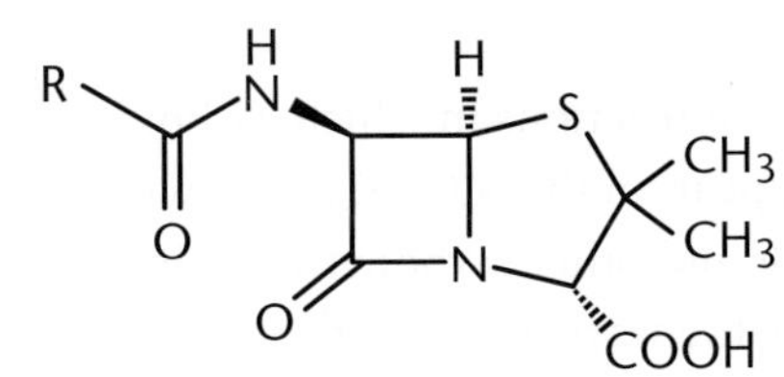


**Figure 9.15** Penicillin, a $\beta$-Lactam-Containing Antibiotic

### REAL WORLD

Many antibiotic families contain $\beta$-lactams, including the penicillin family, cephalosporins, carbapenems, and monobactams. Many bacteria have developed $\beta$-lactamases, which break $\beta$-lactam rings, as a resistance mechanism against these antibiotics. Therefore, $\beta$-lactams are sometimes given with $\beta$-lactamase inhibitors to increase their efficacy.

### MCAT CONCEPT CHECK 9.2

Before you move on, assess your understanding of the material with these questions.

1. Rank the following molecules by decreasing reactivity to $OR^-$: acetamide, acetic anhydride, and ethyl acetate.

    1. ______________________________
    2. ______________________________
    3. ______________________________

2. What is responsible for the increased rate of hydrolysis in $\beta$-lactams?

    ______________________________

3. What properties account for the differences in reactivity seen between anhydrides, esters, and amides with nucleophiles?

    ______________________________

## 9.3 Nucleophilic Acyl Substitution Reactions High Yield

### LEARNING OBJECTIVES

After Chapter 9.3, you will be able to:

- Describe the mechanism for transesterification reactions
- Explain how strong acid and strong base conditions would impact the mechanism of hydrolysis of an amide
- Identify the nucleophile and electrophile within nucleophilic acyl substitution reactions such as:

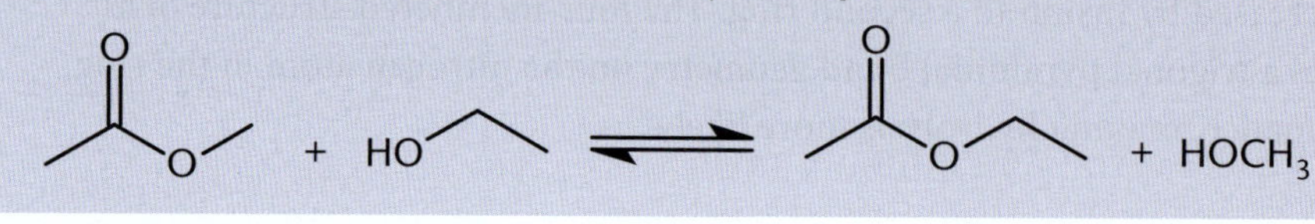


Although there are a seemingly infinite number of reactions in which carboxylic acid derivatives can participate, a much smaller group of reactions will appear on the MCAT. As we will observe, these reactions have much in common with those of carboxylic acids and other carbonyl-containing compounds. Many of the properties we have already discussed determine the ways in which these reactions proceed.

## Anhydride Cleavage

As with carboxylic acids, nucleophilic acyl substitution involves nucleophilic attack of the carbonyl carbon with displacement of a leaving group. All carboxylic acid derivatives can participate in nucleophilic substitution reactions at different relative rates. Specifically, anhydrides are most reactive toward nucleophiles, followed by esters, and finally amides. One example of this is the formation of amides from the nucleophilic substitution reaction between ammonia and any carboxylic acid or derivative. The example shown in Figure 9.16 is not only a nucleophilic substitution reaction, but also a **cleavage reaction** because it splits an anhydride in two. In this reaction, ammonia acts as the nucleophile, one of the carbonyl carbons acts as the electrophile, and a carboxylic acid is the leaving group.

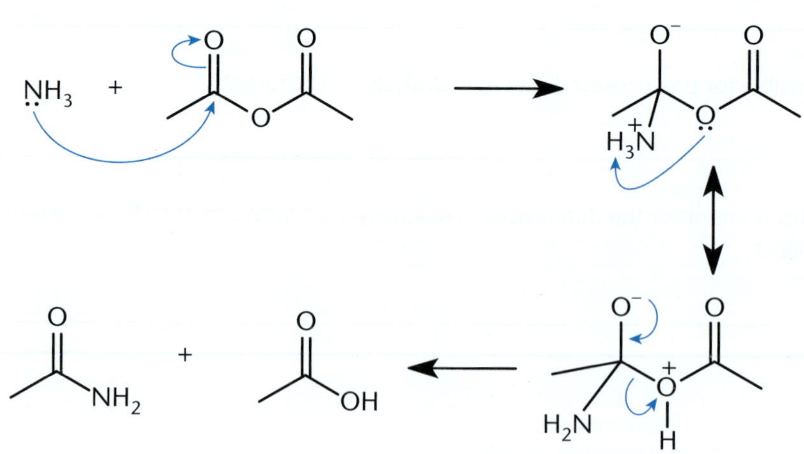


**Figure 9.16** Nucleophilic Acyl Substitution: Anhydride to Amide and Carboxylic Acid

Alcohols can also act as nucleophiles toward anhydrides; this nucleophilic substitution reaction will result in the formation of esters and carboxylic acids, as shown in Figure 9.17.

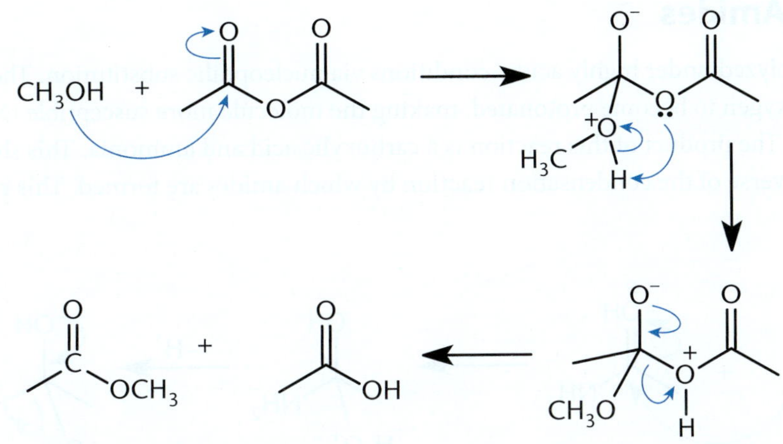


**Figure 9.17** Nucleophilic Acyl Substitution: Anhydride to Ester and Carboxylic Acid

Anhydrides can also be reverted to carboxylic acids by exposing them to water, as shown in Figure 9.18. For these reactions to be useful, the anhydride should be symmetric; otherwise, one forms a mixture of products.

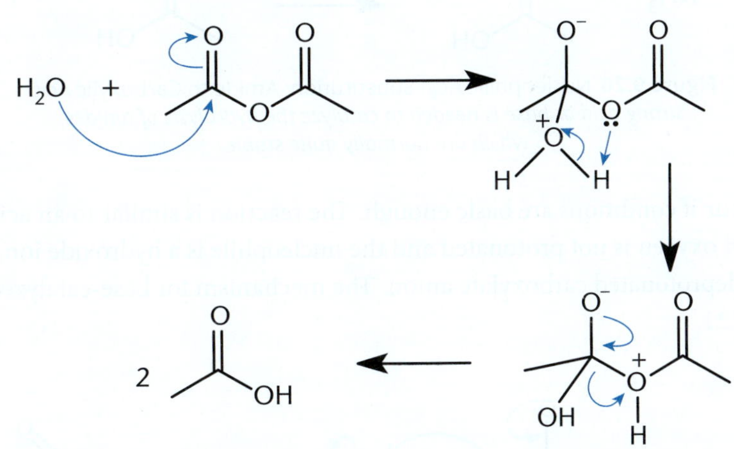


**Figure 9.18** Nucleophilic Acyl Substitution: Anhydride to Carboxylic Acids

## Transesterification

Alcohols can act as nucleophiles and displace the esterifying group on an ester. This process is called **transesterification**. In this reaction, one ester is simply transformed into another, as shown in Figure 9.19.

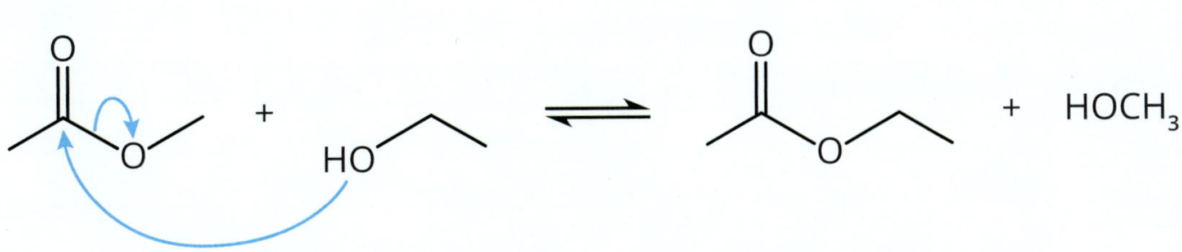


**Figure 9.19** Nucleophilic Acyl Substitution: Transesterification
*Different alcohol chains are swapped into and out of the esterifying group position.*

## Hydrolysis of Amides

Amides can be hydrolyzed under highly acidic conditions via nucleophilic substitution. The acidic conditions allow the carbonyl oxygen to become protonated, making the molecule more susceptible to nucleophilic attack by a water molecule. The product of this reaction is a carboxylic acid and ammonia. This should be no surprise because this is the reverse of the condensation reaction by which amides are formed. This reaction is shown in Figure 9.20.

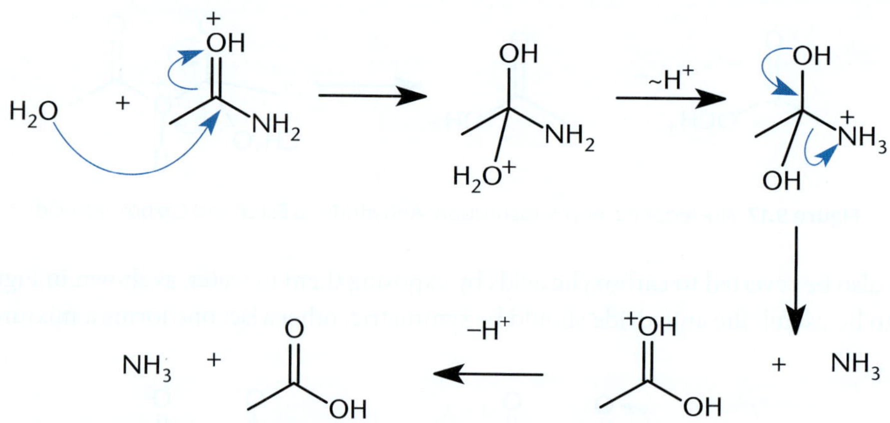


**Figure 9.20** Nucleophilic Acyl Substitution: Amide to Carboxylic Acid
*Strong acid or base is needed to catalyze the hydrolysis of amides, which are normally quite stable.*

Hydrolysis can also occur if conditions are basic enough. The reaction is similar to an acid-catalyzed reaction, except that the carbonyl oxygen is not protonated and the nucleophile is a hydroxide ion. The product of this reaction would be the deprotonated carboxylate anion. The mechanism for base-catalyzed amide hydrolysis can be seen in Figure 9.21.

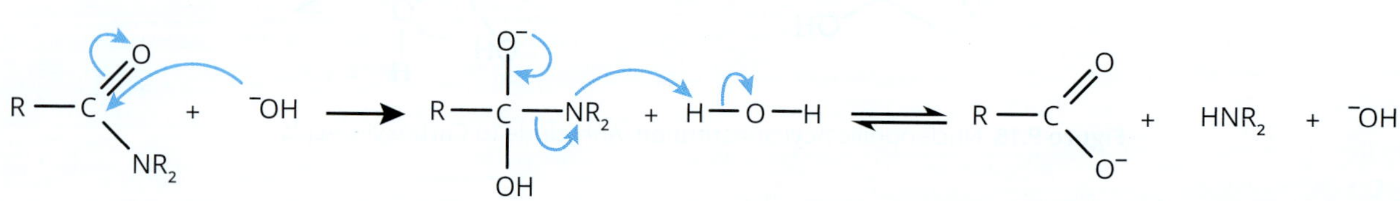


**Figure 9.21** Amide Hydrolysis under Basic Conditions

**MCAT CONCEPT CHECK 9.3**

Before you move on, assess your understanding of the material with these questions.

1. In the formation of an amide from ammonia and an anhydride, what serves as the nucleophile? The electrophile?
   - Nucleophile:

   ______________________________

   - Electrophile:

   ______________________________

2. What are the products of the transesterification reaction between isopropyl butanoate and ethanol?

   ______________________________

3. How do strongly acidic and strongly basic conditions catalyze the hydrolysis of an amide?
   - Strongly acidic conditions:

   ______________________________

   - Strongly basic conditions:

   ______________________________

## Conclusion

We're sure you've noticed that this chapter covers only a few reactions happening in a wide variety of contexts. The MCAT test makers don't want you to memorize all the possible reactions; they simply want you to truly understand the trends and the underlying reasons for these reactions. Make sure you know the order of reactivity of the derivatives (from anhydrides, the most, to amides, the least). Also, learn the special reactions of esters and amides. Your study of amides will pay off right away as we explore amino acids and other nitrogen- and phosphorus-containing compounds in the next chapter.

**▶ GO ONLINE**

**You've reviewed the content, now test your knowledge and critical thinking skills by completing a test-like passage set in your online resources!**

# CONCEPT SUMMARY

## Amides, Esters, and Anhydrides

- **Amides** are the condensation products of carboxylic acids and ammonia or amines.
  - Amides are given the suffix –**amide**. The alkyl groups on a substituted amide are written at the beginning of the name with the prefix ***N***–.
  - Cyclic amides are called **lactams**. Lactams are named by the Greek letter of the carbon forming the bond with the nitrogen ($\beta$-lactam, $\gamma$-lactam, and so on).
- **Esters** are the condensation products of carboxylic acids with alcohols (**Fischer esterification**).
  - Esters are given the suffix –**oate**. The **esterifying group** is written as a substituent, without a number.
  - Cyclic esters are called **lactones**. Lactones are named by the number of carbons in the ring and the Greek letter of the carbon forming the bond with the oxygen ($\alpha$-acetolactone, $\beta$-propiolactone, and so on).
  - **Triacylglycerols**, which are a form of fat storage, include three ester bonds between glycerol and fatty acids. **Saponification** is the breakdown of fat using a strong base to form **soap** (salts of long-chain carboxylic acids).
- **Anhydrides** are the condensation dimers of carboxylic acids.
  - Symmetric anhydrides are named for the parent carboxylic acid, followed by **anhydride**. Asymmetric anhydrides are named by listing the parent carboxylic acids alphabetically, followed by **anhydride**.
  - Some cyclic anhydrides can be synthesized by heating dioic acids. Five- or six-membered rings are generally stable.

## Reactivity Principles

- In nucleophilic substitution reactions, anhydrides are more reactive than esters, which are more reactive than amides.
- **Steric hindrance** describes when a reaction cannot proceed (or significantly slows) because of substituents crowding the reactive site. **Protecting groups**, such as acetals, can be used to increase steric hindrance or otherwise decrease the reactivity of a particular portion of a molecule.
- **Induction** refers to uneven distribution of charge across a $\sigma$ bond because of differences in electronegativity. The more electronegative groups in a carbonyl-containing compound, the greater its reactivity.
- **Conjugation** refers to the presence of alternating single and multiple bonds, which creates delocalized $\pi$ electron clouds above and below the plane of the molecule. Electrons experience **resonance** through the unhybridized $p$-orbitals, increasing stability. Conjugated carbonyl-containing compounds are more reactive because they can stabilize their transition states.
- Increased strain in a molecule can make it more reactive. ***β*-lactams** are prone to hydrolysis because they have significant ring strain. **Ring strain** is due to torsional strain from eclipsing interactions and angle strain from compressing bond angles below 109.5°.

## Nucleophilic Acyl Substitution Reactions

- All carboxylic acid derivatives can undergo nucleophilic substitution reactions. The rates at which they do so are determined by their relative reactivities.
- Anhydrides can be **cleaved** by the addition of a nucleophile.
  - Addition of ammonia or an amine results in an amide and a carboxylic acid.
  - Addition of an alcohol results in an ester and a carboxylic acid.
  - Addition of water results in two carboxylic acids.
- **Transesterification** is the exchange of one esterifying group for another on an ester. The attacking nucleophile is an alcohol.
- **Amides** can be hydrolyzed to carboxylic acids under strongly acidic or basic conditions. The attacking nucleophile is water or the hydroxide anion.

## ANSWERS TO CONCEPT CHECKS

### 9.1

1.

| Carboxylic Acid Derivative | Formed from –COOH by... | Suffix | Cyclic Naming |
|---|---|---|---|
| **Amide** | Ammonia or an amine | –amide | Lactam |
| **Ester** | An alcohol | –oate | Lactone |
| **Anhydride** | Another carboxylic acid | anhydride | Anhydride |

2. A condensation reaction is one in which two molecules are joined with the loss of a small molecule. In all of the examples in this section, the small molecule lost was water.

### 9.2

1. Anhydrides are the most reactive to nucleophiles, followed by esters, and then amides. Therefore, acetic anhydride will be the most reactive, followed by ethyl acetate, and finally acetamide.
2. $\beta$-lactams are susceptible to hydrolysis due to the high level of ring strain, which is due to both torsional strain (eclipsing interactions) and angle strain (deviation from 109.5°).
3. Electronic effects like induction have some effect on the reactivity of the carbonyl in these three functional groups. Differences in resonance also explain the increased reactivity of anhydrides, in particular. Steric effects could also be significant, depending on the specific leaving group present.

### 9.3

1. Ammonia acts as the nucleophile. One of the carbonyl carbons of the anhydride serves as the electrophile.
2. Transesterification is the exchange of one esterifying group for another in an ester. This reaction requires an alcohol as a nucleophile. In this case, the ethyl group of ethanol will replace the isopropyl group of isopropyl butanoate, resulting in ethyl butanoate and 2-propanol.
3. Strongly acidic conditions catalyze amide hydrolysis by protonating the oxygen in the carbonyl. This increases the electrophilicity of the carbon, making it more susceptible to nucleophilic attack. Strongly basic conditions greatly increase the concentration of $OH^-$, which can act as a nucleophile on amide carbonyls.

## SCIENCE MASTERY ASSESSMENT EXPLANATIONS

1. **A**

Methyl propanoate is an ester; it can be synthesized by reacting a carboxylic acid with an alcohol in the presence of acid. Here, the parent chain is propanoate, and the esterifying group is a methyl group. **(B)** reverses the nomenclature and would form propyl methanoate. The other reactions listed would not form esters.

2. **D**

This question asks for the products when ammonia reacts with acetic anhydride. Recall from the chapter that an amide and a carboxylic acid will be formed. However, the carboxylic acid—an acid—is in the same environment as ammonia—a base. The two will react, forming the ammonium carboxylate shown.

3. **A**

A Fischer esterification involves reacting a carboxylic acid and an alcohol with an acid catalyst. Under these conditions, the carbonyl carbon is open to attack by the nucleophilic alcohol. The rate of this reaction depends on the amount of steric hindrance around the carbonyl carbon because there must be room for the alcohol to approach the carboxylic acid substrate. **(B)**, **(C)**, and **(D)** all have more crowding around the carbonyl carbon, which will decrease reactivity. The additional alkyl groups in these other choices also donate electron density to the carbonyl carbon, making it slightly less electrophilic.

4. **C**

This question requires knowledge of the nomenclature of cyclic molecules. A $\delta$-lactam, **(A)**, has a bond between the nitrogen and the fourth carbon away from the carbonyl carbon. This ring will have six elements: the nitrogen, the carbonyl carbon, and the four carbons in between. Cyclohexane carboxylic acid, **(B)**, has cyclohexane, a six-membered cycloalkane. The anhydride formed from pentanedioic acid, **(D)**, will have the five carbons in the parent chain and one oxygen atom closing the ring, meaning there are still six elements. $\gamma$-butyrolactone will have five elements because it contains a bond between the ester oxygen and the third carbon away from the carbonyl carbon. The five elements will be the oxygen, the carbonyl carbon, and the three carbons in between.

5. **D**

With the same R groups, steric influence is the same in each case, so we can therefore rely solely on electronic effects. When this is all that is taken into account, reactivity toward nucleophiles is highest for anhydrides, followed by esters and carboxylic acids, then amides.

6. **C**

Anhydrides, particularly cyclic anhydrides, will form spontaneously from dicarboxylic acids when heated.

7. **A**

Methylamine would react readily to form an amide. The less substituted the nucleophile, the easier it will be for the nucleophile to attack the carbonyl carbon and form the amide. In fact, triethylamine, **(B)**, would not be able to form an amide at all because it does not have a hydrogen to lose while attaching to the carbonyl carbon.

8. **A**

Propanamide is an amide; as such, it is the least reactive of the carboxylic acid derivatives discussed in this chapter. Without a strong acid or base, propanamide will not be able to undergo nucleophilic acyl substitution and no reaction will occur.

9. **D**

$\beta$-lactams are amides in the form of four-membered rings; amides are generally the least reactive type of carboxylic acid derivative. $\beta$-lactams experience significant ring strain from both eclipsing interactions (torsional strain) and angle strain and are therefore more susceptible to hydrolysis than the linear form of the same molecule.

10. **C**

As far as we can tell, we are converting one ester to another in this reaction. The fact that this reaction is acid-catalyzed should confirm the suspicion that this is a transesterification reaction.

11. **B**

This reaction, which is the hydrolysis of an amide, is favored in strong acid. Acid protonates the carbonyl oxygen, which increases the electrophilicity of the carbonyl carbon. This allows water to serve as the nucleophile, attacking the bond and hydrolyzing the molecule.

12. **D**

This molecule is more stable with a positive charge than a straight-chain alkane due to the conjugation of the benzene ring. This permits delocalization of the charge through resonance. Although induction, **(C)**, does have an effect on the stabilization of the molecule, this effect is much less significant than the impact of having a conjugated system. The electronegativity of nitrogen, **(B)**, which primarily affects induction, is also not a vital component of the stabilization by this molecule of a positive charge because oxygen is more electronegative. Steric hindrance, **(A)**, would affect the reactivity of a molecule, but not its ability to stabilize charge.

13. **D**

The molecule shown, $\gamma$-nonalactone, is a cyclic ester, also called a lactone. This molecule could arise from intramolecular attack in a $\gamma$-hydroxycarboxylic acid.

14. **A**

In order to prepare butyl acetate from butanol, we need to perform a nucleophilic acyl substitution reaction. If the product is an ester, we need to start with a reactant that is more reactive than the ester itself, or the reaction will not proceed. Anhydrides are more reactive than esters, but amides are less reactive, eliminating **(C)** and **(D)**. Reaction with propanoic anhydride, as in **(B)**, would result in butyl propanoate.

15. **D**

The presence of water in an esterification reaction would likely revert some of the desired esters back into carboxylic acids. Small carboxylic acids, like formic or acetic acid, are easily dissolved in water, eliminating **(A)**. The polarity of water plays little role in affecting the leaving group; if anything, water can be used to increase the electrophilicity of the carbonyl carbon by protonating the carbonyl oxygen—eliminating **(B)**. Finally, this is a nucleophilic substitution mechanism, not a nucleophilic addition mechanism, as mentioned in **(C)**. Further, hydrogen bonding would likely augment the reaction.

**GO ONLINE**
**Consult your online resources for additional practice.**

## SHARED CONCEPTS

**Biochemistry Chapter 11**
Lipid and Amino Acid Metabolism

**Organic Chemistry Chapter 1**
Nomenclature

**Organic Chemistry Chapter 3**
Bonding

**Organic Chemistry Chapter 4**
Analyzing Organic Reactions

**Organic Chemistry Chapter 6**
Aldehydes and Ketones I

**Organic Chemistry Chapter 8**
Carboxylic Acids

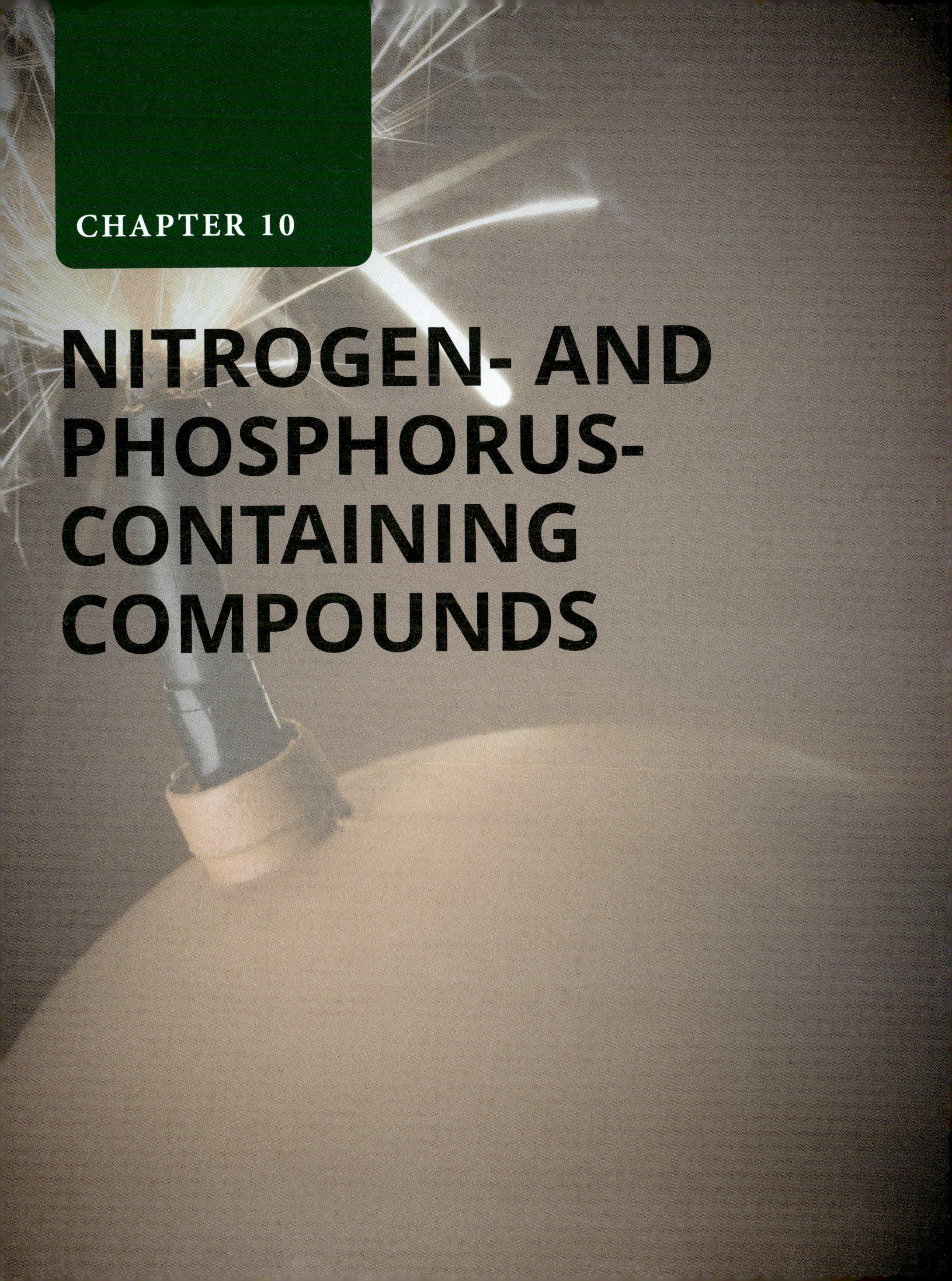

CHAPTER 10

# NITROGEN- AND PHOSPHORUS-CONTAINING COMPOUNDS

# SCIENCE MASTERY ASSESSMENT

Every pre-med knows this feeling: there is so much content I have to know for the MCAT! How do I know what to do first or what's important?

While the high-yield badges throughout this book will help you identify the most important topics, this Science Mastery Assessment is another tool in your MCAT prep arsenal. This quiz (which can also be taken in your online resources) and the guidance below will help ensure that you are spending the appropriate amount of time on this chapter based on your personal strengths and weaknesses. Don't worry though—skipping something now does not mean you'll never study it. Later on in your prep, as you complete full-length tests, you'll uncover specific pieces of content that you need to review and can come back to these chapters as appropriate.

## How to Use This Assessment

**If you answer 0–7 questions correctly:**

Spend about 1 hour to read this chapter in full and take limited notes throughout. Follow up by reviewing **all** quiz questions to ensure that you now understand how to solve each one.

**If you answer 8–11 questions correctly:**

Spend 20–40 minutes reviewing the quiz questions. Beginning with the questions you missed, read and take notes on the corresponding subchapters. For questions you answered correctly, ensure your thinking matches that of the explanation and you understand why each choice was correct or incorrect.

**If you answer 12–15 questions correctly:**

Spend less than 20 minutes reviewing all questions from the quiz. If you missed any, then include a quick read-through of the corresponding subchapters, or even just the relevant content within a subchapter, as part of your question review. For questions you got correct, ensure your thinking matches that of the explanation and review the Concept Summary at the end of the chapter.

1. Which of the following amino acids does not have an l-enantiomer?
   - **A.** Cysteine
   - **B.** Threonine
   - **C.** Glutamic acid
   - **D.** Glycine

2. Which of the following would be formed if methyl bromide were reacted with phthalimide and followed by hydrolysis with an aqueous base?
   - **A.** $C_2H_5NH_2$
   - **B.** $CH_3NH_2$
   - **C.** $(C_2H_5)_3N$
   - **D.** $(CH_3)_4N^+Br^-$

3. Which of the following amino acids contain(s) sulfur?
   - **I.** Cysteine
   - **II.** Serine
   - **III.** Methionine
   - **A.** I only
   - **B.** I and III only
   - **C.** II and III only
   - **D.** I, II, and III

4. Nylon, a polyamide, is produced from hexanediamine and a substance, *X*. This substance, *X*, is most probably a(n):
   - **A.** amine.
   - **B.** carboxylic acid.
   - **C.** ketone.
   - **D.** alcohol.

5. Intermediates in the Strecker synthesis include all of the following nitrogen-containing functional groups EXCEPT a(n):
   - **A.** nitrile.
   - **B.** imine.
   - **C.** amide.
   - **D.** amine.

6. A biochemist is synthesizing valine, shown below, using the Strecker synthesis. Which of the following carbonyl-containing compounds would be an appropriate starting reactant in this synthesis?

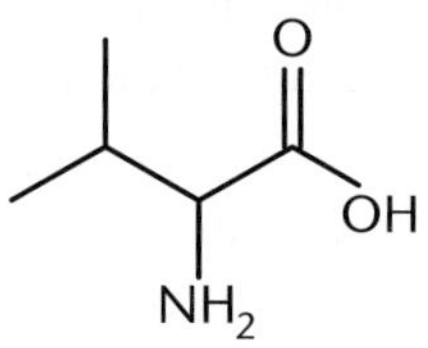


   - **A.** 2-Propanone
   - **B.** Propanal
   - **C.** 2-Methylpropanal
   - **D.** Butanal

7. Why is the C–N bond of an amide planar?
   - **I.** It has partial double-bond character.
   - **II.** It is $sp^3$-hybridized.
   - **III.** It has some $sp^2$ character.
   - **A.** I only
   - **B.** II only
   - **C.** I and II only
   - **D.** I and III only

8. Which of the primary methods of amino acid synthesis results in an optically active solution?
   - **A.** The Strecker synthesis only
   - **B.** The Gabriel synthesis only
   - **C.** Both the Strecker and Gabriel syntheses
   - **D.** Neither the Strecker nor the Gabriel syntheses

9. During the Gabriel synthesis, phthalimide serves as the:
   - **A.** nucleophile.
   - **B.** base.
   - **C.** leaving group.
   - **D.** electrophile.

10. Each of the following reaction types occurs during the Gabriel synthesis EXCEPT:
    - **A.** decarboxylation.
    - **B.** nucleophilic substitution.
    - **C.** dehydration.
    - **D.** hydrolysis.

11. At physiological pH, which two forms of phosphoric acid have the highest concentrations?
    - **A.** $H_3PO_4$ and $H_2PO_4^-$
    - **B.** $H_2PO_4^-$ and $HPO_4^{2-}$
    - **C.** $HPO_4^{2-}$ and $PO_4^{3-}$
    - **D.** $PO_4^{3-}$ and $H_3PO_4$

12. In aqueous solution, pyrophosphate will likely:
    - **A.** form insoluble complexes.
    - **B.** be stable and inert.
    - **C.** degrade into inorganic phosphate.
    - **D.** decrease the polarity of the solvent.

13. What would be the charge of aspartic acid at pH 7?
    - **A.** Neutral
    - **B.** Negative
    - **C.** Positive
    - **D.** There is not enough information to answer the question.

14. When a bond is created between two nucleotide triphosphates in DNA synthesis, the small molecule released from this reaction is:
    - **A.** pyrophosphate.
    - **B.** inorganic phosphate.
    - **C.** ATP.
    - **D.** organic phosphate.

15. The hydrogens of phosphoric acid have $pK_a$ values that:
    - **A.** allow high buffering capacity over a small pH range.
    - **B.** allow moderate buffering capacity over a large pH range.
    - **C.** allow low buffering capacity over a small pH range.
    - **D.** do not allow buffering.

## Answer Key

1. **D** (See section 10.1)
2. **B** (See section 10.2)
3. **B** (See section 10.1)
4. **B** (See section 10.2)
5. **C** (See section 10.2)
6. **C** (See section 10.1)
7. **D** (See section 10.1)
8. **D** (See section 10.2)
9. **A** (See section 10.2)
10. **C** (See section 10.2)
11. **B** (See section 10.3)
12. **C** (See section 10.3)
13. **B** (See section 10.1)
14. **A** (See section 10.3)
15. **B** (See section 10.3)

*The relevant section of the chapter to review for each question is given in parentheses after the correct answer. Detailed explanations can be found at the end of the chapter.*

CHAPTER 10

# NITROGEN- AND PHOSPHORUS-CONTAINING COMPOUNDS

## In This Chapter



### CHAPTER PROFILE

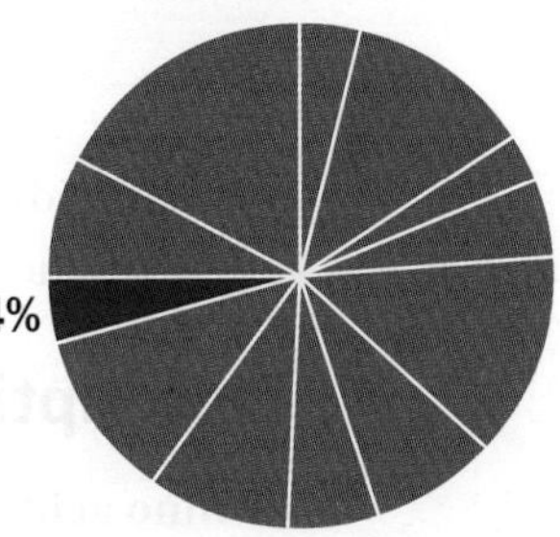

4%

The content in this chapter should be relevant to about 4% of all questions about organic chemistry on the MCAT.

This chapter covers material from the following AAMC content categories:

**1A:** Structure and function of proteins and their constituent amino acids

**5D:** Structure, function, and reactivity of biologically-relevant molecules

## Introduction

Organic chemistry is the study of carbon-containing molecules. But as you've seen, carbon is not the only element that plays a role in organic molecules; many of the functional groups we've explored up until this point also include hydrogen and oxygen. Together, these three elements make up 93% of the composition of the human body by weight. But other atoms also contribute to biomolecules: nitrogen comprises 3.2% of body weight and phosphorus 1.0%.

In this chapter, we'll take a look at some biologically important molecules that contain nitrogen and phosphorus. In addition to the amides explored in the previous chapter, amino acids also contain nitrogen. These building blocks of proteins are discussed in depth in Chapter 1 of *MCAT Biochemistry Review*; in this chapter, we review their structure and focus on laboratory methods for synthesizing amino acids. Finally, we turn our attention to phosphorus-containing molecules, which often are used to transfer energy—or store genetic information.

### MCAT EXPERTISE

Note that, even though biological molecules—amino acids, proteins, and DNA—are called out in this chapter, the low percentage rating for this chapter only applies to non-biochemical reactions of these molecules. Mastery of these molecules in biological settings is still very important for Test Day success; that content is found in Chapters 1, 2, 3, 6, and 7 of *MCAT Biochemistry Review*.

## 10.1 Amino Acids, Peptides, and Proteins

**LEARNING OBJECTIVES**

After Chapter 10.1, you will be able to:

- Identify the functional groups that make amino acids amphoteric
- Recall the mechanisms for forming and cleaving peptide bonds
- Explain why the C–N bond of an amide is planar
- Recall the unique properties of glycine:

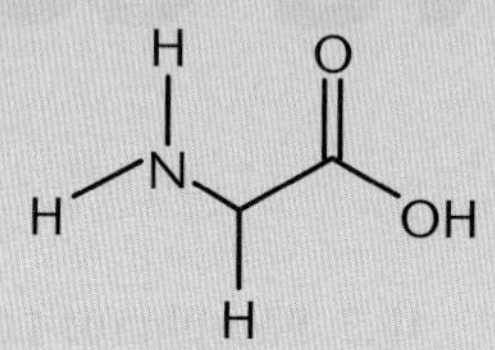

Amino acids are dipolar molecules that come together through a condensation reaction, forming peptides. Larger, folded peptide chains are considered proteins.

### Description

**Amino acids** contain an amino group and a carboxyl group attached to a single carbon atom (the $\alpha$-carbon). The other two substituents of the $\alpha$-carbon are a hydrogen atom and a side chain referred to as the **R group**. This structure is shown in Figure 10.1.

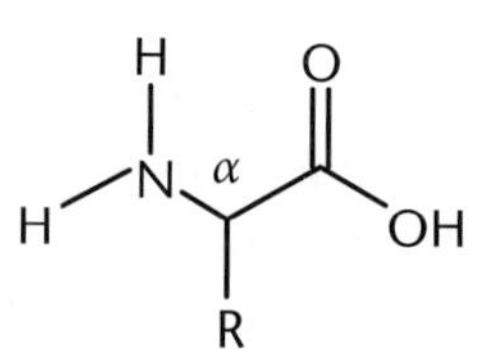

**Figure 10.1** Amino Acid Structure

The $\alpha$-carbon, with its four different groups, is a chiral (stereogenic) center. **Glycine**, the simplest amino acid, is an exception to this rule because its R group is a hydrogen atom. All naturally occurring amino acids in eukaryotes—except for glycine—are optically active, and all are l-isomers. Therefore, by convention, the Fischer projection for an amino acid is drawn with the amino group on the left, as shown in Figure 10.2. l-amino acids have (*S*) configurations, except for **cysteine**, which is (*R*) because of the change in priority caused by the sulfur in its R group.

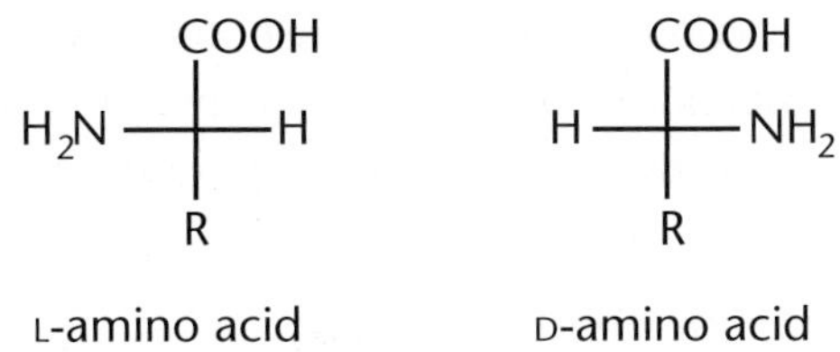


**Figure 10.2** L- and D-Amino Acids

## Properties

Amino acids, with their acidic carboxyl group and basic amino group, are **amphoteric** molecules. That is, they can act as both acids and bases. Amino groups can take on a positive charge by being protonated, and carboxyl groups can take on negative charges by being deprotonated. When an amino acid is put into solution, it will take on both of these charges, forming a dipolar ion or **zwitterion,** as shown in Figure 10.3. How an amino acid acts depends on the pH of the environment. In basic solutions, the amino acid can become fully deprotonated; in acidic solutions, it can become fully protonated.

**BRIDGE**

Amino acids are amphoteric molecules, just like water—they can act as both acids and bases. These acid–base characteristics (and titrations of amino acids) are discussed thoroughly in Chapter 1 of *MCAT Biochemistry Review.*

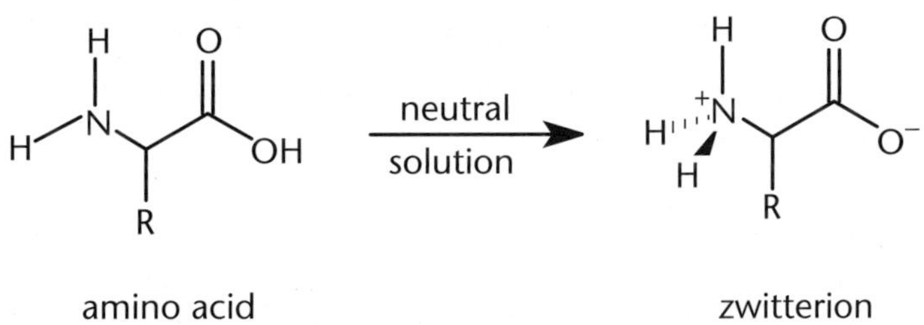


**Figure 10.3** Amino Acids Exist as Zwitterions (Dipolar Ions) at Neutral pH

Aside from the zwitterionic properties common to every amino acid, each one has properties defined by its R group, or side chain. The 20 eukaryotic proteogenic amino acids are grouped into five categories: **nonpolar nonaromatic**, **aromatic**, **polar**, **negatively charged** (**acidic**), and **positively charged** (**basic**). Nonpolar nonaromatic amino acids tend to have side chains that are saturated hydrocarbons, like alanine, valine, leucine, and isoleucine; they also include glycine, proline (which is cyclic, with a secondary amine), and methionine (which contains sulfur). Aromatic amino acids include tryptophan, phenylalanine, and tyrosine. Nonpolar amino acids—both nonaromatic and aromatic—are also hydrophobic and tend to be sequestered in the interior of proteins. Polar amino acids tend to have terminal groups containing oxygen, nitrogen, or sulfur. These include serine, threonine, asparagine, glutamine, and cysteine. Negatively charged (acidic) amino acids include aspartic acid and glutamic acid. These amino acids have terminal carboxylate anions in their R groups. Finally, positively charged (basic) amino acids, including arginine, lysine, and histidine, have a protonated amino group in their R groups. Polar, acidic, and basic amino acids are all hydrophilic and tend to form hydrogen bonds with water in aqueous solution.

Amino acids undergo condensation reactions to form **peptide bonds**. The molecules these bonds form, called **polypeptides**, are the base unit of **proteins**. The reverse reaction, hydrolysis of the peptide bond, is catalyzed by a strong acid or base. Both of these reactions are shown in Figure 10.4.

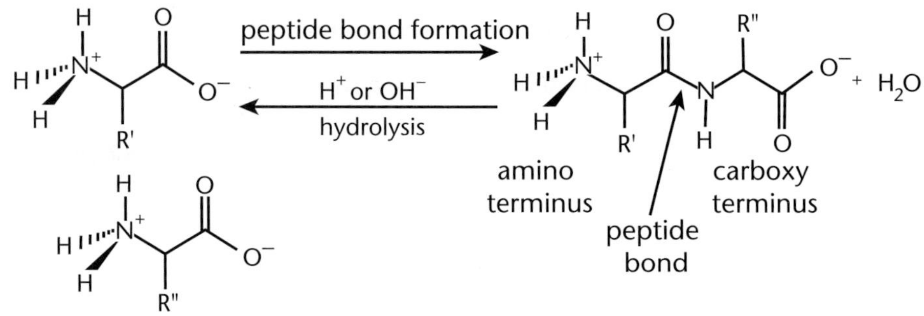


**Figure 10.4** Peptide Bond Formation and Cleavage

Like other carbonyl-containing functional groups, amides have two resonance structures, as shown in Figure 10.5. The true structure of the amide bond is therefore a hybrid of these two structures, with partial double-bond character between the nitrogen atom and the carbonyl carbon. This double-bond character limits rotation about the C—N bond, which adds to the rigidity and stability of the backbone of proteins. The single bonds on either side of the peptide bond, on the other hand, permit free rotation.

**KEY CONCEPT**

Rotation is limited around the peptide bond because resonance gives the C—N bond partial double-bond character.

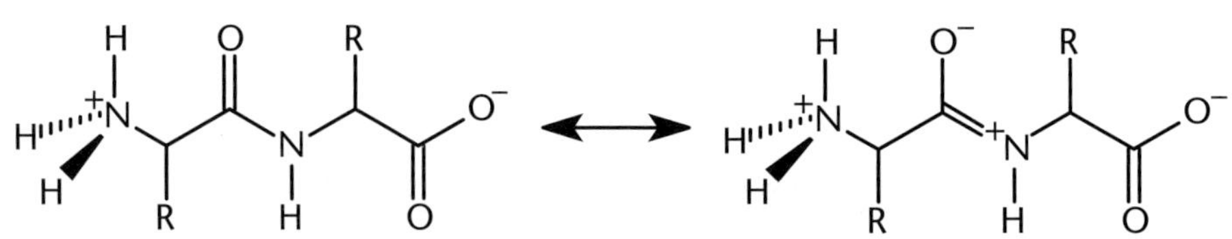

**Figure 10.5** Resonance in the Peptide Bond

## Heterocyclic Compounds

While not confined to amino acids and proteins, heterocyclic compounds are another class of molecules to know for Test Day that often contains nitrogen. Heterocyclic compounds are cyclic organic compounds containing atoms of at least two different elements in their ring(s), with at least one non-carbon atom in the ring. This is typically nitrogen (N), oxygen (O), or sulfur (S). Several examples of heterocyclic compounds can be seen in Figure 10.6 with a description of these compounds in the following paragraphs.

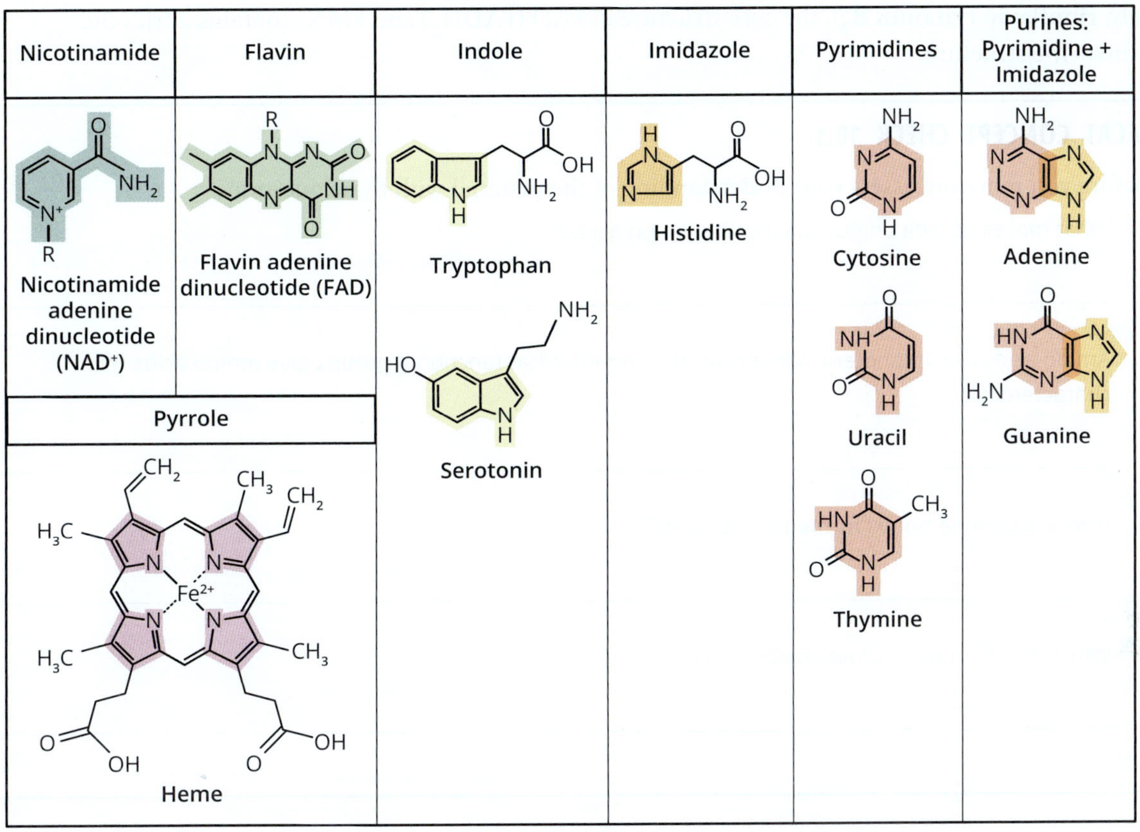


**Figure 10.6** Heterocyclic Ring Structures Found in Biological Molecules

## Nitrogenous Bases in DNA and RNA

The most important heterocycles for the MCAT form the nitrogenous bases of DNA and RNA, the purines and pyrimidines. These are biological aromatic heterocycles.

**Purines** contain a bicyclic structure—a six-membered ring fused to a five-membered ring—and include adenine (A) and guanine (G).

**Pyrimidines** contain a single six-membered ring and include cytosine (C) and thymine (T), both of which are found in DNA, along with uracil (U), found in RNA.

## Other Heterocycles

**Imidazole** is a five-membered ring with 2 N atoms, found in the amino acid histidine. Classified as a basic amino acid, histidine's side chain contains an imidazole ring, which can be protonated at physiological pH. However, for MCAT purposes, histidine is considered neutral. Imidazole is also found in histamine and **biotin (vitamin $B_7$)**, which contains fused tetrahydrothiophene and imidazole rings.

**Pyrrole** is a five-membered ring with 1 N atom. Four pyrrole rings linked together form the **porphyrin** macrocycle, which chelates a metal ion. **Heme** (in hemoglobin) is a porphyrin that contains $Fe^{2+}$.

**Indole** is a bicyclic compound containing benzene and pyrrole. The indole ring forms the side chain of the aromatic amino acid tryptophan and is also found in serotonin.

**Pyridine** is a six-membered ring with 1 N atom. The pyridine ring is part of the nicotinamide structure in $NAD^+$.

Finally, **riboflavin (vitamin $B_2$)**, the core structure of FAD ($FADH_2$) and FMN, contains a tricyclic **isoalloxazine** structure.

### MCAT CONCEPT CHECK 10.1

Before you move on, assess your understanding of the material with these questions.

1. What makes glycine unique among the amino acids?

 ___

2. Amino acids are amphoteric. What does this mean? What functional groups give amino acids this characteristic?

 ___

3. How are peptide bonds formed and cleaved?

 ___

4. Why is the C—N bond of an amide planar?

 ___

## 10.2 Synthesis of α-Amino Acids

### LEARNING OBJECTIVES

After Chapter 10.2, you will be able to:

- Recall the required reactants and product types for the Strecker and Gabriel synthesis reactions
- Identify the reaction types found in the Strecker and Gabriel synthesis reactions

Synthesis of amino acids occurs by an astonishing variety of mechanisms *in vivo*. In the lab, several simple reaction mechanisms are exploited to make amino acids neatly and efficiently.

### Strecker Synthesis

In the **Strecker synthesis**, one starts with an aldehyde, ammonium chloride ($NH_4Cl$), and potassium cyanide (KCN), as shown in Figure 10.7. The carbonyl oxygen is protonated, increasing the electrophilicity of the carbonyl carbon. Then, as seen in Chapter 6 of *MCAT Organic Chemistry Review*, ammonia can attack the carbonyl carbon, forming an **imine**. The imine carbon is also susceptible to nucleophilic addition reactions; thus, the $CN^-$ anion from KCN attacks, forming a **nitrile** group ($-C{\equiv}N$). The final molecule at the end of Step 1 is an **aminonitrile**—a compound containing an amino group ($-NH_2$) and a nitrile group.

**MNEMONIC**

Ni**tri**les have a **tri**ple bond between nitrogen and carbon.

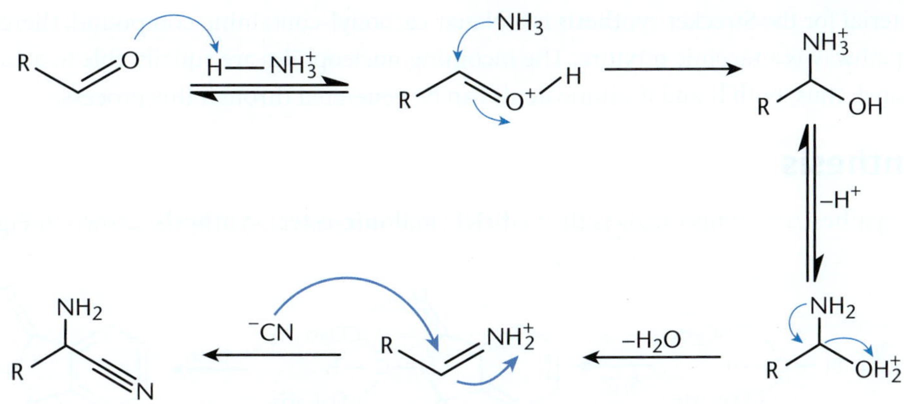


**Figure 10.7** Strecker Synthesis: Step 1
*An aminonitrile is generated from an aldehyde or ketone.*

In Step 2, the nitrile nitrogen is protonated, increasing the electrophilicity of the nitrile carbon. This is similar to protonating the oxygen of a carbonyl. A water molecule attacks, leading to the creation of a molecule with both imine and hydroxyl moieties on the same carbon. This imine is attacked by another equivalent of water. A carbonyl is formed, kicking off ammonia and creating the carboxylic acid functionality. This step, shown in Figure 10.8, is performed in aqueous acid and can be accelerated by the use of heat.

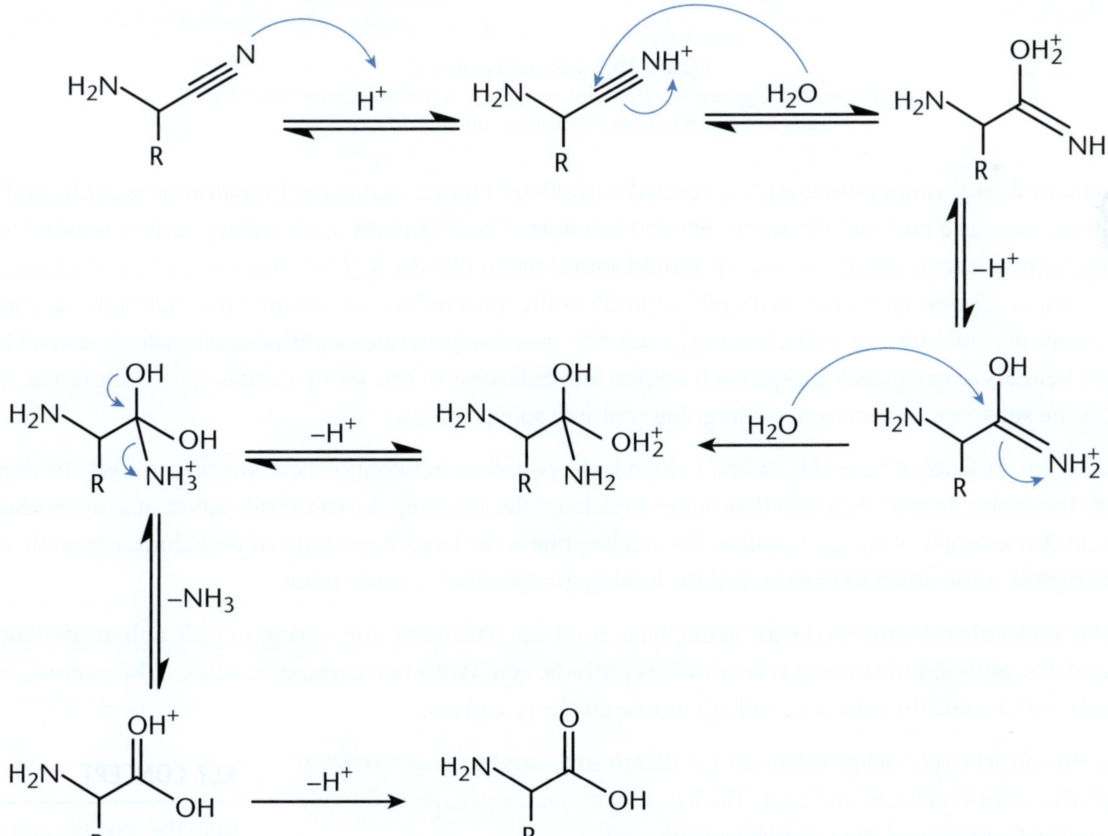


**Figure 10.8** Strecker Synthesis: Step 2
*An amino acid is generated from the aminonitrile.*

The starting material for the Strecker synthesis is a planar carbonyl-containing compound; therefore, the product of this pathway is a racemic mixture. The incoming nucleophiles are equally able to attack from either side of the carbonyl; thus, both l- and d-amino acids can be generated through this process.

## Gabriel Synthesis

Another way of synthesizing amino acids is the **Gabriel (malonic-ester) synthesis**, shown in Figure 10.9.

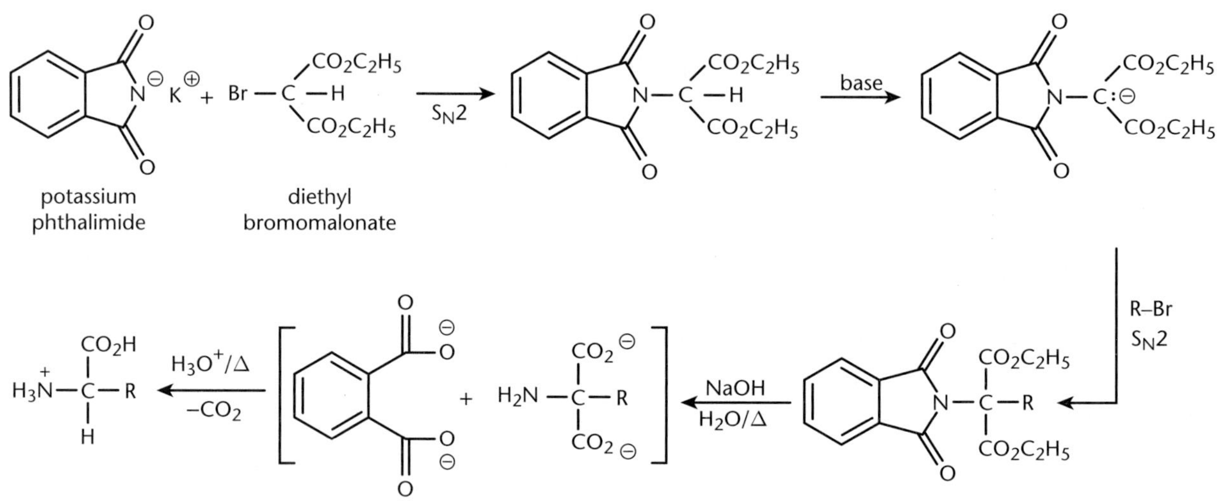


**Figure 10.9** Gabriel Synthesis
*An amino acid is generated from phthalimide and diethyl bromomalonate, using two $S_N2$ reactions, hydrolysis, and decarboxylation.*

In this method, potassium phthalimide is reacted with diethyl bromomalonate. Phthalimide is acidic and exists in solution as a nucleophilic anion. Diethyl bromomalonate contains a secondary carbon bonded to bromine, a good leaving group. This setup should sound much like the $S_N2$ reactions discussed in Chapter 4 of *MCAT Organic Chemistry Review*. With phthalimide as the nucleophile, the (secondary) substrate carbon as the electrophile, and bromine as the leaving group, this reaction generates a phthalimidomalonic ester. Consider the benefits of using such a large nucleophile. The bulkiness of this group creates steric hindrance, which prevents the substrate carbon from undergoing multiple substitutions.

Instead, in the presence of base, this carbon (which is the $\alpha$-carbon between two carbonyls) can easily be deprotonated. The molecule as a whole can then act as a nucleophile, attacking the substrate carbon of a bromoalkane. This is another example of an $S_N2$ reaction. The nucleophile is the large, deprotonated phthalimidomalonic ester, the electrophile is the substrate carbon, and the leaving group is the bromide anion.

Next, this molecule is hydrolyzed with strong base and heat. Much like converting a cyclic anhydride into a dioic acid, the phthalimide moiety is removed as phthalic acid (with two carboxylic acids). The malonic ester is hydrolyzed to a dicarboxylic acid with an amine on the $\alpha$-carbon.

Finally, this dicarboxylic acid, which is a 1,3-dicarbonyl, can be decarboxylated through the addition of acid and heat. The loss of a molecule of carbon dioxide results in the formation of the complete amino acid.

Like the Strecker synthesis, the Gabriel synthesis starts with a planar molecule; thus, the product is a racemic mixture of l- and d-amino acids.

**KEY CONCEPT**

Both the Strecker and Gabriel synthesis methods result in a racemic mixture of amino acids.

## MCAT CONCEPT CHECK 10.2

Before you move on, assess your understanding of the material with these questions.

1. What are the four reactant in the Strecker synthesis of an amino acid?

    - ______________________________
    - ______________________________
    - ______________________________
    - ______________________________

2. What are the reaction types used in the Strecker synthesis?

    ______________________________

3. What are the four main reactants in the Gabriel synthesis of an amino acid?

    - ______________________________
    - ______________________________
    - ______________________________
    - ______________________________

4. What are the reactions types used in the Gabriel synthesis?

    ______________________________

## 10.3 Phosphorus-Containing Compounds

### LEARNING OBJECTIVES

After Chapter 10.3, you will be able to:

- Recognize the traits that make inorganic phosphate a useful molecule for energy transfer
- Explain why phosphoric acids are good buffers
- Recall what makes a molecule an organic phosphate

**Phosphoric acid** is an extremely important molecule biochemically. This molecule forms the high-energy bonds that carry energy in adenosine triphosphate (ATP).

## Description

In a biochemical context, phosphoric acid is sometimes referred to as a **phosphate group** or **inorganic phosphate**, denoted $\mathbf{P_i}$. At physiological pH, inorganic phosphate includes molecules of both hydrogen phosphate ($HPO_4^{2-}$) and dihydrogen phosphate ($H_2PO_4^-$).

In addition to the energy-carrying nucleotide phosphates, phosphorus is also found in the backbone of DNA in **phosphodiester** bonds linking the sugar moieties of the nucleotides, as shown in Figure 10.10.

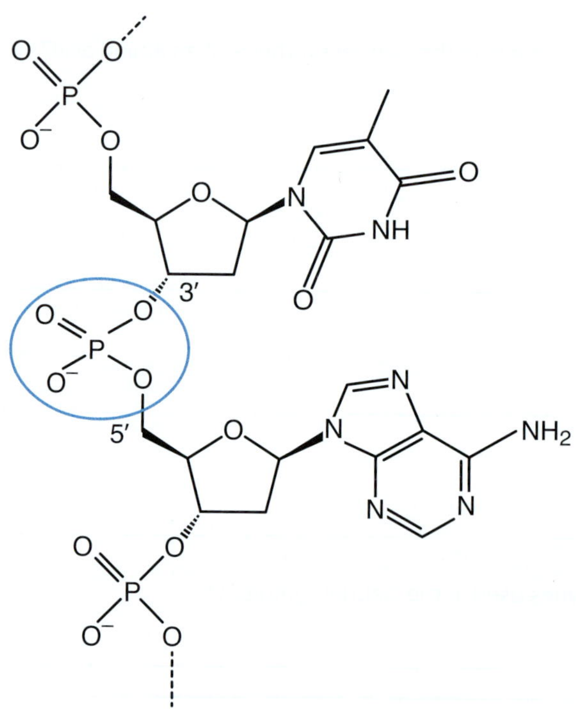


**Figure 10.10** Phosphodiester Bond in DNA

When a new nucleotide is joined to a growing strand of DNA by a *DNA polymerase*, it releases an ester dimer of phosphate, referred to as **pyrophosphate** ($P_2O_7^{4-}$), denoted **$PP_i$**, and shown in Figure 10.11.

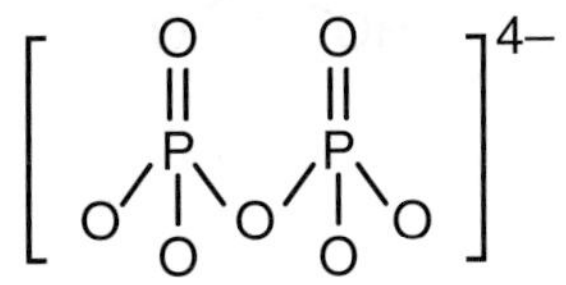

**Figure 10.11** Pyrophosphate Anion

The hydrolytic release of this molecule provides the energy for the formation of the new phosphodiester bond. Pyrophosphate is unstable in aqueous solution and is hydrolyzed to form two molecules of inorganic phosphate (Figure 10.12), which can then be recycled to form high-energy bonds in ATP or for other purposes.

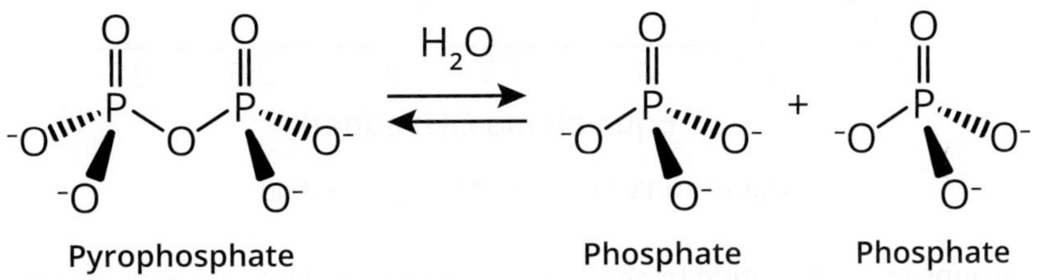


**Figure 10.12** Hydrolysis of Phosphate

Nucleotides, such ATP, GTP, and those in DNA, are referred to as **organic phosphates** due to the presence of the phosphate group bonded to a carbon-containing molecule.

## Properties

Phosphoric acid is unique in that it has three acidic hydrogens, each with its own p$K_a$. Phosphoric acid most properly refers to the form that predominates in strongly acidic conditions, $H_3PO_4$. In mildly acidic conditions, it loses a proton to become dihydrogen phosphate, $H_2PO_4^-$; it will readily lose a second proton to become hydrogen phosphate, $HPO_4^{2-}$ in weakly basic solutions. The form that exists in strongly basic solutions is phosphate, $PO_4^{3-}$. The p$K_a$ for the loss of the first hydrogen is 2.15; for the second, 7.20; and for the third, 12.32 (see Figure 10.13). At a physiological pH of 7.4, this means that dihydrogen phosphate and hydrogen phosphate predominate in nearly equal proportions. This variety of p$K_a$ values also makes phosphates good buffers because they can pick up or give off protons depending on the pH of the solution.

**BRIDGE**

DNA replication is an important process for the MCAT. Nucleotide triphosphates are added to the growing daughter strand with the release of pyrophosphate, $PP_i$. The process of DNA synthesis is described in Chapter 6 of *MCAT Biochemistry Review*.

**KEY CONCEPT**

Phosphoric acid is an excellent buffer because it has three hydrogens with p$K_a$ values that span nearly the entire pH scale.

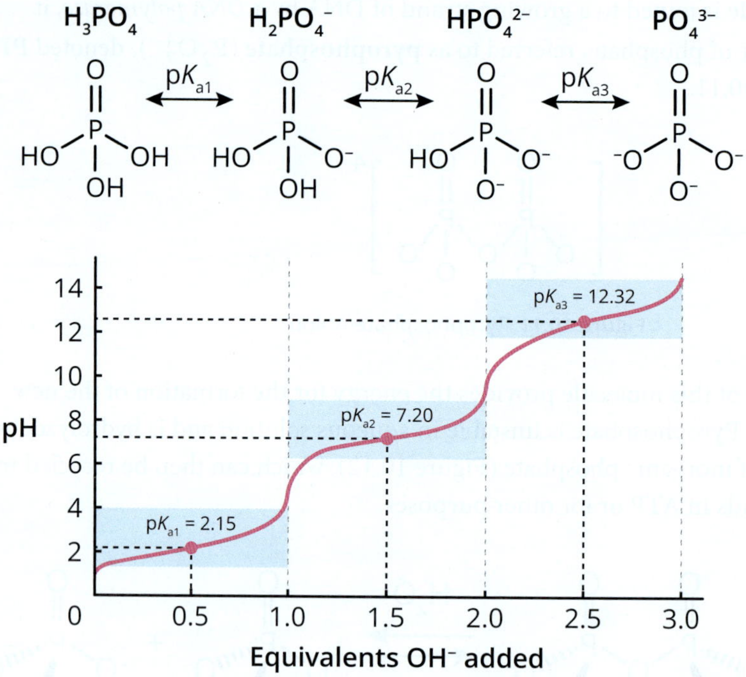


**Figure 10.13** Titration of Phosphoric Acid

Adjacent phosphate groups on a nucleotide triphosphate experience a large amount of repulsion because they are negatively charged. This, combined with the ability of phosphate to stabilize up to three negative charges by resonance, means that the energy released when a phosphate or pyrophosphate is cleaved is quite high.

## MCAT CONCEPT CHECK 10.3

Before you move on, assess your understanding of the material with these questions.

1. What characteristics make inorganic phosphate so useful for energy transfer biologically?

_______________

2. What is an organic phosphate?

_______________

3. What characteristics of phosphoric acids make them good buffers?

_______________

## Conclusion

In this chapter, we spent a lot of time looking at biologically active molecules—but did you notice that these molecules are simply applications of the general principles that we have been learning throughout the chapters of this book? By applying your knowledge of the reactions and properties of different types of molecules, you can understand how biological processes work and how complex organic chemistry mechanisms work, like those of the Strecker and Gabriel syntheses. Many of these processes will fall into categories of reactions that we've seen before over and over—nucleophilic substitution, nucleophilic addition, and condensation reactions are just a few examples. The MCAT doesn't require you to memorize tables of reactants or regurgitate hundreds of named reactions from scratch. Instead, the MCAT asks you to look at the bigger picture and understand the trends—which you've now learned!

**GO ONLINE**

**You've reviewed the content, now test your knowledge and critical thinking skills by completing a test-like passage set in your online resources!**

# CONCEPT SUMMARY

## Amino Acids, Peptides, and Proteins

- The $\alpha$-carbon of an amino acid is attached to four groups: an amino group, a carboxyl group, a hydrogen atom, and an **R group**. It is a chiral stereocenter in all amino acids except **glycine**.
- All amino acids in eukaryotes are l-amino acids. They all have (*S*) stereochemistry except **cysteine**, which is (*R*).
- Amino acids are **amphoteric**, meaning they can act as acids or bases.
  - Amino acids get their acidic characteristics from carboxylic acids and their basic characteristics from amino groups.
  - In a neutral solution, amino acids tend to exist as **zwitterions** (dipolar ions).
- Amino acids can be classified by their R groups.
  - **Nonpolar nonaromatic amino acids** include alanine, valine, leucine, isoleucine, glycine, proline, and methionine.
  - **Aromatic amino acids** include tryptophan, phenylalanine, and tyrosine. Both nonpolar nonaromatic and aromatic amino acids tend to be hydrophobic and reside in the interior of proteins.
  - **Polar amino acids** include serine, threonine, asparagine, glutamine, and cysteine.
  - **Negatively charged amino acids** contain carboxylic acids in their R groups and include aspartic acid and glutamic acid.
  - **Positively charged amino acids** contain amines in their R groups and include arginine, lysine, and histidine.
  - Nonpolar nonaromatic and aromatic amino acids tend to be hydrophobic and reside in the interior of proteins.
  - Polar, negatively charged (acidic), and positively charged (basic) amino acids tend to be hydrophilic and reside on the surface of proteins, making hydrogen bonds with the aqueous environment.
- **Peptide bonds** form by condensation reactions and can be cleaved hydrolytically.
  - Resonance of the peptide bond restricts motion about the C—N bond, which takes on partial double-bond character.
  - Strong acid or base is needed to cleave a peptide bond.
- **Polypeptides** are made up of multiple amino acids linked by peptide bonds. **Proteins** are large, folded, functional polypeptides.

## Synthesis of α-Amino Acids

- Biologically, amino acids are synthesized in many ways. In the lab, certain standardized mechanisms are used.
- The **Strecker synthesis** generates an amino acid from an aldehyde.
  - An aldehyde is mixed with ammonium chloride ($NH_4Cl$) and potassium cyanide. The ammonia attacks the carbonyl carbon, generating an imine. The imine is then attacked by the cyanide, generating an aminonitrile.
  - The aminonitrile is hydrolyzed by two equivalents of water, generating an amino acid.
- The **Gabriel synthesis** generates an amino acid from potassium phthalimide, diethyl bromomalonate, and an alkyl halide.
  - Phthalimide attacks the diethyl bromomalonate, generating a phthalimidomalonic ester.
  - The phthalimidomalonic ester attacks an alkyl halide, adding an alkyl group to the ester.
  - The product is hydrolyzed, creating phthalic acid (with two carboxyl groups) and converting the esters into carboxylic acids.
  - One carboxylic acid of the resulting 1,3-dicarbonyl is removed by decarboxylation.

## Phosphorus-Containing Compounds

- Phosphorus is found in **inorganic phosphate ($P_i$)**, a buffered mixture of hydrogen phosphate ($HPO_4^{2-}$) and dihydrogen phosphate ($H_2PO_4^-$).
- Phosphorus is found in the backbone of DNA, which uses **phosphodiester bonds**. In forming these bonds, a **pyrophosphate ($PP_i$**, $P_2O_7^{4-}$) is released. Pyrophosphate can then be hydrolyzed to two inorganic phosphates.
- Phosphate bonds are high energy because of large negative charges in adjacent phosphate groups and resonance stabilization of phosphates.
- **Organic phosphates** are carbon-containing compounds that also have phosphate groups. The most notable examples are nucleotide triphosphates (such as ATP or GTP) and DNA.
- Phosphoric acid has three hydrogens, each with a unique p$K_a$. This wide variety in p$K_a$ values allows phosphoric acid to act as a buffer over a large range of pH values.

# ANSWERS TO CONCEPT CHECKS

## 10.1

1. All amino acids, except glycine, have chiral $\alpha$-carbons. Because the R group of glycine is a hydrogen atom, it is not chiral and therefore is not optically active.
2. Amphoteric molecules can act as acids or bases. Carboxylic acids give amino acids their acidic properties because they can be deprotonated. Amino groups give amino acids their basic properties because they can be protonated.
3. Peptide bonds are formed by a condensation reaction, in which water is lost, and cleaved hydrolytically by strong acid or base.
4. The C–N bond of an amide is planar because it has partial double-bond character due to resonance. Double bonds exist in a planar conformation and restrict movement.

## 10.2

1. An aldehyde, ammonium chloride ($NH_4Cl$), and potassium cyanide (KCN) are used to make the aminonitrile; water is used to hydrolyze the aminonitrile to form the amino acid.
2. Strecker synthesis is a condensation reaction (formation of an imine from a carbonyl-containing compound and ammonia, with loss of water), followed by nucleophilic addition (addition of the nitrile group), followed by hydrolysis.
3. Gabriel synthesis begins with potassium phthalimide and diethyl bromomalonate, followed by an alkyl halide. Water is then used to hydrolyze the resulting compound to form the amino acid. While acids and bases are used at various times as catalysts, they are not main reactants.
4. Gabriel synthesis proceeds through two $S_N2$ reactions, hydrolysis, and decarboxylation.

## 10.3

1. Inorganic phosphate contains a very negative charge. When bonded to other phosphate groups in a nucleotide triphosphate, this creates repulsion with adjacent phosphate groups, increasing the energy of the bond. Further, inorganic phosphate can be resonance-stabilized.
2. Organic phosphates are carbon-containing molecules with phosphate groups; the most common examples are nucleotides, like those in DNA, ATP, or GTP.
3. The three hydrogens in phosphoric acid have very different $pK_a$ values. This allows phosphoric acid to pick up or give off protons in a wide pH range, making it a good buffer over most of the pH scale.

## SCIENCE MASTERY ASSESSMENT EXPLANATIONS

1. **D**

Glycine's R group is a hydrogen atom; this amino acid is therefore achiral because the central carbon is not bonded to four different substituents. The other amino acids are all chiral and therefore have both l- and d-enantiomers.

2. **B**

This reaction is similar to the Gabriel synthesis. Phthalimide acts as a nucleophile, the methyl carbon acts as an electrophile, and bromide acts as the leaving group. Therefore, the reaction between methyl bromide and phthalimide results in the formation of methyl phthalimide. Subsequent hydrolysis then yields methylamine.

3. **B**

Cysteine is well known for containing a sulfur atom because it is able to form disulfide bridges; however, methionine also contains a sulfur atom in its R group.

4. **B**

An amide is formed from an amine and a carboxyl group or its acyl derivatives. In this question, an amine is already given; the compound to be identified must be an acyl compound. The only acyl compound among the choices given is a carboxylic acid.

5. **C**

During the Strecker synthesis, ammonia attacks a carbonyl, forming an imine, **(B)**. This imine is attacked by cyanide, forming an amine, **(D)**, and a nitrile, **(A)**. Amide bonds are formed between amino acids but do not appear during the Strecker synthesis.

6. **C**

The Strecker synthesis creates an amino acid from an aldehyde. The carbonyl carbon ultimately becomes the $\alpha$-carbon of the amino acid. Any remaining alkyl chain becomes the R group, as shown below. The starting compound is therefore 2-methylpropanal (isobutyraldehyde).

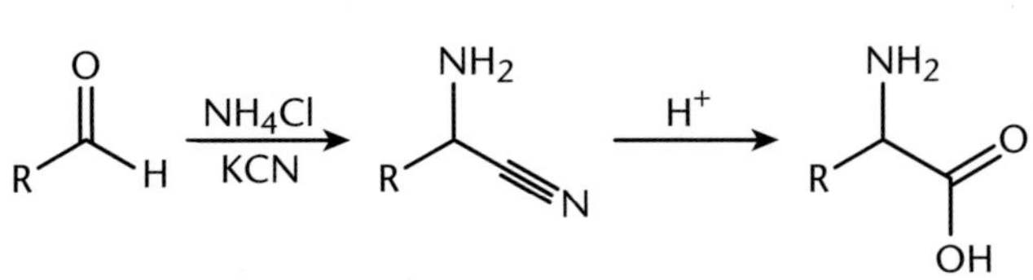


7. **D**

One resonance structure of a C—N bond in an amide has the double bond between the C and N, not between the C and O. Thus, the C—N bond of an amide has some $sp^2$ character, and $sp^2$-hybridized atoms exhibit planar geometry.

8. **D**

Both the Strecker and Gabriel syntheses contain planar intermediates, which can be attacked from either side by a nucleophile. This results in a racemic mixture of enantiomers, and the solution will therefore be optically inactive.

9. **A**

During the Gabriel synthesis, phthalimide attacks a secondary carbon in diethyl bromomalonate. The secondary carbon is the electrophile, **(D)**, and bromide is the leaving group, **(C)**.

10. **C**

The Gabriel synthesis includes two nucleophilic substitution steps, followed by hydrolysis and decarboxylation. Dehydration—the loss of a water molecule—is not a part of this reaction.

11. **B**

The $pK_{a2}$ of phosphoric acid is close to physiological pH; therefore, $[H_2PO_4^-] \approx [HPO_4^{2-}]$ at this pH.

12. **C**

Pyrophosphate is unstable in aqueous solution and will degrade to form two equivalents of inorganic phosphate. The solvent is water, which should retain its polarity regardless of the presence of solutes, eliminating **(D)**. Pyrophosphate and inorganic phosphate are small, charged molecules which are relatively soluble, eliminating **(A)**.

13. **B**

The amino acid in question is aspartic acid, which is an acidic amino acid because it contains an extra carboxyl group. At neutral pH, both of the carboxyl groups are ionized, so there are two negative charges on the molecule. Only one of the charges is neutralized by the positive charge on the amino group, so the molecule has an overall negative charge.

14. **A**

As DNA is synthesized, it forms phosphodiester bonds, releasing pyrophosphate, $PP_i$. Pyrophosphate is an inorganic phosphate-containing molecule, but it is not the single phosphate group commonly referred to as inorganic phosphate, **(B)**. The DNA molecule itself is referred to as an organic phosphate, **(D)**.

15. **B**

Phosphoric acid has three hydrogens with $pK_a$ values spread across the pH range. This allows some degree of buffering over almost the entire standard pH range from 0 to 14.

**GO ONLINE**

**Consult your online resources for additional practice.**

## SHARED CONCEPTS

**Biochemistry Chapter 1**
Amino Acids, Peptides, and Proteins

**Biochemistry Chapter 6**
DNA and Biotechnology

**Biochemistry Chapter 9**
Carbohydrate Metabolism I

**General Chemistry Chapter 10**
Acids and Bases

**Organic Chemistry Chapter 4**
Analyzing Organic Reactions

**Organic Chemistry Chapter 8**
Carboxylic Acids

CHAPTER 11

# SPECTROSCOPY

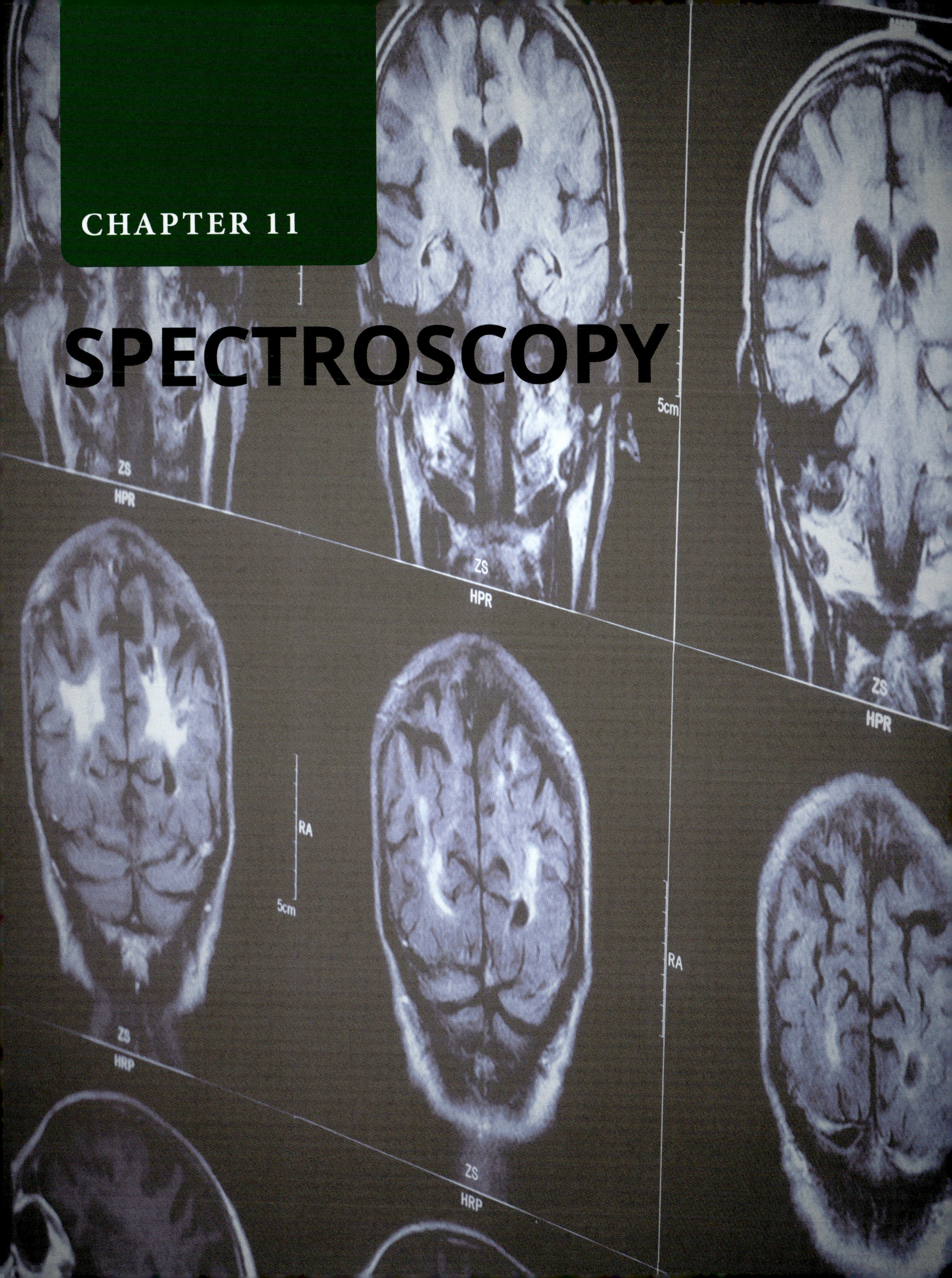

# SCIENCE MASTERY ASSESSMENT

Every pre-med knows this feeling: there is so much content I have to know for the MCAT! How do I know what to do first or what's important?

While the high-yield badges throughout this book will help you identify the most important topics, this Science Mastery Assessment is another tool in your MCAT prep arsenal. This quiz (which can also be taken in your online resources) and the guidance below will help ensure that you are spending the appropriate amount of time on this chapter based on your personal strengths and weaknesses. Don't worry though—skipping something now does not mean you'll never study it. Later on in your prep, as you complete full-length tests, you'll uncover specific pieces of content that you need to review and can come back to these chapters as appropriate.

## How to Use This Assessment

### If you answer 0–7 questions correctly:

Spend about 1 hour to read this chapter in full and take limited notes throughout. Follow up by reviewing **all** quiz questions to ensure that you now understand how to solve each one.

### If you answer 8–11 questions correctly:

Spend 20–40 minutes reviewing the quiz questions. Beginning with the questions you missed, read and take notes on the corresponding subchapters. For questions you answered correctly, ensure your thinking matches that of the explanation and you understand why each choice was correct or incorrect.

### If you answer 12–15 questions correctly:

Spend less than 20 minutes reviewing all questions from the quiz. If you missed any, then include a quick read-through of the corresponding subchapters, or even just the relevant content within a subchapter, as part of your question review. For questions you got correct, ensure your thinking matches that of the explanation and review the Concept Summary at the end of the chapter.

1. IR spectroscopy is most useful for distinguishing:
   **A.** double and triple bonds.
   **B.** C–H bonds.
   **C.** chirality of molecules.
   **D.** relative percentage of enantiomers in mixtures.

2. Oxygen ($O_2$) does not exhibit an IR spectrum because:
   **A.** it has no molecular motions.
   **B.** it is not possible to record IR spectra of a gaseous molecule.
   **C.** molecular vibrations do not result in a change in the dipole moment.
   **D.** molecular oxygen contains four lone pairs overall.

3. If IR spectroscopy were employed to monitor the oxidation of benzyl alcohol to benzaldehyde, which of the following would provide the best evidence that the reaction was proceeding as planned?
   **A.** Comparing the fingerprint region of the spectra of starting material and product
   **B.** Noting the change in intensity of the peaks corresponding to the benzene ring
   **C.** Noting the appearance of a broad absorption peak in the region of 3100–3500 $cm^{-1}$
   **D.** Noting the appearance of a strong absorption in the region of 1750 $cm^{-1}$

4. Which of the following chemical shifts could correspond to an aldehydic proton signal in a $^{1}H$–NMR spectrum?
   **A.** 9.5 ppm
   **B.** 7.0 ppm
   **C.** 11.0 ppm
   **D.** 1.0 ppm

5. The isotope $^{12}C$ is not useful for NMR because:
   **A.** it is not abundant in nature.
   **B.** its resonances are not sensitive to the presence of neighboring atoms.
   **C.** it has no magnetic moment.
   **D.** the signal-to-noise ratio in the spectrum is too low.

6. In $^{1}H$–NMR, splitting of spectral lines is due to:
   **A.** coupling between a carbon atom and protons attached to that carbon atom.
   **B.** coupling between a carbon atom and protons attached to adjacent carbon atoms.
   **C.** coupling between adjacent carbon atoms.
   **D.** coupling between protons on adjacent carbon atoms.

7. Compared to IR and NMR spectroscopy, UV spectroscopy is preferred for detecting:
   **A.** aldehydes and ketones.
   **B.** unconjugated alkenes.
   **C.** conjugated alkenes.
   **D.** aliphatic acids and amines.

8. Considering only the 0 to 4.5 ppm region of a $^1H$–NMR spectrum, how could ethanol and isopropanol be distinguished?
   - **A.** They cannot be distinguished from $^1H$–NMR alone.
   - **B.** A triplet and quartet are observed for ethanol, whereas a doublet and septet are observed for isopropanol.
   - **C.** A triplet and quartet are observed for isopropanol, whereas a doublet and septet are observed for ethanol.
   - **D.** The alcohol hydrogen in ethanol will appear within that region, whereas the alcohol hydrogen in isopropanol will appear downfield of that region.

9. Before absorbing an ultraviolet photon, electrons can be found in:
   - **A.** the HOMO only.
   - **B.** the LUMO only.
   - **C.** both the HOMO and the LUMO.
   - **D.** neither the HOMO nor the LUMO.

10. In an IR spectrum, how does extended conjugation of double bonds affect the absorbance band of carbonyl (C=O) stretches compared with normal absorption?
   - **A.** The absorbance band will occur at a lower wavenumber.
   - **B.** The absorbance band will occur at a higher wavenumber.
   - **C.** The absorbance band will occur at the same wavenumber.
   - **D.** The absorbance band will disappear.

11. Wavenumber is directly proportional to:
   - **A.** wavelength.
   - **B.** frequency.
   - **C.** percent transmittance.
   - **D.** absorbance.

12. Two enantiomers will:
   - **A.** have identical IR spectra because they have the same functional groups.
   - **B.** have identical IR spectra because they have the same specific rotation.
   - **C.** have different IR spectra because they are structurally different.
   - **D.** have different IR spectra because they have different specific rotations.

13. In a molecule containing a carboxylic acid group, what would be expected in a $^1H$–NMR spectrum?
   - **A.** A deshielded hydrogen peak for the hydroxyl hydrogen, shifted left
   - **B.** A deshielded hydrogen peak for the hydroxyl hydrogen, shifted right
   - **C.** A shielded hydrogen peak for the hydroxyl hydrogen, shifted left
   - **D.** A shielded hydrogen peak for the hydroxyl hydrogen, shifted right

14. The coupling constant, *J*, is:
   - **A.** the value of $n + 1$ when determining splitting in NMR spectra.
   - **B.** measured in parts per million (ppm).
   - **C.** corrected for by calibration with tetramethylsilane.
   - **D.** a measure of the degree of splitting caused by other atoms in the molecule.

15. The IR spectrum of a fully protonated amino acid would likely contain which of the following peaks?
   - **I.** A sharp peak at 1750 $cm^{-1}$
   - **II.** A sharp peak at 3300 $cm^{-1}$
   - **III.** A broad peak at 3300 $cm^{-1}$
   - **A.** I only
   - **B.** I and II only
   - **C.** II and III only
   - **D.** I, II, and III

## Answer Key

1. **A** (See section 11.1)
2. **C** (See section 11.1)
3. **D** (See section 11.1)
4. **A** (See section 11.3)
5. **C** (See section 11.3)
6. **D** (See section 11.3)
7. **C** (See section 11.2)
8. **B** (See section 11.3)
9. **A** (See section 11.2)
10. **A** (See section 11.1)
11. **B** (See section 11.2)
12. **A** (See section 11.1)
13. **A** (See section 11.3)
14. **D** (See section 11.3)
15. **B** (See section 11.1)

*The relevant section of the chapter to review for each question is given in parentheses after the correct answer. Detailed explanations can be found at the end of the chapter.*

CHAPTER 11

# SPECTROSCOPY

## In This Chapter



**CHAPTER PROFILE**

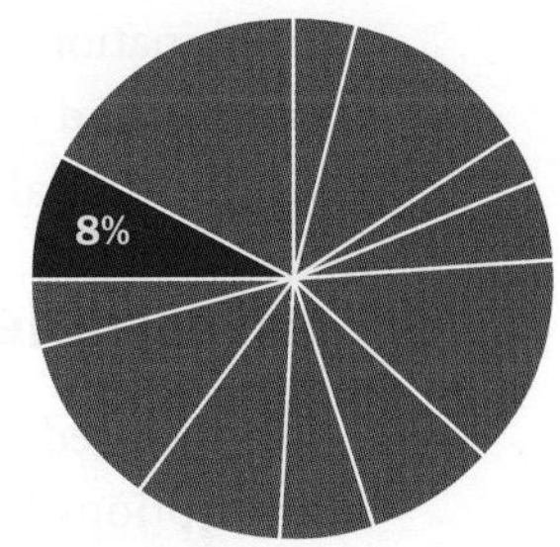


The content in this chapter should be relevant to about 8% of all questions about organic chemistry on the MCAT.

This chapter covers material from the following AAMC content category:

**4D:** How light and sound interact with matter

## Introduction

If we are given an unknown compound, one of the most efficient ways to identify it and determine its properties is by using spectroscopy. **Spectroscopy** measures the energy differences between the possible states of a molecular system by determining the frequencies of electromagnetic radiation absorbed by the molecules. These possible states are quantized energy levels associated with different types of molecular motion, such as molecular rotation, vibration of bonds, electron absorption, and nuclear spin transitions. Different types of spectroscopy measure different types of molecular properties, allowing us to identify the presence of specific functional groups and to detect the connectivity (backbone) of a molecule.

In a medical context, spectroscopy is important in magnetic resonance imaging (MRI). MRI scanners actually measure $^1$H–NMR spectra of water molecules in different environments in the body. They then convert these signals into greyscale, allowing excellent visualization of the body, especially soft tissue.

One of the big advantages of laboratory spectroscopy is that only a small quantity of a sample is needed. Also, the sample may be reused after a test is performed. The downside of spectroscopy is that it's difficult to do without special equipment—but as long as you have a chemistry lab available, these are some of the best techniques to identify compounds.

# 11.1 Infrared Spectroscopy

**LEARNING OBJECTIVES**

After Chapter 11.1, you will be able to:

- Predict the IR peaks for common organic functional groups, including ketones, carboxylic acids, and alcohols
- Recall the conditions in which IR spectroscopy is generally used, and what it is used to measure

**Infrared (IR) spectroscopy** measures molecular vibrations, which can be seen as bond stretching, bending, or combinations of different vibrational modes. To record an IR spectrum, infrared light is passed through a sample, and the absorbance is measured. By determining what bonds exist within a molecule, we hope to infer the functional groups in the molecule.

## Intramolecular Vibrations and Rotations

The infrared light range runs from $\lambda = 700$ nm to 1 mm, but the useful absorptions for spectroscopy occur at wavelengths of 2500 to 25,000 nm. On an IR spectrum, we use an analog of frequency called **wavenumber**. The standard range corresponding to 2500 to 25,000 nm is 4000 to 400 cm$^{-1}$. When light of these wavenumbers is absorbed, the molecules enter excited vibrational states. Four types of vibration that can occur are shown in Figure 11.1. Others include twisting and folding.

**KEY CONCEPT**

Wavenumbers (cm$^{-1}$) are an analog of frequency. $f = \frac{c}{\lambda}$, whereas wavenumber $= \frac{1}{\lambda}$.

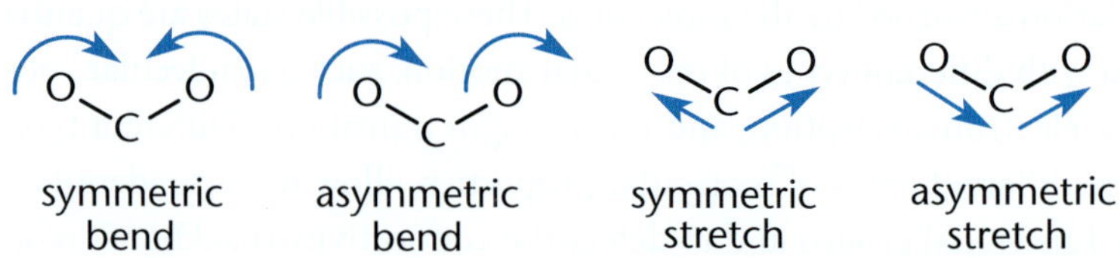


**Figure 11.1** Molecular Vibrations Measured by Infrared (IR) Spectroscopy
*Bond bending and stretching; twisting and folding can also occur.*

More complex vibration patterns, caused by the motion of the molecule as a whole, can be seen in the 1500 to 400 cm$^{-1}$ range. This is called the **fingerprint region** because the specific absorbance pattern is characteristic of each individual molecule. Spectroscopy experts can use this region to identify a substance, but you won't ever need to use it on the MCAT.

**KEY CONCEPT**

Symmetric stretches do not show up in IR spectra because they involve no net change in dipole movement.

For an absorption to be recorded, the vibration must result in a change in the bond dipole moment. For example, we cannot get an absorption from $O_2$ or $Br_2$, but we can from HCl or CO, as seen in Figure 11.2.

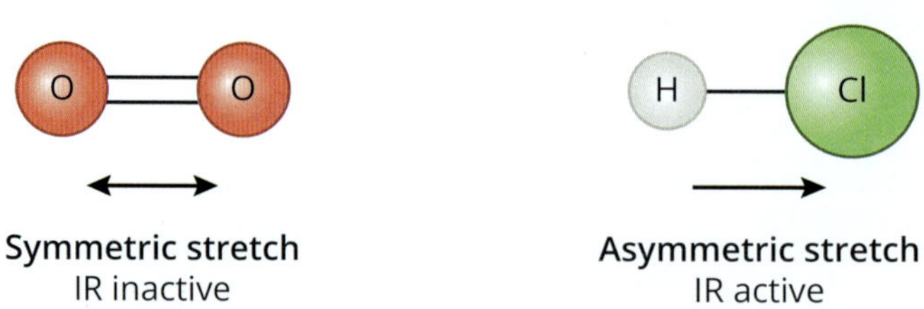


**Figure 11.2** IR Stretch

## Characteristic Absorptions

For the MCAT, you only need to memorize a few absorptions. The first is the hydroxyl group, O–H, which absorbs with a broad (wide) peak at around one of two frequencies: 3300 $cm^{-1}$ for alcohols, and 3000 $cm^{-1}$ for carboxylic acids. The carbonyl of a carboxylic acid pulls some of the electron density out of the O–H bond, shifting the absorption to a lower wavenumber. The second is the carbonyl, which absorbs around 1700 $cm^{-1}$ with a sharp (deep) peak. In Table 11.1, notice how the bond between any atom and hydrogen always has a relatively high absorption frequency and how, as we add more bonds between carbon atoms, the absorption frequency increases. N–H bonds are in the same region as O–H bonds (around 3300 $cm^{-1}$), but have a sharp peak instead of a broad one. You should be able to identify these three peaks in an IR spectrum. If you need to identify other peaks on Test Day, a list or table of peak wavenumbers will be provided.

| Functional Group | Wavenumber ($cm^{-1}$) | Vibration |
|---|---|---|
| Alkanes | 2800–3000<br>1200 | C–H<br>C–C |
| Alkenes | 3080–3140<br>1645 | =C–H<br>C=C |
| Alkynes | 3300<br>2200 | ≡C–H<br>C≡C |
| Aromatic | 2900–3100<br>1475–1625 | C–H<br>C–C |
| Alcohols | 3100–3500 | O–H (broad) |
| Ethers | 1050–1150 | C–O |
| Aldehydes | 2700–2900<br>1700–1750 | (O)C–H<br>C=O |
| Ketones | 1700–1750 | C=O |
| Carboxylic Acids | 1700–1750<br>2800–3200 | C=O<br>O–H (broad) |
| Amines | 3100–3500 | N–H (sharp) |

**Table 11.1** Absorption Frequencies

### MCAT EXPERTISE

Infrared spectroscopy is best used for identification of functional groups. The most important peaks to know are:

- O–H (broad around 3300 $cm^{-1}$)
- N–H (sharp around 3300 $cm^{-1}$)
- C=O (sharp around 1750 $cm^{-1}$)

We can learn a great deal of information from an IR spectrum; for the MCAT, all of the information comes from the frequencies between 1400 and 4000 $cm^{-1}$. Everything lower (in the fingerprint region) is out of scope. IR spectra are plotted as percent **transmittance**, the amount of light that passes through the sample and reaches the detector, vs. wavenumber.

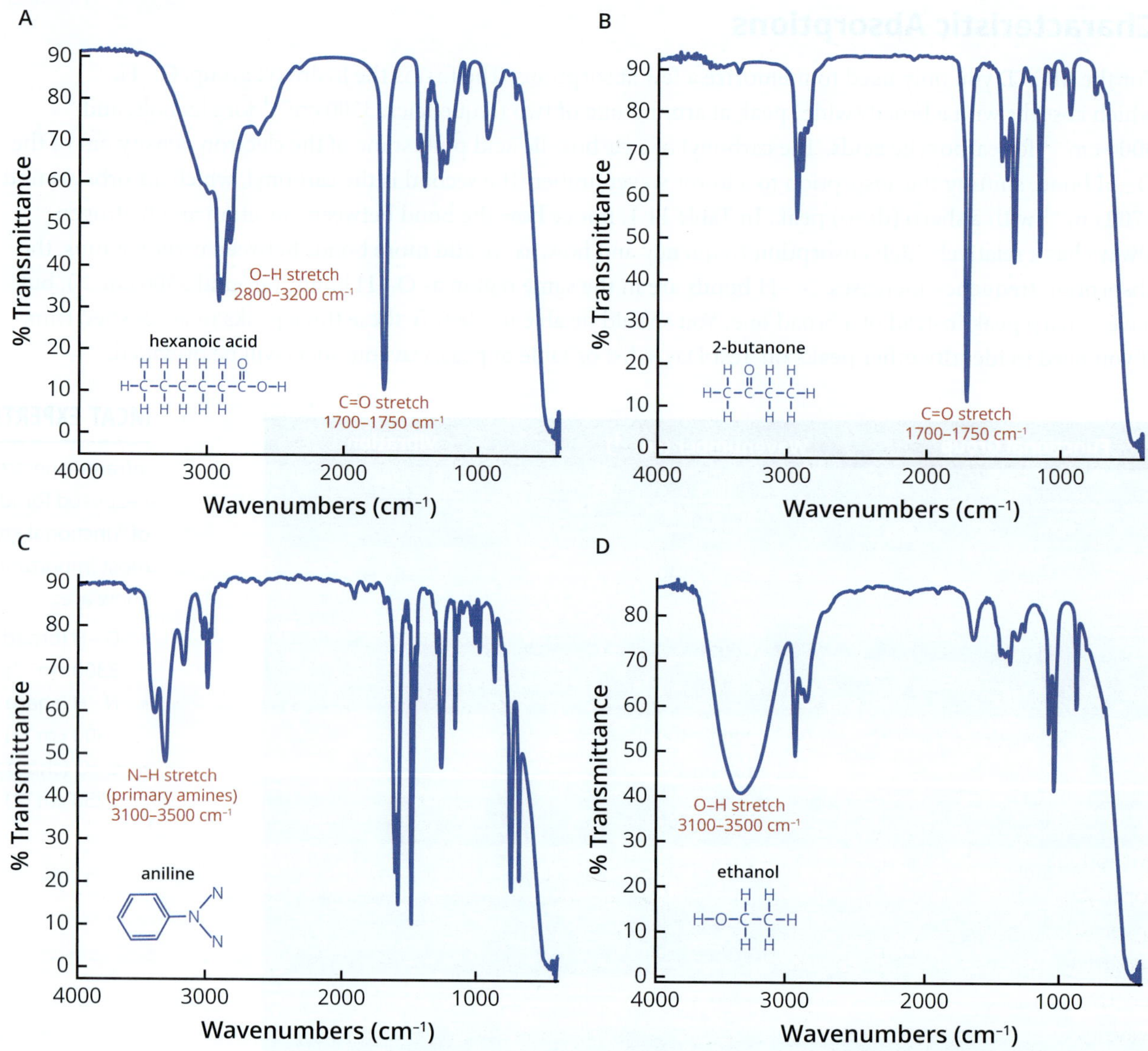


**Figure 11.3** Key Peaks in IR Spectra

Figure 11.3 displays representative IR spectra. Spectrum A (hexanoic acid) features a sharp C=O stretch (1700–1750 $cm^{-1}$) and a very broad O–H stretch (2800–3200 $cm^{-1}$). Spectrum B (2-butanone) has the sharp C=O stretch but lacks the O-H stretch. Spectrum C (aniline) is identified by its two sharp N–H stretches (3100–3500 $cm^{-1}$). Finally, Spectrum D shows the IR spectrum for an aliphatic alcohol: the large broad peak centered around 3300 $cm^{-1}$ is due to the presence of a hydroxyl group, whereas the sharper peak at 3000 $cm^{-1}$ is due to the carbon–hydrogen bonds in the molecule, as listed in Table 11.1.

## KEY CONCEPT

In an IR spectrum, percent transmittance is plotted vs. frequency. The equation relating absorbance, $A$, and percent transmittance, $\% T$, is $A = 2 - \log \%T$; this means that maximum absorptions appear as the bottoms of valleys on the spectrum.

### MCAT CONCEPT CHECK 11.1

Before you move on, assess your understanding of the material with these questions.

1. What does infrared (IR) spectroscopy measure? What is IR spectroscopy generally used for?

_______________________________________________

2. What two peaks would you expect to see in the IR spectrum of a carboxylic acid?

- _______________________________________________
- _______________________________________________

## 11.2 Ultraviolet Spectroscopy

### LEARNING OBJECTIVES

After Chapter 11.2, you will be able to:

- Predict whether a given molecule can be detected via UV spectroscopy
- Describe the relationship between HOMO, LUMO, and absorption wavelength

Although you will never have to interpret **ultraviolet (UV) spectroscopy** data on the MCAT, it is fair game for discussion. A basic understanding of how it works and when it is used will suffice. UV spectra are obtained by passing ultraviolet light through a sample that is usually dissolved in an inert, nonabsorbing solvent, and recording the absorbance. The absorbance is then plotted against wavelength. The absorbance is caused by electronic transitions between orbitals. The biggest piece of information we get from this technique is the wavelength of maximum absorbance, which tells us the extent of conjugation within conjugated systems: the more conjugated the compound, the lower the energy of the transition and the greater the wavelength of maximum absorbance.

### Electron Transitions

UV spectroscopy works because molecules with $\pi$-electrons or nonbonding electrons can be excited by ultraviolet light to higher-energy antibonding orbitals, as depicted in Figure 11.4. Molecules with a lower energy gap between **highest occupied molecular orbital** (**HOMO**) and **lowest unoccupied molecular orbital** (**LUMO**) are more easily excited and can absorb longer wavelengths (lower frequencies) with lower energy.

#### MCAT EXPERTISE

UV spectroscopy is most useful for studying compounds containing double bonds or heteroatoms with lone pairs that create conjugated systems. For the MCAT, that is all you need to know.

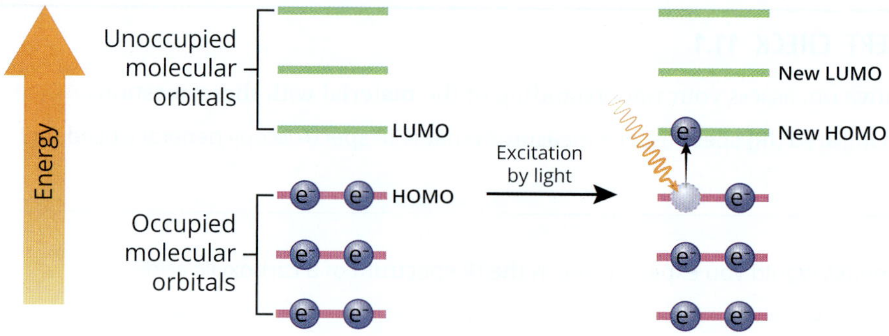


**Figure 11.4** Electron Excitation

## Conjugated Systems

**Conjugated** molecules, or molecules with unhybridized *p*-orbitals, can also be excited by ultraviolet light (see Figure 11.5). Conjugation shifts the absorption spectrum, resulting in higher maximum wavelengths (lower frequencies).

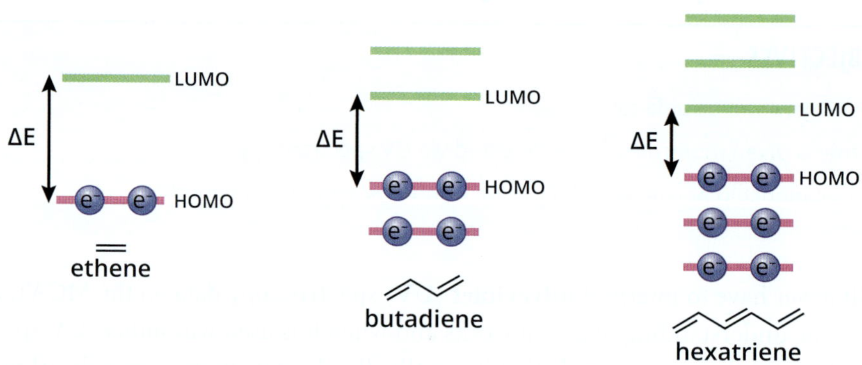


**Figure 11.5** Excitation in Conjugated Systems

For example, a simple aromatic ring like benzene shows characteristic UV absorbances around 180, 200, and 255 nm. As the degree of conjugation increases (that is, more double bonds separated by a single bond), the energy difference between the highest occupied molecular orbital (HOMO) and the lowest unoccupied molecular orbital (LUMO) decreases. This drop in the HOMO-LUMO energy gap allows the molecule to absorb lower-energy (longer-wavelength) light. Very large conjugated molecules absorb light in the visible range (400 to 750 nm), which is why many colored organic compounds contain extensive conjugation. Because the principle is the same across both regions, the technique is often called *UV–Vis spectroscopy*. Figure 11.6 illustrates how the degree of conjugation in amino acids affects their UV absorption spectra, with more conjugated aromatic rings absorbing at longer wavelengths and with greater molar absorptivity.

### REAL WORLD

Because aromatic amino acids like tryptophan and tyrosine absorb UV light, biochemists can measure absorbance at 280 nm to track protein concentration during purification. This absorbance is also sensitive to the local environment of the residues, allowing researchers to monitor conformational changes as a protein folds.

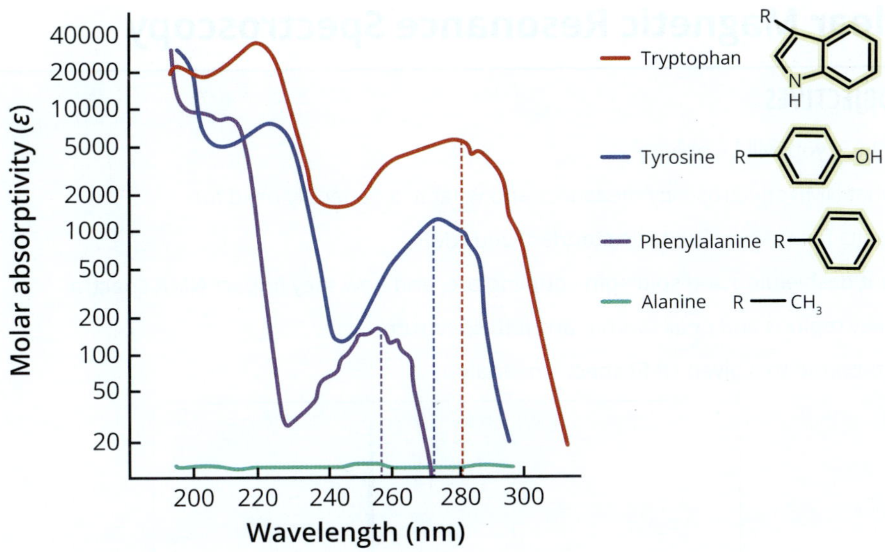


**Figure 11.6** UV Spectra of Conjugated vs. Unconjugated Molecules

## MCAT CONCEPT CHECK 11.2

Before you move on, assess your understanding of the material with these questions.

1. Which of the following molecules are detectable by UV spectroscopy: propane, propene, propanone?

 ______________________________

2. In UV spectroscopy, what is the HOMO? What is the LUMO? How are they related to absorption wavelength?
    - HOMO:

      ______________________________

    - LUMO:

      ______________________________

    - Relation to absorption wavelength:

      ______________________________

# 11.3 Nuclear Magnetic Resonance Spectroscopy

## LEARNING OBJECTIVES

After Chapter 11.3, you will be able to:

- Describe what NMR spectroscopy measures and what it is generally used for
- Recall the units for chemical shift on standardized NMR
- Identify what deshielding and spin-spin coupling are, and how they impact NMR spectra
- Recognize key regions and peaks within an NMR spectrum
- Match a compound to a given NMR spectrum analysis:

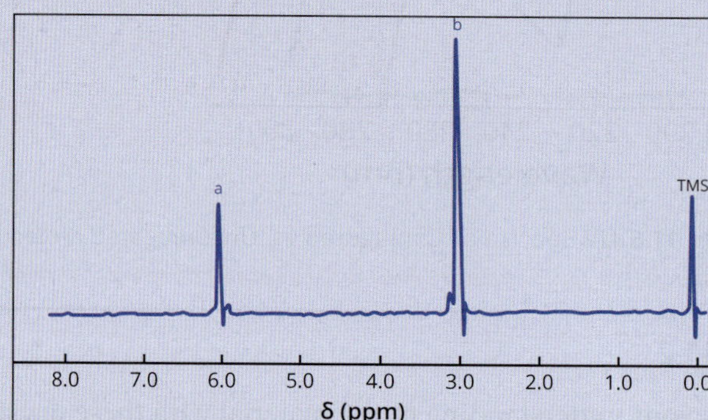


**Nuclear magnetic resonance (NMR)** spectroscopy is the most important spectroscopic technique to understand for the MCAT. NMR spectroscopy is based on the fact that certain atomic nuclei have magnetic moments that are oriented at random. When such nuclei are placed in a magnetic field, their magnetic moments tend to align either with or against the direction of this applied field, as can be seen in Figure 11.7. Nuclei with magnetic moments that are aligned with the field are said to be in the **$\alpha$-state** (lower energy). The nuclei can then be irradiated with radiofrequency pulses that match the energy gap between the two states, which will excite some lower-energy nuclei into the **$\beta$-state** (higher energy). The absorption of this radiation leads to excitation at different frequencies, depending on an atom's magnetic environment. In addition, the nuclear magnetic moments of atoms are affected by nearby atoms that also possess magnetic moments.

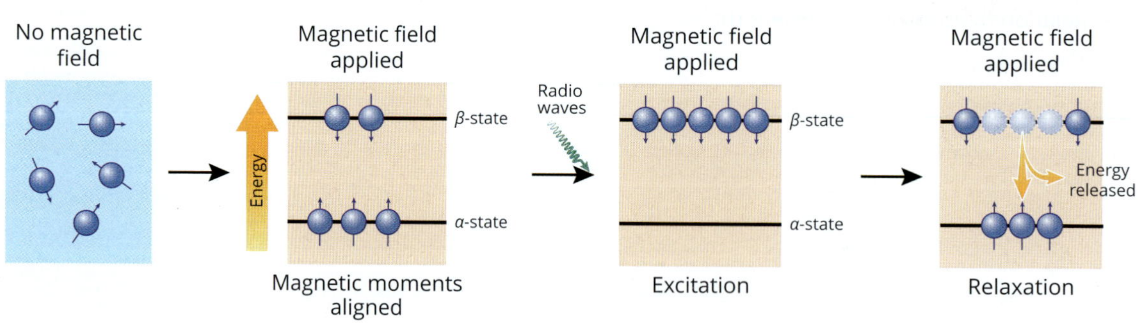


**Figure 11.7** Principle of Nuclear Magnetic Resonance (NMR) Spectroscopy

**Magnetic resonance imaging (MRI)** is a noninvasive diagnostic tool that uses proton NMR, as shown in Figure 11.8. Multiple cross-sectional scans of the patient's body are taken, and the various chemical shifts of absorbing protons are translated into specific shades of grey. This produces a picture that shows the relative density of specific types of protons; for instance, a dark area on a T1-weighted MRI tends to correspond to water, whereas a light area indicates fattier tissue. Comparison with a normal MRI then allows the diagnostician to detect abnormalities in the scanned region. We mention this to explain the relevance of NMR spectroscopy to medicine; the MCAT will not test you on the details of how MRI works.

An MRI machine combines a variety of NMR data to produce views of internal body tissues such as the brain.

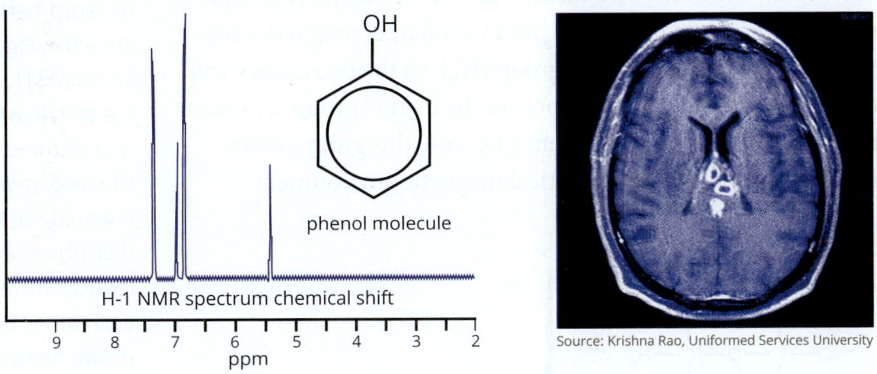


Source: Krishna Rao, Uniformed Services University

Image adapted from source: sdbs.db.aist.go.jp
(National Institute of Advanced Industrial Science and Technology)

**Figure 11.8** Magnetic Resonance Imaging (MRI)

A typical NMR spectrum is a plot of frequency vs. absorption of energy. Because different NMR spectrometers operate at different magnetic field strengths, a standardized method of plotting the NMR spectrum has been adopted. This standardized method, which is the only one seen on the MCAT, uses an arbitrary variable called **chemical shift** ($\delta$), with units of **parts per million (ppm)** of spectrometer frequency. The chemical shift is plotted on the $x$-axis, and it increases toward the left (referred to as **downfield**) and decreases toward the right (referred to as **upfield**), as seen in Figure 11.9. To make sure that we know just how far downfield compounds are, we use **tetramethylsilane (TMS)** as the calibration standard to mark 0 ppm; when counting peaks, make sure to skip the TMS peak.

## KEY CONCEPT

TMS provides a reference peak. The signal for its $^1H$ atoms is assigned $\delta = 0$.

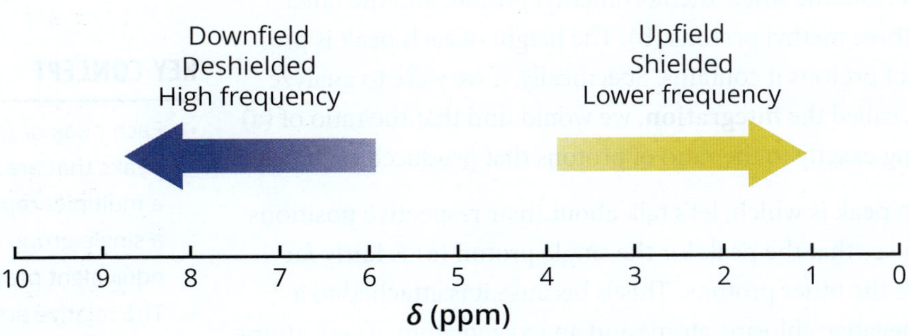


**Figure 11.9** Chemical Shift in NMR Spectra

Nuclear magnetic resonance is most commonly used to study $^1H$ nuclei (protons), although any atom possessing a nuclear spin (with an odd atomic number, odd mass number, or both) can be studied, such as $^{13}C$, $^{19}F$, $^{17}O$, $^{31}P$, and $^{59}Co$. The MCAT, however, only tests knowledge of $^1H$–NMR.

## BRIDGE

Nuclei with odd mass numbers, odd atomic numbers, or both, will have a magnetic moment when placed in a magnetic field. Not all nuclei have magnetic moments ($^{12}C$, for example). Atomic numbers and mass numbers are discussed in more detail in Chapter 1 of *MCAT General Chemistry Review.*

## Proton NMR ($^1H-NMR$)

Most hydrogen ($^1H$) nuclei come into resonance 0 to 10 ppm downfield from TMS. Each distinct set of nuclei gives rise to a separate peak. This means that if multiple protons are **chemically equivalent**, having the same magnetic environment, they will lead to the same peak. For example, Figure 11.10 depicts the $^1H-NMR$ of dichloromethyl methyl ether, which has two distinct sets of $^1H$ nuclei. The single proton attached to the dichloromethyl group ($H_a$) is in a different magnetic environment from the three protons on the methyl group ($H_b$), so the two classes will resonate at different frequencies. The three protons on the methyl group are chemically equivalent and resonate at the same frequency because this group rotates freely, and, on average, each proton sees an identical magnetic environment.

### MCAT EXPERTISE

To determine how many peaks will be in the spectrum, see if you can describe protons differently using words. In the dichloromethyl methyl ether shown in Figure 11.10, one could call $H_a$ the *hydrogen on the carbon with two chlorides* and all three $H_b$ hydrogens the *ones in the methyl group*. It would not be possible to describe each of these three hydrogens as distinct from each other because they rotate freely in space.

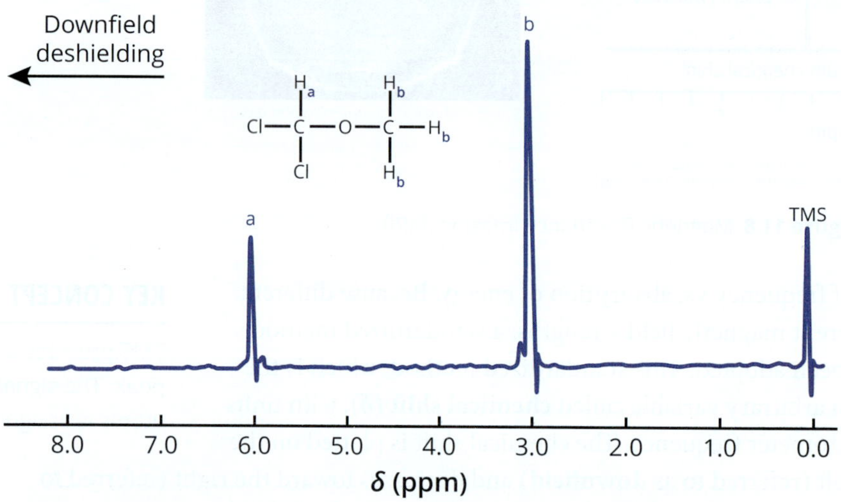


**Figure 11.10** $^1H-NMR$ Spectrum of Dichloromethyl Methyl Ether
*Peak a: Dichloromethyl proton; Peak b: Methyl protons.*

The peak on the left (a) is from the single dichloromethyl proton, and the taller middle peak is from the three methyl protons (b). The height of each peak is proportional to the number of protons it contains. Specifically, if we were to analyze the area under the peaks, called the **integration**, we would find that the ratio of (a) to (b) is 1:3, corresponding exactly to the ratio of protons that produced each peak.

Now that we know which peak is which, let's talk about their respective positions on the spectrum. We can see that the peak for the single proton (a) is fairly far downfield compared with the other protons. This is because it is attached to a carbon with two electronegative chlorine atoms and an oxygen atom. These atoms pull electron density away from the surrounding atoms, thus **deshielding** the proton from the magnetic field. The more the proton's electron density is pulled away, the less it can shield itself from the applied magnetic field (see Figure 11.11), resulting in a reading further downfield. With this same reasoning, we know that if we had an electron-donating group, such as the silicon atom in TMS, it would help shield the $^1H$ nuclei and give it a position further upfield. This is why tetramethylsilane is used as the reference or calibration peak; everything else in proton NMR will be more deshielded than it.

### KEY CONCEPT

- Each peak or group of peaks that are part of a multiplet represents a single group of equivalent protons
- The relative area of each peak reflects the ratio of the protons producing each peak
- The position of the peak (upfield or downfield) is due to shielding or deshielding effects and reflects the chemical environment of the protons

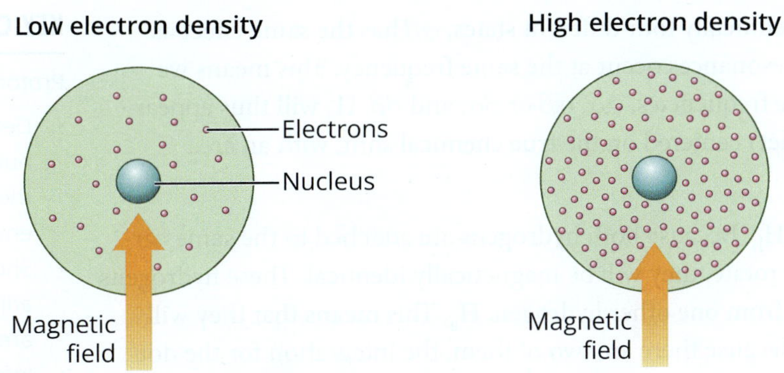


**Figure 11.11** Electronic Shielding and Deshielding

Now, let's make it a little more interesting. Consider a compound containing protons that are within three bonds of each other: in other words, a compound in which there are hydrogens on two adjacent atoms. When we have two protons in such close proximity to each other that are not magnetically identical, **spin–spin coupling (splitting)** occurs. Let's use the molecule in Figure 11.12 to demonstrate this concept.

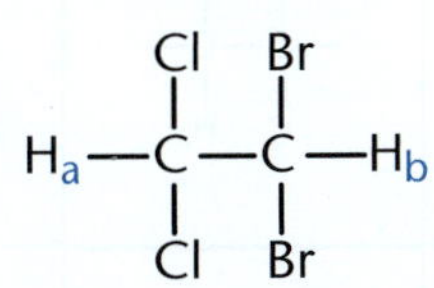


**Figure 11.12** 1,1-Dibromo-2,2-dichloroethane

Notice the two protons, $H_a$ and $H_b$, on 1,1-dibromo-2,2-dichloroethane. Because of their proximity, the magnetic environment of $H_a$ can be affected by $H_b$, and vice-versa. Thus, at any given time, $H_a$ can experience two different magnetic environments because $H_b$ can be in either the $\alpha$- or the $\beta$-state. The different states of $H_b$ influence the nucleus of $H_a$, causing slight upfield and downfield shifts. There is approximately a 50% chance that $H_b$ will be in either of the two states, so the resulting absorption is a **doublet**: two peaks of identical intensity, equally spaced around the true chemical shift of $H_a$. $H_a$ and $H_b$ will both appear as doublets because each one is coupled with one other hydrogen. To determine the number of peaks present (as doublets, triplets, and so on), we use the ***n* + 1 rule***:* if a proton has *n* protons that are three bonds away, it will be split into $n + 1$ peaks. (One caveat: do *not* include protons attached to oxygen or nitrogen.) The magnitude of this splitting, measured in hertz, is called the **coupling constant, *J*.**

Let's try a molecule that has even more coupled protons. In 1,1-dibromo-2-chloroethane, shown in Figure 11.13, the $H_a$ nucleus is affected by two nearby $H_b$ nuclei, which together can be in one of four different states: $\alpha\alpha$, $\alpha\beta$, $\beta\alpha$, or $\beta\beta$.

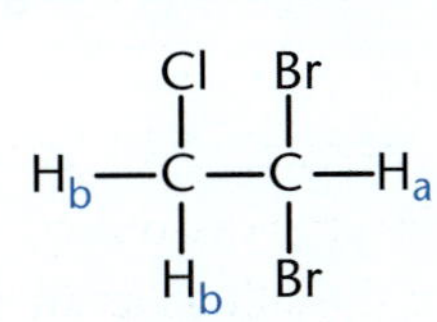


**Figure 11.13** 1,1-Dibromo-2-chloroethane

## MNEMONIC

When dealing with $^1$H–NMR on the MCAT, think of a proton as being surrounded by a shield of electrons. As we add electronegative atoms or have resonance structures that pull electrons away from the proton, we **D**eshield and move **D**ownfield.

## KEY CONCEPT

The splitting of the peak represents the number of adjacent hydrogens. A peak will be split into $n + 1$ subpeaks, where *n* is the number of adjacent hydrogens.

Although there are technically four different states, $\alpha\beta$ has the same effect as $\beta\alpha$, so both of these resonances occur at the same frequency. This means we will have three unique frequencies, $\alpha\alpha$, $\alpha\beta$ or $\beta\alpha$, and $\beta\beta$. $H_a$ will thus appear as three peaks (a **triplet**) centered on the true chemical shift, with an area ratio of 1:2:1.

Now let's move on to $H_b$. Because both hydrogens are attached to the same carbon, which can freely rotate, they will be magnetically identical. These hydrogens are three bonds away from one other hydrogen, $H_a$. This means that they will appear as a doublet. Because there are two of them, the integration for the doublet representing $H_b$ will be larger than the triplet for $H_a$. Different variations of this molecule and the splitting that results can be seen in Figure 11.14, which can serve as practice reading $^1$H-NMR.

## KEY CONCEPT

Proton NMR is good for:

- Determining the relative number of protons and their relative chemical environments
- Showing how many adjacent protons there are by splitting patterns
- Inferring certain functional groups

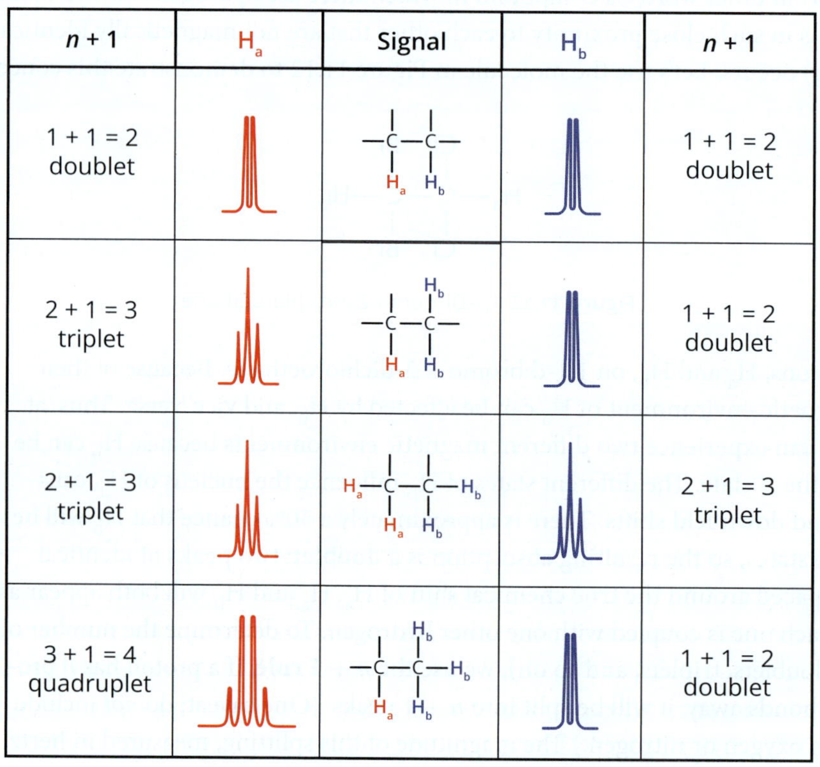


**Figure 11.14** $^1$H-NMR Peak Splitting

Table 11.2 shows the ratios for up to seven adjacent hydrogens, but it isn't necessary to memorize this table for the MCAT. Just remember to follow the $n + 1$ rule for the proton of interest to determine the number of peaks. In addition, peaks that have more than four shifts will generally be referred to generically as a **multiplet**.

| Number of Adjacent Hydrogens | Total Number of Peaks | Area Ratios |
|---|---|---|
| 0 | 1 | 1 |
| 1 | 2 | 1:1 |
| 2 | 3 | 1:2:1 |
| 3 | 4 | 1:3:3:1 |
| 4 | 5 | 1:4:6:4:1 |
| 5 | 6 | 1:5:10:10:5:1 |
| 6 | 7 | 1:6:15:20:15:6:1 |
| 7 | 8 | 1:7:21:35:35:21:7:1 |

**Table 11.2** Area Ratios for Peaks Split by Adjacent Hydrogens

Figure 11.15 indicates the chemical shift ranges of several different types of protons. Although this is fairly low-yield information, the values that are useful to know are the outliers like the deshielded aldehyde at 9 to 10 ppm, and the even more deshielded carboxylic acid between 10.5 and 12 ppm. Another popular peak on the MCAT is the hydrogen of an aromatic ring, which lies between 6.0 and 8.5 ppm. It is also worthwhile to know the general ranges for hydrogens on $sp^3$-hybridized carbons (1.0 to 3.0 ppm; higher if electron-withdrawing groups are present), $sp^2$-hybridized carbons (4.6 to 6.0 ppm), and $sp$-hybridized carbons (2.0 to 3.0 ppm). When electronegative groups are present, they pull electron density away from the protons. The more electron density that is pulled away from the proton, the more deshielded it will be and the further downfield the proton will appear. As always for the MCAT, it is better to understand the trends than to memorize specific values.

## MCAT EXPERTISE

On Test Day, just counting the number of peaks and unique hydrogens may be enough to get you the correct answer. (Remember *not* to count the peak for TMS, though!) If you need to consider shifts, the main ones for Test Day are:

- Alkanes: 1 to 3 ppm
- Alkynes: 2 to 3 ppm
- Alkenes: 4.6 to 6 ppm
- Aromatics: 6 to 8.5 ppm
- Aldehydes: 9 to 10 ppm
- Carboxylic acids: 10.5 to 12 ppm

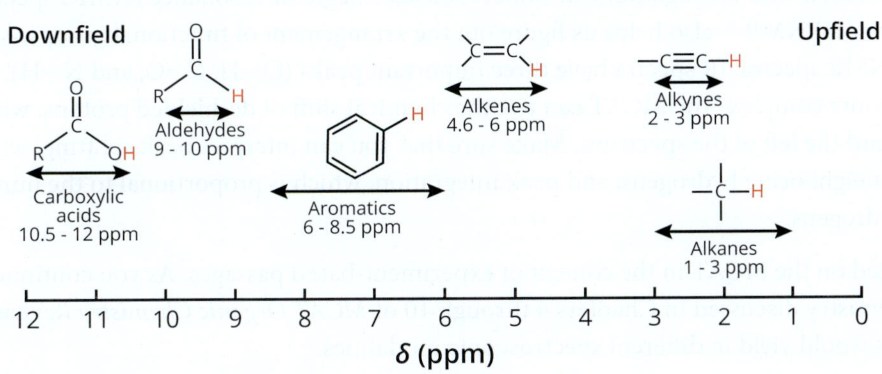


**Figure 11.15** Proton Chemical Shift Ranges

## MCAT CONCEPT CHECK 11.3

Before you move on, assess your understanding of the material with these questions.

1. What does nuclear magnetic resonance (NMR) spectroscopy measure? What is NMR spectroscopy generally used for?

    ____________________________________________

2. What are the units for chemical shift on a standardized NMR spectrum?

    ____________________________________________

3. What does it mean for a proton to be deshielded? How does this affect its peak in NMR spectroscopy?

    ____________________________________________

4. What is spin–spin coupling?

    ____________________________________________

# Conclusion

This chapter was full of numbers and values, but the most important thing to know about spectroscopy on the MCAT is that you don't need to know a lot of numbers. The numbers that you *do* need to know have already been stressed heavily in this chapter. Know that infrared (IR) spectroscopy is best for identifying the presence (or, more importantly, the absence) of functional groups. A cursory understanding of ultraviolet (UV) spectroscopy and its association with conjugation will suffice. Nuclear magnetic resonance (NMR) spectroscopy—specifically, proton ($^1H$) NMR— also helps us figure out the arrangement of functional groups. Know how to interpret IR and NMR spectra: IR spectra have three important peaks (O–H, C=O, and N–H), but NMR spectra can be far more complex. The MCAT can test the chemical shift of deshielded protons, which will be downfield, or toward the left of the spectrum. Make sure that you can interpret peak splitting, which is due to interference from neighboring hydrogens, and peak integration, which is proportional to the number of magnetically identical hydrogens.

Spectroscopy is often tested on the MCAT in the context of experiment-based passages. As you continue studying the reaction chemistry discussed in Chapters 4 through 10 of *MCAT Organic Chemistry Review*, consider what these products would yield in different spectroscopic modalities.

This chapter focused on one method of identifying compounds based on structural characteristics and interactions with electromagnetic energy, but spectroscopy is not the only method for characterizing organic molecules. In the next chapter, we explore another side of laboratory techniques: separation and purification schemes. These utilize physical differences between molecules to allow us to isolate and describe them.

**GO ONLINE**

**You've reviewed the content, now test your knowledge and critical thinking skills by completing a test-like passage set in your online resources!**

# CONCEPT SUMMARY

## Infrared Spectroscopy

- **Infrared** (**IR**) **spectroscopy** measures **absorption** of infrared light, which causes molecular vibration (stretching, bending, twisting, and folding).
- IR spectra are generally plotted as **percent transmittance** vs. **wavenumber** $\left(\frac{1}{\lambda}\right)$.
  - The normal range of a spectrum is 4000 to 400 $cm^{-1}$.
  - The **fingerprint region** is between 1500 and 400 $cm^{-1}$. It contains a number of peaks that can be used by experts to identify a compound.
- To appear on an IR spectrum, vibration of a bond must change the bond dipole moment. Certain bonds have characteristic absorption frequencies, which allow us to infer the presence (or absence) of particular functional groups.
  - The O–H peak is a broad peak around 3300 $cm^{-1}$. Molecules with O–H include alcohols, water, and carboxylic acids; the carboxylic acid O–H peak will be shifted around 3000 $cm^{-1}$.
  - The N–H peak is a sharp peak around 3300 $cm^{-1}$. Molecules with N–H include some amines, imines, and amides.
  - The C=O peak is a sharp peak around 1750 $cm^{-1}$. Molecules with C=O include aldehydes, ketones, carboxylic acids, amides, esters, and anhydrides.

## Ultraviolet Spectroscopy

- Ultraviolet (UV) spectroscopy measures absorption of ultraviolet light, which causes movement of electrons between molecular orbitals.
- UV spectra are generally plotted as percent transmittance or absorbance vs. wavelength.
- To appear on a UV spectrum, a molecule must have a small enough energy difference between its **highest occupied molecular orbital** (**HOMO**) and its **lowest unoccupied molecular orbital** (**LUMO**) to permit an electron to move from one orbital to the other.
  - The smaller the difference between HOMO and LUMO, the longer the wavelengths a molecule can absorb.
  - **Conjugation** occurs in molecules with unhybridized *p*-orbitals. Conjugation shifts the absorption spectrum to higher maximum wavelengths (lower frequencies).

## Nuclear Magnetic Resonance Spectroscopy

- **Nuclear magnetic resonance (NMR) spectroscopy** measures alignment of nuclear spin with an applied magnetic field, which depends on the magnetic environment of the nucleus itself. It is useful for determining the structure (connectivity) of a compound, including functional groups.
  - Nuclei may be in the lower-energy **$\alpha$-state** or higher-energy **$\beta$-state**; radiofrequency pulses push the nucleus from the $\alpha$-state to the $\beta$-state, and these frequencies can be measured.
- Magnetic resonance imaging (MRI) is a medical application of NMR spectroscopy.
- NMR spectra are generally plotted as frequency vs. absorption of energy. They are standardized by using **chemical shift** ($\delta$), measured in parts per million (ppm) of spectrophotometer frequency.
  - NMR spectra are calibrated using **tetramethylsilane (TMS)**, which has a chemical shift of 0 ppm.
  - Higher chemical shifts are located to the left (**downfield**); lower chemical shifts are located to the right (**upfield**).
- Proton ($^1H$) NMR is the most common.
  - Each unique group of protons has its own peak.
  - The **integration** (area under the curve) of this peak is proportional to the number of protons contained under the peak.
  - **Deshielding** of protons occurs when electron-withdrawing groups pull electron density away from the nucleus, allowing it to be more easily affected by the magnetic field. Deshielding moves a peak further downfield.
  - When hydrogens are on adjacent atoms, they interfere with each other's magnetic environment, causing **spin–spin coupling (splitting)**. A proton's (or group of protons') peak is split into $n + 1$ subpeaks, where $n$ is the number of protons that are three bonds away from the proton of interest.
  - Splitting patterns include **doublets**, **triplets**, and **multiplets**.
  - Protons on $sp^3$-hybridized carbons are usually in the 1 to 3 ppm range (but higher if electron-withdrawing groups are present). Protons on $sp^2$-hybridized carbons are usually in the 4.6 to 6.0 ppm range. Protons on $sp$-hybridized carbons are usually in the 2.0 to 3.0 ppm range.
  - Aldehydic hydrogens tend to appear between 9 and 10 ppm.
  - Carboxylic acid hydrogens tend to appear between 10.5 and 12 ppm.
  - Aromatic hydrogens tend to appear between 6.0 and 8.5 ppm.

# ANSWERS TO CONCEPT CHECKS

## 11.1

1. IR spectroscopy measures absorption of infrared light by specific bonds that vibrate. These vibrations cause changes in the dipole moment of the molecule that can be measured. Once the bonds in a molecule are determined, one can infer the presence of a number of functional groups to determine the identity of the molecule.
2. A carboxylic acid would have a broad O–H peak around 2800–3200 $cm^{-1}$ and a sharp carbonyl peak at 1700–1750 $cm^{-1}$.

## 11.2

1. Conjugated systems and other molecules with $\pi$ or nonbonding electrons can give absorbances on a UV spectroscopy plot. Therefore, propane would not be detectable, but propene and propanone would.
2. HOMO is the highest occupied molecular orbital; LUMO is the lowest unoccupied molecular orbital. The smaller the difference in energy between the two, the longer the wavelengths that can be absorbed by the molecule.

## 11.3

1. NMR measures alignment of the spin of a nucleus with an applied magnetic field. It is most often used for identifying the different types and magnetic environments of protons in a molecule, which allows us to infer the connectivity (backbone) of a molecule.
2. The units for chemical shift on a standardized NMR spectrum are parts per million (ppm).
3. Deshielding occurs in molecules that have electronegative atoms that pull electron density away from the hydrogens being measured. This results in a downfield (leftward) shift of the proton peak.
4. Spin–spin coupling occurs when two protons close to one another have an effect on the other's magnetic environment. This results in the splitting of peaks into doublets, triplets, or multiplets, depending on the environment.

# SCIENCE MASTERY ASSESSMENT EXPLANATIONS

1. **A**

Infrared spectroscopy is most useful for distinguishing between different functional groups. Almost all organic compounds have C—H bonds, **(B)**, so except for fingerprinting a compound, these absorptions are not useful. Little information about the optical properties of a compound, such as **(C)** and **(D)**, can be obtained by IR spectroscopy.

2. **C**

Because molecular oxygen is homonuclear (composed of only one element) and diatomic, there is no net change in its dipole moment during vibration or rotation; in other words, the compound does not absorb in a measurable way in the infrared region. IR spectroscopy is based on the principle that, when the molecule vibrates or rotates, there is a change in dipole moment. **(A)** is incorrect because oxygen does have molecular motions; they are just not detectable in IR spectroscopy. **(B)** is incorrect because it is possible to record the IR of a gaseous molecule as long as it shows a change in its dipole moment when it vibrates. **(D)** is incorrect because lone pairs do not have an effect on the ability to generate an IR spectrum of a compound.

3. **D**

In this reaction, the functional group is changing from a hydroxyl to an aldehyde. This means that a sharp peak will appear around 1750 $cm^{-1}$, which corresponds to the carbonyl functionality. **(C)** is the opposite of what occurs; the reaction will be characterized by the disappearance of the O—H peak at 3100 to 3500 $cm^{-1}$, not its appearance. Comparing the fingerprint regions, as in **(A)**, will provide evidence that a reaction is occurring, but it is not as useful for knowing that the reaction that occurred was indeed the one that was desired.

4. **A**

The peak at 9.5 ppm corresponds to an aldehydic proton. This signal lies downfield because the carbonyl oxygen is electron-withdrawing and deshields the proton. **(C)** corresponds to a carboxyl proton and is even further downfield because the acidic proton is deshielded to a greater degree than the aldehydic proton. **(B)** corresponds to aromatic protons. **(D)** is characteristic of an alkyl proton on an $sp^3$-hybridized carbon.

5. **C**

This isotope has no magnetic moment and will therefore not exhibit resonance with an applied magnetic field. Nuclei with odd mass numbers ($^1H$, $^{11}B$, $^{13}C$, $^{15}N$, $^{19}F$, and so on) or those with an even mass number but an odd atomic number ($^2H$, $^{10}B$) will have a nonzero magnetic moment.

6. **D**

Spin–spin coupling (splitting) is due to influence on the magnetic environment of one proton by protons on the adjacent atom. These protons are three bonds away from each other. Splitting in other NMR spectra can include coupling with carbon atoms, but not in $^1H$—NMR.

7. **C**

Most conjugated alkenes have an intense ultraviolet absorption. Aldehydes, ketones, acids, and amines, mentioned in **(A)** and **(D)**, all absorb in the ultraviolet range. However, other forms of spectroscopy (mainly IR and NMR) are more useful for precise identification. Isolated alkenes, **(B)**, can rarely be identified by UV spectroscopy.

8. **B**

The region in question often gives information about the types of alkyl groups present. Specifically, ethanol will give a characteristic triplet for the methyl group (which is coupled to $-CH_2-$) and a quartet for $-CH_2-$ (which is coupled to the methyl group). Isopropanol will have a septet for the $-CH-$ group (which is coupled to both methyl groups combined) and a doublet for the two methyl groups (which are coupled to $-CH-$). In both cases, the proton in the alcohol does not participate in coupling. The alcohol hydrogen likely lies downfield for both compounds because it is bonded to such an electronegative element.

9. **A**

The HOMO is the highest occupied molecular orbital. Only after absorbing ultraviolet light is an electron is excited from the HOMO to the LUMO, the lowest unoccupied molecular orbital.

10. **A**

Carbonyl groups (C=O) in conjugation with double bonds tend to absorb at lower wavenumbers because the delocalization of $\pi$ electrons causes the C=O bond to lose double-bond character, shifting the stretching frequency closer to C–O stretches. Remember that higher-order bonds tend to have higher absorption frequencies, so loss of double-bond character should decrease the absorption frequency of the group.

11. **B**

Wavenumber $\left(\frac{1}{\lambda}\right)$ is directly proportional to frequency $\left(\frac{c}{\lambda}\right)$. It is inversely proportional to wavelength, **(A)**, and has no proportionality to percent transmittance or absorbance, **(C)** and **(D)**.

12. **A**

Enantiomers will have identical IR spectra because they have the same functional groups and will therefore have the exact same absorption frequencies. Enantiomers have opposite specific rotations, but specific rotation actually has no effect on the IR spectrum.

13. **A**

The oxygen of the hydroxyl group will deshield the hydroxyl hydrogen, shifting it downfield, or leftward. Hydrogens in carboxylic acids can have some of the most downfield absorbances, around 10.5 to 12 ppm.

14. **D**

The coupling constant is a measure of the degree of splitting introduced by other atoms in a molecule, and is the frequency of the distance between subpeaks. It is measured in hertz, eliminating **(B)**. The coupling constant is independent of the value of $n + 1$ and is not changed by calibration with tetramethylsilane, eliminating **(A)** and **(B)**.

15. **B**

Amino acids in their fully protonated form contain all three of the peaks that should be memorized for Test Day: C–O, N–H, and O–H. While statements I and II correctly give the peaks for the C=O bond (sharp peak at 1750 $cm^{-1}$) and the N–H bond (sharp peak at 3300 $cm^{-1}$), the peak for the O–H bond is in the wrong place. In a carboxylic acid, the C=O bond withdraws electron density from the O–H bond, shifting the absorption frequency down to about 3000 $cm^{-1}$. Statement III is therefore incorrect.

**GO ONLINE**

**Consult your online resources for additional practice.**

## SHARED CONCEPTS

**General Chemistry Chapter 1**
Atomic Structure

**General Chemistry Chapter 3**
Bonding and Chemical Interactions

**Organic Chemistry Chapter 3**
Bonding

**Organic Chemistry Chapter 12**
Separations and Purifications

**Physics and Math Chapter 8**
Light and Optics

**Physics and Math Chapter 9**
Atomic and Nuclear Phenomena

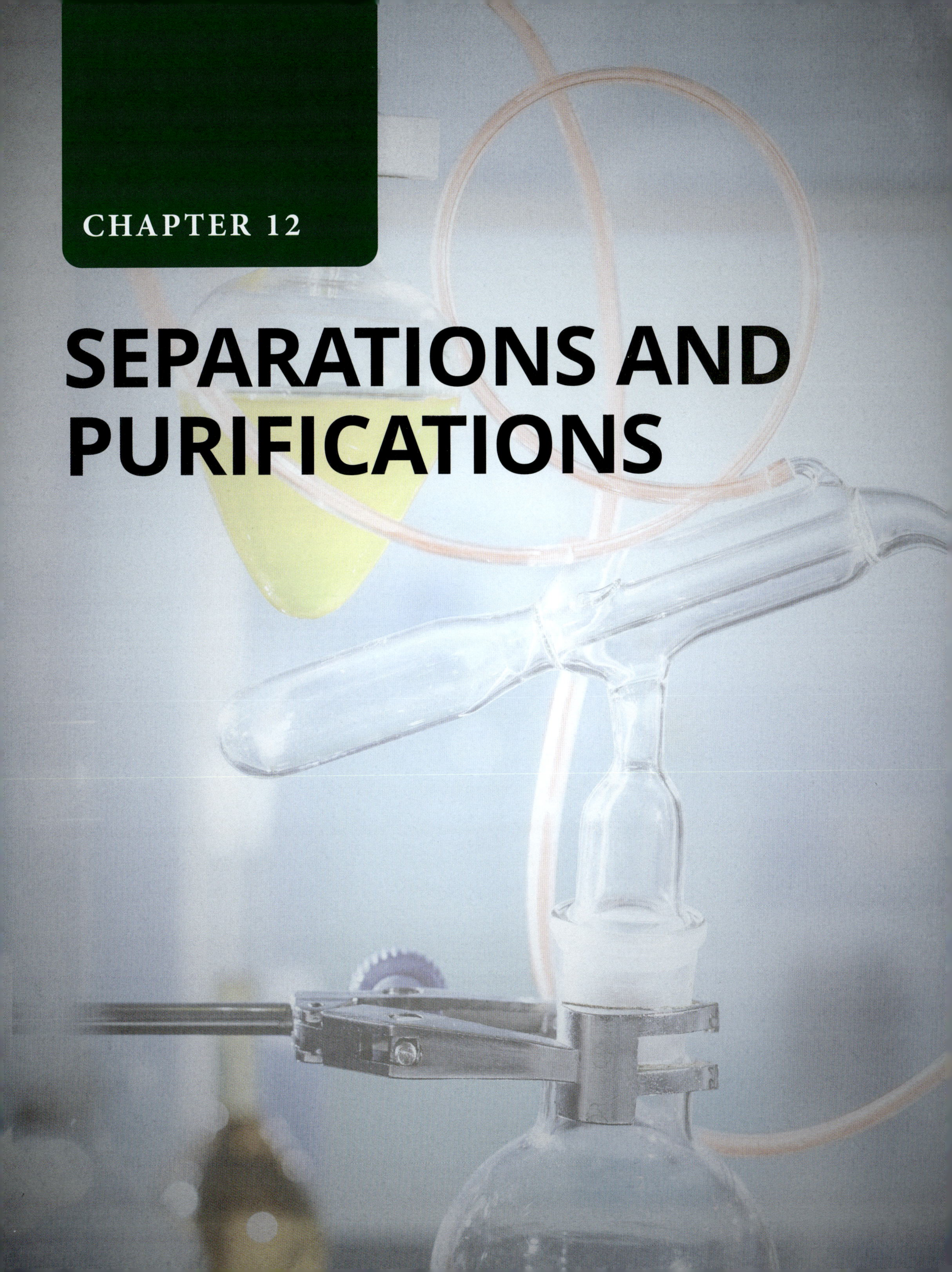

CHAPTER 12

# SEPARATIONS AND PURIFICATIONS

# SCIENCE MASTERY ASSESSMENT

Every pre-med knows this feeling: there is so much content I have to know for the MCAT! How do I know what to do first or what's important?

While the high-yield badges throughout this book will help you identify the most important topics, this Science Mastery Assessment is another tool in your MCAT prep arsenal. This quiz (which can also be taken in your online resources) and the guidance below will help ensure that you are spending the appropriate amount of time on this chapter based on your personal strengths and weaknesses. Don't worry though—skipping something now does not mean you'll never study it. Later on in your prep, as you complete full-length tests, you'll uncover specific pieces of content that you need to review and can come back to these chapters as appropriate.

## How to Use This Assessment

**If you answer 0–7 questions correctly:**

Spend about 1 hour to read this chapter in full and take limited notes throughout. Follow up by reviewing **all** quiz questions to ensure that you now understand how to solve each one.

**If you answer 8–11 questions correctly:**

Spend 20–40 minutes reviewing the quiz questions. Beginning with the questions you missed, read and take notes on the corresponding subchapters. For questions you answered correctly, ensure your thinking matches that of the explanation and you understand why each choice was correct or incorrect.

**If you answer 12–15 questions correctly:**

Spend less than 20 minutes reviewing all questions from the quiz. If you missed any, then include a quick read-through of the corresponding subchapters, or even just the relevant content within a subchapter, as part of your question review. For questions you got correct, ensure your thinking matches that of the explanation and review the Concept Summary at the end of the chapter.

1. Fractional distillation under atmospheric pressure would most likely be used to separate which of the following compounds?
   - **A.** Methylene chloride (boiling point of 40°C) and water (boiling point of 10°C)
   - **B.** Ethyl acetate (boiling point of 77°C) and ethanol (boiling point of 80°C)
   - **C.** Aniline (boiling point of 184°C) and benzyl alcohol (boiling point of 205°C)
   - **D.** Aniline (boiling point of 184°C) and water (boiling point of 100°C)

2. Which of the following compounds would be most effective in extracting benzoic acid from a diethyl ether solution?
   - **A.** Tetrahydrofuran
   - **B.** Aqueous hydrochloric acid
   - **C.** Aqueous sodium hydroxide
   - **D.** Water

3. Which of the following would be the best procedure for extracting acetaldehyde from an aqueous solution?
   - **A.** A single extraction with 100 mL of ether
   - **B.** Two successive extractions with 50 mL portions of ether
   - **C.** Three successive extractions with 33.3 mL portions of ether
   - **D.** Four successive extractions with 25 mL portions of ether

Questions 4 and 5 refer to the following table:

| Compound | Retardation Factor in Ether |
|---|---|
| benzyl alcohol | 0.10 |
| benzyl acetate | 0.26 |
| *p*-nitrophenol | 0.23 |
| 1-naphthalenemethanol | 0.40 |

4. What would be the effect on the $R_f$ values if thin-layer chromatography (TLC) were run with hexane rather than ether as the eluent?
   - **A.** No effect
   - **B.** Increase tenfold
   - **C.** Double
   - **D.** Decrease

5. If these compounds were separated by column chromatography with ether on silica gel, which would elute first?
   - **A.** Benzyl alcohol
   - **B.** Benzyl acetate
   - **C.** *p*-Nitrophenol
   - **D.** 1-Naphthalenemethanol

6. Four compounds, I, II, III, and IV, are separated by chromatographic techniques. Compound III is the most polar, II the least polar, and I and IV have intermediate polarity. The solvent system is 85:15 ethanol:methylene chloride. Which spot on the card below likely belongs to compound III?

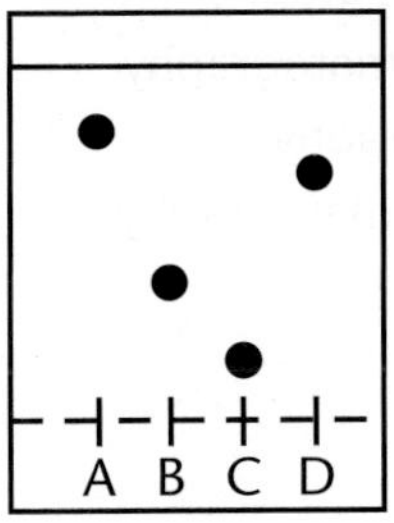


   **A.** A
   **B.** B
   **C.** C
   **D.** D

7. Suppose an extraction with methylene chloride $\left(\rho = 1.33 \frac{g}{mL}\right)$ is performed, with the desired compound initially in brine $\left(\rho = 1.04 \frac{g}{mL}\right)$. In a separatory funnel, which layer will be the organic layer?
   **A.** The top layer
   **B.** The bottom layer
   **C.** No layers are observed; methylene chloride and brine are miscible.
   **D.** More information is needed to answer the question.

8. Silica gel is often used in thin-layer chromatography. What property does silica gel probably possess that makes it useful for this purpose?
   **A.** Acidity
   **B.** Polarity
   **C.** Specifically sized pores
   **D.** Aqueous solubility

9. A mixture of sand, benzoic acid, and naphthalene in ether is best separated by:
   **A.** filtration, followed by acidic extraction, followed by recrystallization.
   **B.** filtration, followed by basic extraction, followed by evaporation.
   **C.** extraction, followed by distillation, followed by gas chromatography.
   **D.** filtration, followed by size-exclusion column chromatography, followed by extraction.

10. Simple distillation could be used to separate which of the following compounds?
   **A.** Toluene (boiling point of 111°C) and water (boiling point of 100°C)
   **B.** Naphthalene (boiling point of 218°C) and butyric acid (boiling point of 163°C)
   **C.** Propionaldehyde (boiling point of 50°C) and acetic acid (boiling point of 119°C)
   **D.** Benzene (boiling point of 80°C) and isopropyl alcohol (boiling point of 83°C)

11. In order to separate a biological effector from solution, which chromatographic technique would be the most effective?
   **A.** Thin-layer chromatography
   **B.** Ion-exchange chromatography
   **C.** Affinity chromatography
   **D.** Size-exclusion chromatography

12. Given a solution of insulin (molecular weight = 5.8 kD) and titin (molecular weight = 3816 kD), which chromatographic technique would be the most effective for separating out usable molecules of titin?
   **A.** Thin-layer chromatography
   **B.** Ion-exchange chromatography
   **C.** Affinity chromatography
   **D.** Size-exclusion chromatography

**13.** The gas eluent in gas chromatography and the liquid eluent in paper chromatography are examples of which component of these systems?

**A.** Stationary phase
**B.** Mobile phase
**C.** Column
**D.** Fraction

**14.** During gravity filtration, a student forgets to heat the solution before running it through the filter. After capturing the filtrate, the student analyzes the sample via infrared (IR) spectroscopy and finds none of the desired product in the filtrate. What likely occurred to the student's product?

**A.** The product degraded because of a prolonged filtration time.
**B.** The product evaporated with collection of the filtrate.
**C.** The product precipitated and is present in the residue.
**D.** The product was dissolved in the solvent.

**15.** Lactoferrin, a milk protein, is a valuable antimicrobial agent that is extracted from pasteurized, defatted milk utilizing a column containing a charged resin. This is an example of which of the following chromatographic techniques?

**A.** Thin-layer chromatography
**B.** Ion-exchange chromatography
**C.** Affinity chromatography
**D.** Size-exclusion chromatography

**Answer Key follows on next page.**

## Answer Key

1. **B** (See section 12.2)
2. **C** (See section 12.1)
3. **D** (See section 12.3)
4. **D** (See section 12.3)
5. **D** (See section 12.1)
6. **A** (See section 12.3)
7. **B** (See section 12.1)
8. **B** (See section 12.3)
9. **B** (See section 12.2)
10. **C** (See section 12.2)
11. **C** (See section 12.3)
12. **D** (See section 12.3)
13. **B** (See section 12.3)
14. **C** (See section 12.1)
15. **B** (See section 12.3)

*The relevant section of the chapter to review for each question is given in parentheses after the correct answer. Detailed explanations can be found at the end of the chapter.*

CHAPTER 12

# SEPARATIONS AND PURIFICATIONS

## In This Chapter



### CHAPTER PROFILE

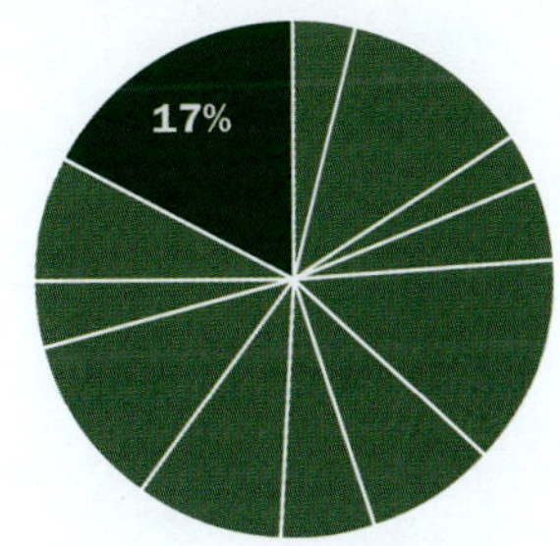


The content in this chapter should be relevant to about 17% of all questions about organic chemistry on the MCAT.

This chapter covers material from the following AAMC content category:

**5C:** Separation and purification methods

## Introduction

We've spent a lot of time discussing how to theoretically get various products from a range of reagents. However, as we're sure you've learned in your organic chemistry labs, chemistry isn't as straightforward in the real world as it is on paper. Much of the time spent in the lab is dedicated to the isolation and purification of the desired product after the reaction has occurred. Throughout this chapter, we will discuss several techniques for this. Good news, though—there isn't a lab practical on the MCAT, of course! All you need to understand is when these techniques are used and how they work.

## 12.1 Solubility-Based Methods

**LEARNING OBJECTIVES**

After Chapter 12.1, you will be able to:

- Recall the conditions required for two solvents to be used together in an extraction
- Explain why repetition is important in extraction procedures
- Predict whether a given solute is more likely to dissolve in the aqueous or organic layer within a separatory funnel

### MCAT EXPERTISE

Purification and separation techniques are procedures that exploit different physical properties. These show up on the MCAT to test your knowledge of the basic principles of each of these techniques.

One of the simplest ways to separate out a desired product is through **extraction**, the transfer of a dissolved compound (the desired product) from a starting solvent into a solvent in which the product is more soluble. Extraction is based on the fundamental concept that *like dissolves like*. This principle tells us that a polar substance will dissolve best in polar solvents, and a nonpolar substance will dissolve best in nonpolar solvents. These characteristics can be taken advantage of in order to extract only the desired product, leaving most of the impurities behind in the first solvent.

### KEY CONCEPT

*Like dissolves like* is a fundamental concept on the MCAT. Remember that polar substances will associate with other polar substances, and nonpolar with nonpolar.

## Extraction

When we perform **extractions**, it is important to make sure that the two solvents are **immiscible**, meaning that they form two layers that do not mix, like water and oil. The two layers are temporarily mixed by shaking so that solute can pass from one solvent to the other. For example, in a solution of isobutyric acid and diethyl ether, shown in Figure 12.1, we can extract the isobutyric acid with water. Isobutyric acid, with its polar carboxyl group, is more soluble in a polar solvent like water than in a nonpolar solvent like ether. When the two solvents are mixed together, isobutyric acid will transfer to the water layer, which is called the **aqueous phase (layer)**. The nonpolar ether layer is called the **organic phase (layer)**.

**MCAT EXPERTISE**

Think of the organic and aqueous layers as being like the oil and water in salad dressings: you can shake the mixture to increase their interaction, but ultimately they will separate again.

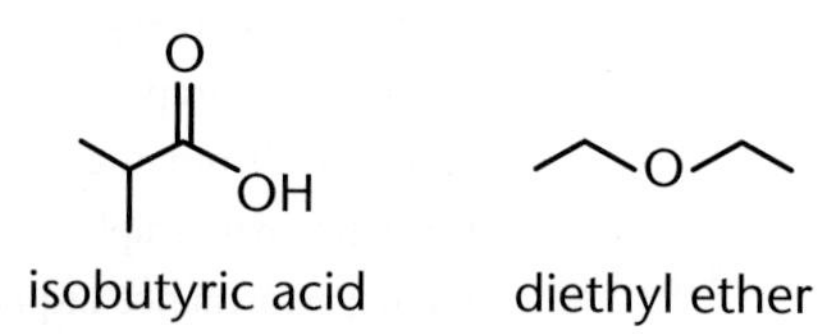


**Figure 12.1** Isobutyric Acid and Diethyl Ether
*Isobutyric acid is more polar than diethyl ether and can exhibit hydrogen bonding, so it will congregate in the aqueous layer; diethyl ether will remain in the organic layer.*

After the two layers are mixed together, how do we then get the desired product out? The water (aqueous) and ether (organic) phases will separate on their own, given time to do so. In order to isolate these two phases, we use a piece of equipment called a **separatory funnel**, as shown in Figure 12.2. Gravitational forces cause the denser layer to sink to the bottom of the funnel, where it can then be removed by turning the stopcock at the bottom. It is more common for the organic layer to be on top, although the opposite can also occur. Remember that the position of the layers is determined by their relative densities.

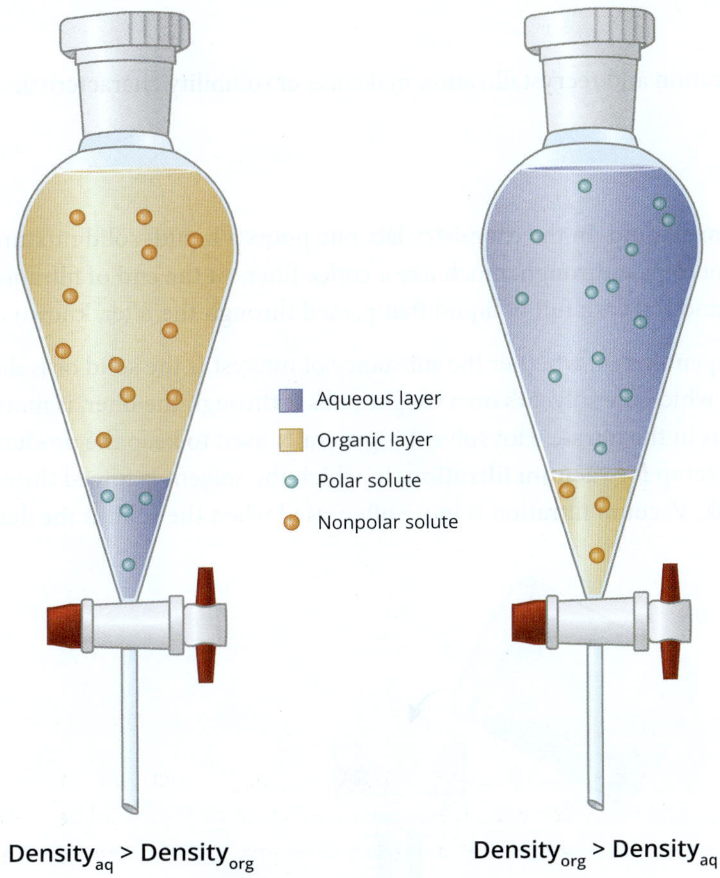


**Figure 12.2** Separatory Funnel
*Used to separate solvents based on their relative densities; the denser solvent is always drained first.*

## KEY CONCEPT

Extraction depends on the rules of solubility and *like dissolves like*. Remember the three intermolecular forces that affect solubility:

1. Hydrogen bonding: Compounds that can do this, such as alcohols or acids, will move most easily into the aqueous layer
2. Dipole–dipole interactions: These compounds are less likely to move into the aqueous layer
3. Van der Waals (London) forces: With only these interactions, compounds are least likely to move into the aqueous layer

In this example, we'll assume that the aqueous layer is more dense and settles to the bottom of the separatory funnel. Once we drain the aqueous layer from the separatory funnel, we repeat the extraction several times. Additional water is added to the separatory funnel, it is shaken and allowed to settle, and the aqueous layer is once again drained off. This is done in order to extract as much of the isobutyric acid from the ether layer as possible because it does not completely transfer with the first extraction. Multiple extractions with fresh water are more effective for obtaining the most product, rather than a single extraction with a larger volume of water. You can imagine this as analogous to laundering dirty clothes several times, rather than laundering them with more water—the cleaner each volume of water is, the less dirt is likely to be left on the clothes afterward.

Once the desired product has been isolated in the solvent, we can obtain the product alone by evaporating the solvent, usually by using a **rotary evaporator (rotovap)**.

Another way to take advantage of solubility properties is to perform the reverse of the extraction we just described in order to remove unwanted impurities. In this case, a small amount of solvent is used to extract and remove impurities, rather than the compound of interest. This process is called a **wash**.

## BRIDGE

You can use the properties of acids and bases to your advantage in extraction:

$$HA + \text{base} \rightarrow A^- + H\text{–base}^+$$

When the acid dissociates, the anion formed will be more soluble in the aqueous layer than the original protonated acid because it is charged. Thus, adding a base will help to extract an acid into the aqueous phase.

## Other Methods

In addition to extraction, filtration and recrystallization make use of solubility characteristics to separate compounds from a mixture.

### Filtration

**Filtration** isolates a solid from a liquid. In the chemistry lab, one pours a liquid–solid mixture onto a paper filter that allows only the solvent to pass through, much like a coffee filter. At the end of filtration, one is left with the solid, called the **residue**, and the flask full of liquid that passed through the filter, known as the **filtrate**.

Filtration can be modified depending on whether the substance of interest is the solid or is dissolved in the filtrate. **Gravity filtration**, in which the solvent's own weight pulls it through the filter, is more commonly used when the product of interest is in the filtrate. Hot solvent is generally used to keep the product dissolved in liquid. Figure 12.3 shows the setup for **vacuum filtration**, in which the solvent is forced through the filter by a vacuum connected to the flask. Vacuum filtration is more often used when the solid is the desired product.

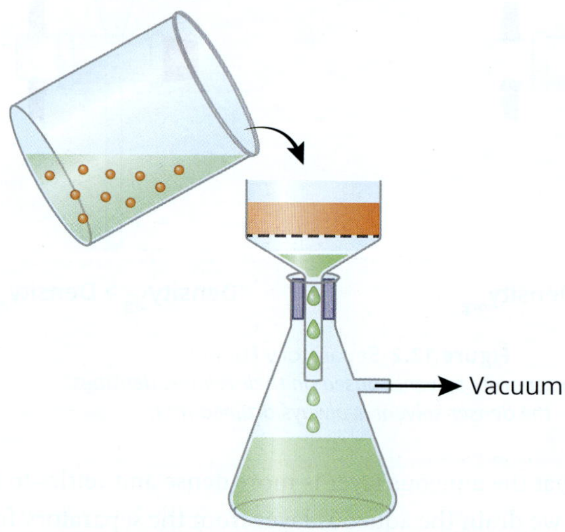


**Figure 12.3** Vacuum Filtration
*Using a vacuum helps to increase the speed of filtration.*

### Recrystallization

**Recrystallization** is a method for further purifying crystals in solution. In this process, shown in Figure 12.4, product is dissolved in a minimum amount of hot solvent and filtered to remove impurities. The solution is then cooled to allow the recrystallization of the product. The solvent chosen for this process should be one in which the product is soluble only at high temperatures. Thus, when the solution cools, only the desired product will recrystallize out of solution, excluding the impurities.

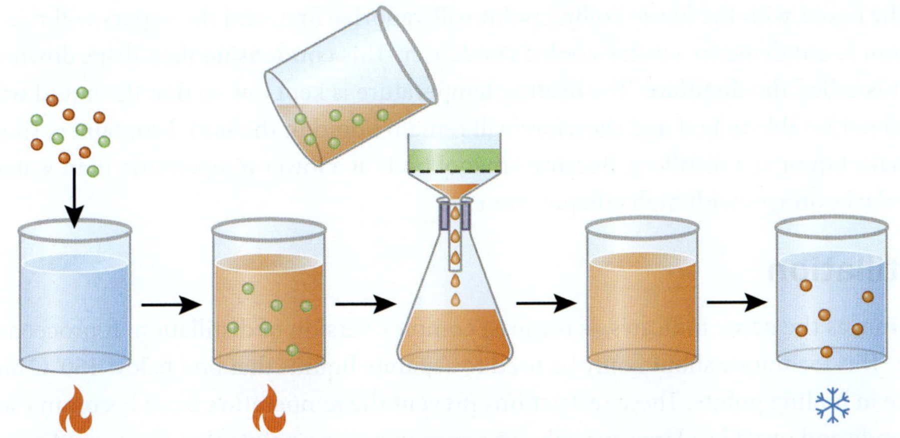


**Figure 12.4** Purification through Recrystallization

### MCAT CONCEPT CHECK 12.1

Before you move on, assess your understanding of the material with these questions.

1. What must be true about the two solvents used for an extraction to work?

______________________________

2. When doing an extraction, would it be better to do three extractions with 10 mL of solvent, or one extraction with 30 mL?

______________________________

3. Would acid dissolve better in an aqueous acid or aqueous base? Why?

______________________________

## 12.2 Distillation

### LEARNING OBJECTIVES

After Chapter 12.2, you will be able to:

- Differentiate between the separatory capabilities of simple, vacuum, and fractional distillation
- Recall the conditions in which distillation is a helpful separatory technique
- Select the best distillation technique for a given solute mixture

Extraction requires two solvents that are immiscible in order to separate the product. But what happens when the product itself is a liquid that is soluble in the solvent? This is where distillation comes in handy. **Distillation** takes advantage of differences in the boiling point to separate two liquids by evaporation and condensation. The liquid with the lower boiling point will vaporize first, and the vapors will rise up the distillation column to condense in a water-cooled condenser. This **condensate** then drips down into a vessel. The end product is called the **distillate**. The heating temperature is kept low so that the liquid with the higher boiling point will not be able to boil and therefore will remain liquid in the initial container. This is the process that is used to make liquor at a distillery. Because ethanol boils at a lower temperature than water, we can use distillation to make beverages with high ethanol contents.

## Simple Distillation

**Simple distillation**, as the name indicates, is the least complex version of distillation. It proceeds precisely as described above. This technique should only be used to separate liquids that boil below 150°C and have at least a 25°C difference in boiling points. These restrictions prevent the temperature from becoming so high that the compounds degrade and provide a large enough difference in boiling points that the second compound won't accidentally boil off into the distillate. The apparatus for this technique consists of a **distilling flask** containing the combined liquid solution, a **distillation column** consisting of a thermometer and a **condenser**, and a **receiving flask** to collect the distillate. The setup is the same as that shown in Figure 12.5, sans the vacuum adapter. Sometimes an additional piece of equipment, such as a boiling chip, ebulliator, or magnetic stirrer, will be introduced to break surface tension and prevent superheating. **Superheating** occurs when a liquid is heated to a temperature above its boiling point without vaporization. Superheating situations occur when gas bubbles within a liquid are unable to overcome the combination of atmospheric pressure and surface tension.

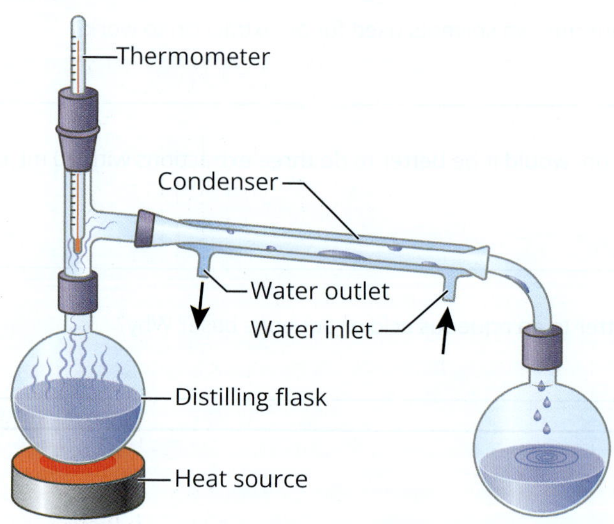


**Figure 12.5** Vacuum Distillation
*The initial solution is placed in the heated distilling flask, where the components of the solution with the lowest boiling points will vaporize first. The vapor then condenses in the water-cooled condenser, and this distillate drips into the receiving flask.*

## Vacuum Distillation

We use **vacuum distillation** whenever we want to distill a liquid with a boiling point over 150°C. By using a vacuum, we lower the ambient pressure, thereby decreasing the temperature that the liquid must reach in order to have sufficient vapor pressure to boil. This allows us to distill compounds with higher boiling points at lower temperatures so that we do not have to worry about degrading the product. The apparatus for vacuum distillation is shown above in Figure 12.5.

**BRIDGE**

Remember from Chapter 7 of *MCAT General Chemistry Review* that liquids boil when their vapor pressure equals ambient pressure. In vacuum distillation, we lower the ambient pressure so that the liquid can boil at lower temperatures.

## Fractional Distillation

To separate two liquids with similar boiling points (less than 25°C apart), we use **fractional distillation**. In this technique, a fractionation column connects the distillation flask to the condenser, as shown in Figure 12.6. A fractionation column is a column in which the surface area is increased by the inclusion of inert objects like glass beads or steel wool. As the vapor rises up the column, it condenses on these surfaces and refluxes back down until rising heat causes it to evaporate again, only to condense again higher in the column. Each time the condensate evaporates, the vapor consists of a higher proportion of the compound with the lower boiling point. By the time the top of the column is reached, only the desired product drips down to the receiving flask.

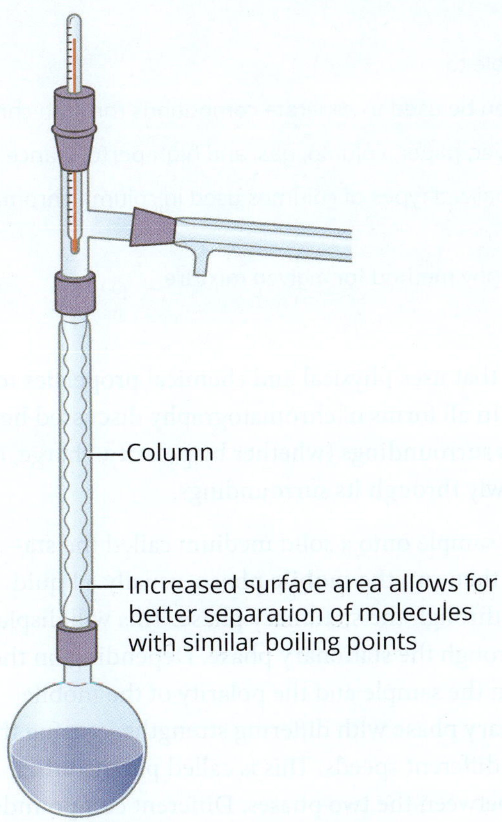


**Figure 12.6** Fractional Distillation
*With increased surface area in the distillation column, the distillate has more places to condense on its way up the column. This allows for more refined separation of liquids with fairly close boiling points.*

## MCAT CONCEPT CHECK 12.2

Before you move on, assess your understanding of the material with these questions.

1. Distillation separates compounds based on what property?

______________________________

2. If we are given a solution of ether, with a boiling point of 308 K, and methylene chloride, with a boiling point of 313 K, which type of distillation should be used to separate them?

______________________________

3. If we are given a solution of bromobenzene, with a boiling point of 156°C, and camphor, with a boiling point of 204°C, which type of distillation should be used to separate them?

______________________________

## 12.3 Chromatography High Yield

### LEARNING OBJECTIVES

After Chapter 12.3, you will be able to:

- Identify the properties that can be used to separate compounds through chromatography
- Differentiate between thin-layer, paper, column, gas, and high-performance liquid chromatography
- Describe the three main specialized types of columns used in column chromatography, and their methods for separation
- Predict the best chromatography method for a given mixture

**Chromatography** is another tool that uses physical and chemical properties to separate and identify compounds from a complex mixture. In all forms of chromatography discussed here, the concept is identical: the more similar a compound is to its surroundings (whether by polarity, charge, or other characteristics), the more it will stick to and move slowly through its surroundings.

The process begins by placing the sample onto a solid medium called the **stationary phase**, or **adsorbent**. We then run the **mobile phase**, usually a liquid (or a gas in gas chromatography) through the stationary phase. This will displace (**elute**) the sample and carry it through the stationary phase. Depending on the characteristics of the substances in the sample and the polarity of the mobile phase, it will adhere to the stationary phase with differing strengths, causing the different substances to migrate at different speeds. This is called **partitioning**, and it represents an equilibrium between the two phases. Different compounds will have different **partitioning coefficients** and will elute at different rates. This results in separation within the stationary phase, allowing us to isolate each substance individually.

### KEY CONCEPT

Chromatography separates compounds based on how strongly they adhere to the solid, or stationary, phase (or in other words, how easily they come off into the mobile phase).

There are many different media that can be used as the stationary phase, each one exploiting different properties that allow us to separate out the desired compound. On the MCAT, the property most commonly used is polarity. For instance, thin-layer chromatography (TLC), which we will shortly discuss, uses silica gel, a highly polar substance, as its stationary phase. Cellulose, another polar substance, may also be used. This means that any polar compound will adhere well to the gel and thus move through (elute) slowly. When using column chromatography, size and charge both have a role in how quickly a compound moves through the stationary phase. Chromatography can use even strong interactions, such as antibody–ligand binding.

As mentioned earlier, chromatography is based on the speed at which compounds move through media. In practice, however, we will measure either how far each substance travels in a given amount of time (such as in TLC) or how long it takes to elute (as in column or gas chromatography).

The types of chromatography that we will discuss include thin-layer and paper chromatography, column chromatography, gas chromatography (also called gas–liquid chromatography), and high-performance liquid chromatography, or HPLC.

## Thin-Layer and Paper Chromatography

**Thin-layer chromatography** and **paper chromatography** are extremely similar techniques, varying only in the medium used for the stationary phase. For thin-layer chromatography, a thin layer of silica gel or alumina adherent to an inert carrier sheet is used. For paper chromatography, as the name suggests, the medium used is paper, which is composed of cellulose.

For these techniques, the sample that we want to separate is placed directly onto the adsorbent itself; this is called **spotting** because we apply a small, well-defined spot of the sample directly onto the silica or paper plate. The plate is then **developed**, which involves placing the adsorbent upright in a developing chamber, usually a beaker with a lid or a wide-mouthed jar. At the bottom of this jar is a shallow pool of solvent, called the **eluent**. The spots of the sample must be above the level of the solvent, or else they will dissolve into the pool of solvent rather than running up the plate. When set up correctly, the solvent will creep up the plate by capillary action, carrying the various compounds in the sample with it at varying rates. When the solvent front nears the top of the plate, the plate is removed from the chamber and allowed to dry.

As mentioned before, TLC is often done with silica gel, which is polar and hydrophilic. The mobile phase, on the other hand, is usually an organic solvent of weak to moderate polarity, so it doesn't bind well to the gel. Because of this, nonpolar compounds dissolve in the organic solvent and move quickly as the solvent moves up the plate, whereas the more polar molecules stick to the gel. Thus, the more nonpolar the sample is, the further up the plate it will move, as shown in Figure 12.7.

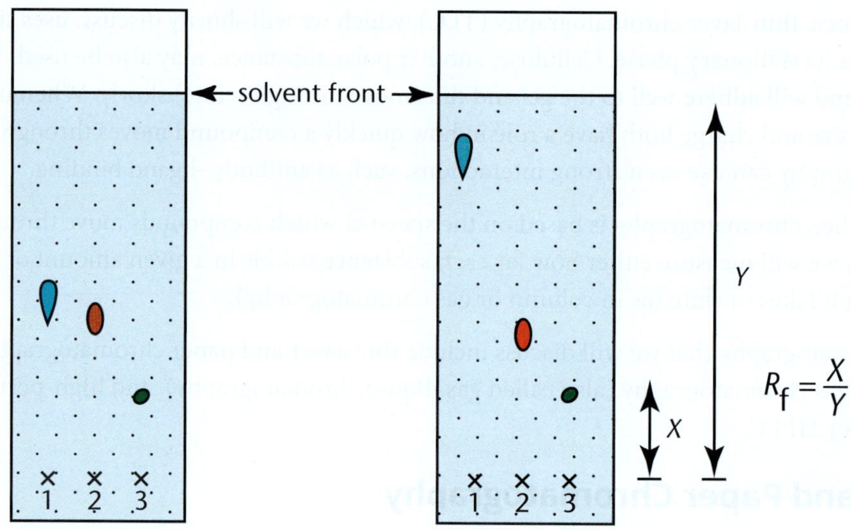


**Figure 12.7** Thin-Layer Chromatography
*Samples are placed at the "x" marks. As the nonpolar solvent moves up the plate via capillary action, the samples that are nonpolar move further up the plate along with the solvent, while the samples that are polar do not move as far.*

**Reverse-phase chromatography** is the exact opposite. In this technique, the stationary phase used is nonpolar, so polar molecules move up the plate quickly, while nonpolar molecules stick more tightly to the stationary phase.

The spots of individual compounds are usually white, which makes them difficult or impossible to see on the white paper or TLC plate. To get around this problem, the developed plate can be placed under ultraviolet light, which will show any compounds that are ultraviolet-sensitive. Alternatively, iodine, phosphomolybdic acid, or vanillin can be used to stain the spots, although this will destroy the compounds such that they cannot be recovered.

When TLC is performed, compounds are generally identified using the **retardation factor ($R_f$)**, which is relatively constant for a particular compound in a given solvent. The $R_f$ is calculated using the equation:

$$R_f = \frac{\text{distance spot moved}}{\text{distance solvent front moved}}$$

**Equation 12.1**

Because its value is relatively constant, the $R_f$ value can be used to identify unknown compounds.

This technique is most frequently performed on a small scale to identify unknown compounds. It can also be used on a larger scale as a means of purification, a technique called **preparative TLC**. As the large plate develops, the larger spot of sample splits into bands of individual compounds, which can then be scraped off and washed to yield pure compounds.

## Column Chromatography

The principles behind column chromatography are the same as for thin-layer chromatography, although there are some differences. First, **column chromatography** uses an entire column filled with silica or aluminum beads as an adsorbent, allowing for much greater separation. The setup for this is shown in Figure 12.8. In addition, thin-layer chromatography uses capillary action to

**BRIDGE**

A more detailed description of chromatography columns can be found in Chapter 3 of *MCAT Biochemistry Review*.

move the solvent up the plate, whereas column chromatography uses gravity to move the solvent and compounds down the column. To speed up the process, one can force the solvent through the column using gas pressure, a technique called flash column chromatography. In column chromatography, the solvent polarity can also be changed to help elute the desired compound.

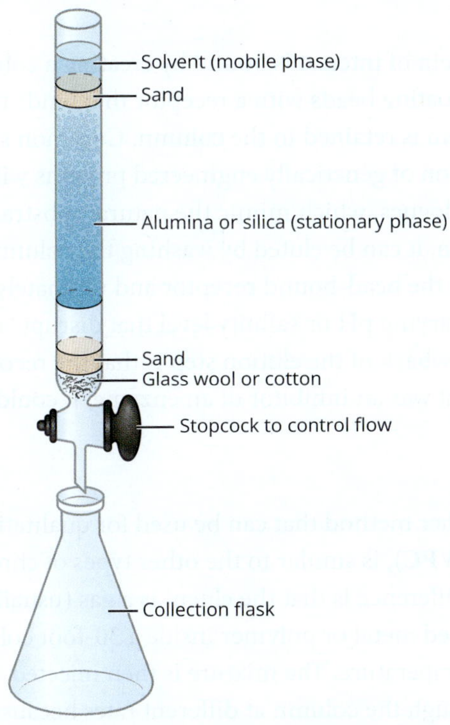


**Figure 12.8** Column Chromatography
*The sample is added to the top of the column, and a solvent is poured over it. The more similar the sample is to the mobile phase, the faster it elutes; the more similar it is to the stationary phase, the more slowly it will elute (if at all).*

Eventually, the solvent drips out of the end of the column, and the different fractions that leave the column can be collected over time. Each fraction will contain different compounds. After collection, the solvent can be evaporated, leaving behind the compounds of interest. Column chromatography is particularly useful in biochemistry because it can be used to separate and collect macromolecules such as proteins or nucleic acids. There are several techniques that can be used to isolate specific materials, which are described in the following paragraphs, as well as in Chapter 3 of *MCAT Biochemistry Review*.

### Ion-Exchange Chromatography

In **ion-exchange chromatography**, the beads in the column are coated with charged substances so that they attract or bind compounds that have an opposite charge. For instance, a positively charged compound will attract and hold a negatively charged backbone of DNA or protein as it passes through the column, either increasing its retention time or retaining it completely. After all other compounds have moved through the column, a salt gradient is used to elute the charged molecules that have stuck to the column.

### Size-Exclusion Chromatography

In **size-exclusion chromatography**, the beads used in the column contain tiny pores of varying sizes. These tiny pores allow small compounds to enter the beads, thus slowing them down. Large compounds can't fit into the pores, so they will move around them and travel through the column faster. It is important to remember that in this type of chromatography, the small compounds are slowed down and retained longer—which may be counterintuitive. The size of the pores may be varied so that molecules with different molecular weights can be fractionated. A common approach in protein purification is to use an ion-exchange column followed by a size-exclusion column.

### Affinity Chromatography

In **affinity chromatography**, a protein of interest is bound by creating a column with high affinity for that protein. This can be accomplished by coating beads with a receptor that binds the protein or a specific antibody to the protein; in either case, the protein is retained in the column. Common stationary phase molecules include nickel, which is used in the separation of genetically engineered proteins with histidine tags, antibodies or antigens, and enzyme substrate analogues, which mimic the natural substrate for an enzyme of interest. Once the protein is retained in the column, it can be eluted by washing the column with a free receptor (or target or antibody), which will compete with the bead-bound receptor and ultimately free the protein from the column. Eluents can also be created with a varying pH or salinity level that disrupts the bonds between the ligand and the protein of interest. The only drawback of the elution step is that the recovered substance can be bound to the eluent. If, for example, the eluent was an inhibitor of an enzyme, it could be difficult to remove.

## Gas Chromatography

**Gas chromatography (GC)** is another method that can be used for qualitative separation. GC, also known as **vapor-phase chromatography** (**VPC**), is similar to the other types of chromatography and is shown in Figure 12.9. The main conceptual difference is that the eluent is a gas (usually helium or nitrogen) instead of a liquid. The adsorbent is a crushed metal or polymer inside a 30-foot column. This column is coiled and kept inside an oven to control its temperature. The mixture is then injected into the column and vaporized. The gaseous compounds travel through the column at different rates because they adhere to the adsorbent in the column to different degrees and will separate in space by the time they reach the end of the column. The injected compounds must be **volatile**: low melting-point, sublimable solids or vaporizable liquids. The compounds are registered by a detector, which records them as a peak on a chart.

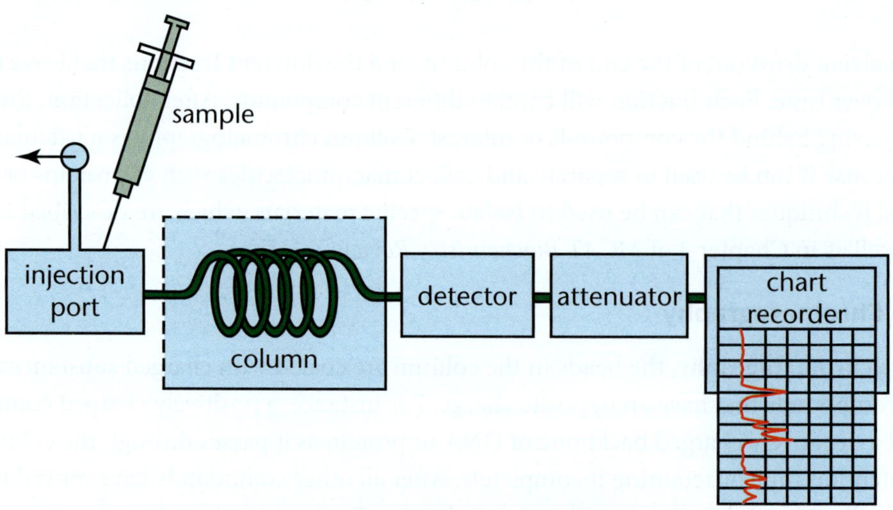


**Figure 12.9** Gas Chromatography
*The sample is injected into the column and moves with the gaseous mobile phase through a stationary liquid or solid phase; a computer identifies the sample components.*

It is common to separate molecules using GC and then to inject the pure molecules into a **mass spectrometer** for molecular weight determination. **Mass spectrometry** involves the ionization and fragmentation of compounds; these fragments are then run through a magnetic field, which separates them by mass-to-charge ratio. The total molecular weight can thus be determined, or the relative concentrations of the different fragments can be calculated and compared against reference values to identify the compound.

## High-Performance Liquid Chromatography

**High-performance liquid chromatography (HPLC)** was previously called high-pressure liquid chromatography. As the name suggests, the eluent is a liquid, and it travels through a column of a defined composition. There is a variety of stationary phases that can be chosen depending on the target molecule and the quantity of material that needs to be purified. This is fairly similar to column chromatography because the various compounds in solution will react differently with the adsorbent material. In the past, very high pressures were used, but recent advances allow for much lower pressures—hence the change in name. As depicted in Figure 12.10, in HPLC, a small sample is injected into the column, and separation occurs as it flows through. The compounds pass through a detector and are collected as the solvent flows out of the end of the apparatus. The interface is similar to that used for GC because the entire process is computerized, but it uses liquid under pressure instead of gas. Because the whole process is under computer control, sophisticated solvent gradients as well as temperature can be applied to the column to help resolve the various compounds in the sample—hence the higher performance of HPLC over regular column chromatography.

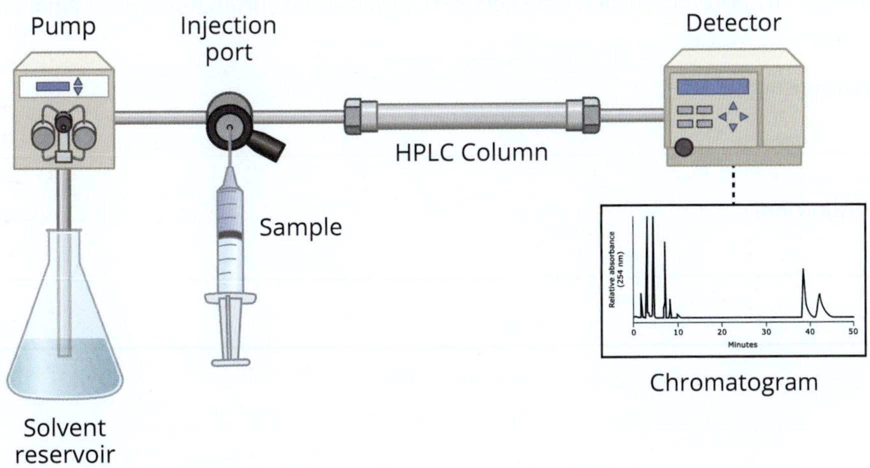


**Figure 12.10** High-Performance Liquid Chromatography (HPLC) Setup
*The sample is injected and passed through a liquid column, where it is separated into its component compounds.*

## MCAT CONCEPT CHECK 12.3

Before you move on, assess your understanding of the material with these questions.

1. What properties of molecules do thin-layer chromatography, paper chromatography, and standard column chromatography take advantage of to separate compounds?

   ______________________________

2. What are the three specialized types of column chromatography? What does each use in order to separate the sample?

| Type of Column Chromatography | Method for Separating Sample |
|---|---|
| | |
| | |
| | |

3. In what way is gas chromatography distinct from all of the other techniques we have discussed?

   ______________________________

4. What is the major historical distinction between HPLC and column chromatography? What is the major distinction now?

   - Historical distinction:

     ______________________________

   - Current distinction:

     ______________________________

## Conclusion

Don't forget, the MCAT won't ask you to get into your lab coat and extract the product of a reaction! As long as you understand the principles governing these techniques and when you should apply them, you'll be in great shape. Table 12.1 summarizes the scientific basis and purpose of the major techniques discussed in this chapter. Remember that separation and purification techniques exploit physical properties of compounds, such as polarity, solubility, size and shape, and charge, to obtain a purified product. These properties can be traced back to intermolecular forces or properties of the molecules themselves. Having a variety of tools and methods to separate and collect a purified product is essential in practical organic chemistry, and choosing the proper techniques often requires knowledge and consideration of the desired product. When you look at the bigger picture, these methods may be easier to conceptualize than to actually apply in the lab!

| Technique | Purpose | Basis for Separation |
| --- | --- | --- |
| **Extraction** | Separate solutes | Solubility in immiscible solvents |
| **Filtration** | Remove solids from liquids | Particle size |
| **Recrystallization** | Purify solids | Solubility at different temperatures |
| **Simple Distillation** | Separate liquids ($\Delta BP \geq 25°C$) | Boiling point |
| **Vacuum Distillation** | Separate high-BP liquids ($BP > 150°C$) | Boling point (reduced pressure) |
| **Fractional Distillation** | Separate liquids ($\Delta BP < 25°C$) | Boiling point (fractionating column) |
| **TLC/Paper Chromatography** | Identify compounds, monitor reactions | Polarity/partitioning ($R_f$) |
| **Column Chromatography** | Separate/purify mixtures | Polarity or mechanism |
| **Ion-Exchange** | Separate charged molecules | Electrostatic interactions |
| **Size-Exclusion** | Separate by molecule size | Molecular size/shape |
| **Affinity** | Separate a protein through specific binding | Ligand–target interactions |
| **Gas Chromatography** | Separate volatile compounds | Volatility/boiling point |
| **HPLC** | Separate complex solvents precisely | Partitioning (column-dependent) |

**Table 12.1** Summary of Separation and Purification Techniques

Despite the subject's compelling relevance to everyday life, college organic chemistry often terrifies and alienates its students. The MCAT, on the other hand, doesn't ask you to memorize tables of reactants or regurgitate hundreds of named reactions from scratch. Instead, the MCAT asks you to look at the bigger picture, to know trends, and to participate in the logic of chemistry. We hope that studying for the MCAT has given you a chance to rediscover organic chemistry—to focus on the *how* and the *why*, instead of the *what*. Organic chemistry, like the MCAT as a whole, should be seen not as an obstacle but as an opportunity. So, work hard, have some fun along the way, and keep thinking about where you're heading—you can almost feel that white coat.

**GO ONLINE**

**You've reviewed the content, now test your knowledge and critical thinking skills by completing a test-like passage set in your online resources!**

# CONCEPT SUMMARY

## Solubility-Based Methods

- **Extraction** combines two immiscible liquids, one of which easily dissolves the compound of interest.
  - The polar (water) layer is called the **aqueous phase** and dissolves compounds with hydrogen bonding or polarity.
  - The nonpolar layer is called the **organic phase** and dissolves nonpolar compounds.
  - Extraction is carried out in a separatory funnel. One phase is collected, and the solvent is then evaporated.
  - Acid–base properties can be used to increase solubility.
- A **wash** is the reverse of extraction, in which a small amount of solvent that dissolves impurities is run over the compound of interest.
- **Filtration** isolates a solid (**residue**) from a liquid (**filtrate**).
  - **Gravity filtration** is used when the product of interest is in the filtrate. Hot solvent is used to maintain solubility.
  - **Vacuum filtration** is used when the product of interest is the solid. A vacuum is connected to the flask to pull the solvent through more quickly.
- In **recrystallization**, the product is dissolved in a minimum amount of hot solvent. If the impurities are more soluble, the crystals will reform while the flask cools, excluding the impurities.

## Distillation

- **Distillation** separates liquids according to differences in their boiling points; the liquid with the lowest boiling point vaporizes first and is collected as the **distillate**.
- **Simple distillation** can be used if the boiling points are under 150°C and are at least 25°C apart.
- **Vacuum distillation** should be used if the boiling points are over 150°C to prevent degradation of the product.
- **Fractional distillation** should be used if the boiling points are less than 25°C apart because it allows more refined separation of liquids by boiling point.

## Chromatography

- All forms of **chromatography** use two phases to separate compounds based on physical or chemical properties.
  - The **stationary phase** or **adsorbent** is usually a polar solid.
  - The **mobile phase** runs through the stationary phase and is usually a liquid or gas. This **elutes** the sample through the stationary phase.
  - Compounds with higher affinity for the stationary phase have smaller **retardation factors** and take longer to pass through, if at all; compounds with higher affinity for the mobile phase elute through more quickly. Compounds, therefore, get separated from each other, which is called **partitioning**.
- **Thin-layer** and **paper chromatography** are used to identify a sample.
  - The stationary phase is a polar material, such as silica, alumina, or paper.
  - The mobile phase is a nonpolar solvent, which climbs the card through capillary action.
  - The card is **spotted** and **developed**; $R_f$ values can be calculated and compared to reference values.
  - **Reverse-phase chromatography** uses a nonpolar card with a polar solvent.
- **Column chromatography** utilizes polarity, size, or affinity to separate compounds based on their physical or chemical properties.
  - The stationary phase is a column containing silica or alumina beads.
  - The mobile phase is a nonpolar solvent, which travels through the column by gravity.
  - In **ion-exchange chromatography**, the beads are coated with charged substances to bind compounds with opposite charge.
  - In **size-exclusion chromatography**, the beads have small pores which trap smaller compounds and allow larger compounds to travel through faster.
  - In **affinity chromatography**, the column is made to have high affinity for a compound by coating the beads with a receptor or antibody to the compound.
- **Gas chromatography** separates vaporizable compounds according to how well they adhere to the adsorbent in the column.
  - The stationary phase is a coil of crushed metal or a polymer.
  - The mobile phase is a nonreactive gas.
  - Gas chromatography may be combined in sequence with **mass spectrometry**, which ionizes and fragments molecules and passes these fragments through a magnetic field to determine molecular weight or structure.
- **High-performance liquid chromatography (HPLC)** is similar to column chromatography but uses sophisticated computer-mediated solvent and temperature gradients. It is used if the sample size is small or if forces such as capillary action will affect results. It was formerly called high-pressure liquid chromatography.

## ANSWERS TO CONCEPT CHECKS

### 12.1

1. The two solvents must be immiscible and must have different polarity or acid–base properties that allow a compound of interest to dissolve more easily in one than the other.
2. It is better to do three washes with 10 mL than to do one with 30 mL; more of the compound of interest would be extracted with multiple sequential extractions than one large one.
3. Acid dissolves better in an aqueous base because it will dissociate to form the conjugate base and, being more highly charged, will become more soluble. Note that *like dissolves like* applies to polarity; acids and bases dissolve more easily in solutions with the opposite acid–base characteristics.

### 12.2

1. Distillation takes advantage of differences in boiling points in order to separate solutions of miscible liquids.
2. A solution of ether and methylene chloride, which have very close boiling points, can be separated by using fractional distillation.
3. Vacuum distillation would be the best technique to separate two chemicals with such high boiling points because the decreased ambient pressure will allow them to boil at a lower temperature.

### 12.3

1. Each of these methods separates compounds using charge and polarity.
2.

| Type of Column Chromatography | Method for Separating Sample |
|---|---|
| **Ion-exchange** | The column is given a charge, which attracts molecules with the opposite charge. |
| **Size-exclusion** | Small pores are used; smaller molecules are trapped, while larger molecules pass through the column. |
| **Affinity** | Specific receptors or antibodies can trap the target in the column; the target must then be washed out using other solutions. |

3. As the name suggests, gas chromatography is simply the same technique of mobile and stationary phases performed with a gaseous eluent (instead of liquid). The stationary phase is usually a crushed metal or polymer.
4. Historically, HPLC was performed at high pressures, whereas column chromatography uses gravity to pull the solution through the column. Now, HPLC is performed with sophisticated and variable solvent and temperature gradients, allowing for much more specific separation of compounds than column chromatography; high pressures are no longer required.

## SCIENCE MASTERY ASSESSMENT EXPLANATIONS

1. **B**

Fractional distillation is the most effective procedure for separating two liquids that boil within a few degrees of each other. Ethyl acetate and ethanol boil well within 25°C of each other and thus would be good candidates for fractional distillation. Fractional distillation could also be used for the liquids in **(C)**, but would require lower pressures because of their high boiling points.

2. **C**

By extracting with sodium hydroxide, benzoic acid will be converted to its sodium salt, sodium benzoate. Sodium benzoate, unlike its conjugate acid, will dissolve in an aqueous solution. The aqueous layer simply has to be acidified afterward to retrieve benzoic acid. **(A)** is incorrect because diethyl ether and tetrahydrofuran are both nonpolar and are miscible. Hydrochloric acid will not transform benzoic acid into a soluble salt, so **(B)** is incorrect. Finally, **(D)** is incorrect because protonated benzoic acid has limited solubility in water.

3. **D**

It is more effective to perform four successive extractions with small amounts of ether than to perform one extraction with a large amount of ether.

4. **D**

Hexane is less polar than ether and, therefore, is less likely to displace polar compounds adsorbed to the silica gel. This would decrease the distance these polar compounds would travel, decreasing $R_f$ values.

5. **D**

In column chromatography, as in TLC, the less polar compound travels most rapidly. This means that 1-naphthalenemethanol, with the highest $R_f$ value, would travel most rapidly and would be the first to elute from the column.

6. **A**

This is an example of reverse-phase chromatography. The solvent system is polar, which means that the most polar compound will travel the furthest up the card, resulting in the largest $R_f$. This gives compound III the largest $R_f$, which corresponds to spot A.

7. **B**

Because methylene chloride is denser than brine (salt water), the organic layer will settle at the bottom of the funnel. Methylene chloride is not soluble in water, eliminating **(C)**.

8. **B**

Silica gels are polar. Polarity is used to selectively attract specific solutes within a nonpolar solvent phase. Although silica gels have other properties, this is the most important to TLC.

9. **B**

In this question, three substances must be separated using a combination of techniques. The first step should be the most obvious: remove the sand by filtration. The remaining compounds—benzoic acid and naphthalene—are still dissolved in ether. If the solution is extracted with an aqueous base, the benzoate anion is formed and becomes dissolved in the aqueous layer, while naphthalene, a nonpolar compound, remains in the ether. Finally, evaporation of the ether will yield purified naphthalene.

10. **C**

This is the only option that would be effectively separated by a simple distillation. **(B)** would require vacuum distillation because the boiling points are over 150°C. In **(A)** and **(D)**, the boiling points are within 25°C of each other and would therefore require fractional distillation in order to be separated.

11. **C**

Affinity chromatography, using the target for the biological effector or a specific antibody, would work best in this case. It will specifically bind the protein of interest and keep it in the column.

12. **D**

Because this solution is composed of a much larger molecule and a much smaller molecule, size-exclusion chromatography would effectively remove the smaller insulin molecule into the fraction retained in the column and allow the titin to be eluted. Affinity chromatography, **(C)**, could also be used, but comes with a risk of rendering the titin unusable; the eluent run through an affinity chromatography column often binds to the target molecule.

13. **B**

Each of these is the mobile phase of the system, in which the solutes are dissolved and move. The stationary phase in gas chromatography is usually a crushed metal or polymer; the stationary phase in paper chromatography is paper.

14. **C**

Warm or hot solvent is generally used in gravity filtration to keep the desired product soluble. This allows the product to remain in the filtrate, which can then be collected. In this case, the student likely used solvent that was too cold, and the product crystallized out. The product should be present in the residue.

15. **B**

Because the lactoferrin proteins are likely to be charged, as is the resin described in the question, this is an example of ion-exchange chromatography. The charged protein molecules will stick to the column, while the remainder of the milk washes through and can later be washed off of the column and collected.

**GO ONLINE**

**Consult your online resources for additional practice.**

## EQUATIONS TO REMEMBER

(12.1) **Retardation factor:** $R_f = \frac{\text{distance spot moved}}{\text{distance solvent front moved}}$

## SHARED CONCEPTS

**Biochemistry Chapter 3**
Nonenzymatic Protein Function and Protein Analysis

**General Chemistry Chapter 7**
Thermochemistry

**General Chemistry Chapter 8**
The Gas Phase

**General Chemistry Chapter 9**
Solutions

**General Chemistry Chapter 10**
Acids and Bases

**Organic Chemistry Chapter 11**
Spectroscopy

# GLOSSARY

**$\alpha$-Carbon**–The carbon adjacent to a carbonyl; in amino acids, the chiral stereocenter in all amino acids except glycine.

**$\alpha$-Hydrogen**–Hydrogen atoms connected to $\alpha$-carbons adjacent to carbonyls.

**$\alpha$-State**–A magnetic state seen in NMR spectroscopy in which nuclei have magnetic moments that are aligned with an incident magnetic field, thus having lower energy.

**Absolute conformation**–The exact spatial arrangement of atoms or groups in a chiral molecule around a single chiral atom, designated by (*R*) or (*S*).

**Acetal**–A functional group that contains a carbon atom bonded to two –OR groups, an alkyl chain, and a hydrogen atom.

**Achiral**–A molecule that either does not contain a chiral center or contains chiral centers and a plane of symmetry; as such, it has a superimposable mirror image.

**Acid dissociation constant ($K_a$)**–A measurement of the strength of an acid in solution; the higher the $K_a$, the lower the p$K_a$ and the stronger the acid.

**Affinity chromatography**–A special type of column chromatography in which a column is customized to bind a substance of interest.

**Aldehyde**–A functional group containing a carbonyl and a hydrogen (RCOH); always found at the end of a chain.

**Aldol condensation**–A reaction in which an aldehyde or ketone acts as both the electrophile and nucleophile, resulting in the formation of a carbon–carbon bond in a new molecule called an aldol.

**Alkane**–A simple hydrocarbon molecule with the formula $C_nH_{2n+2}$.

**Amide**–A functional group containing a carbonyl and an amino group ($RCONR_2$).

**Amino acids**–Dipolar compounds that contain an amine and a carboxylic acid attached to a single carbon (the $\alpha$-carbon); the building blocks of peptides.

**Amphoteric**–Describes molecules that can act as both acids and bases.

**Angle strain**–Increased energy that results when bond angles deviate from their ideal values.

**Anhydride**–A functional group containing two carbonyls separated by an oxygen atom (RCOOCOR); often the condensation dimer of a carboxylic acid.

***Anti* conformation**–A type of staggered conformation in which the two largest groups are antiperiplanar to each other; the most energetically favorable conformation.

**Antibonding orbital**–A higher-energy, less stable orbital that results from the overlap of wave functions with opposite signs.

**Antiperiplanar**–A conformation in which substituents are in the same plane, but on opposite sides of a bond.

**Axial**–Describes groups on a cyclic molecule that are perpendicular to the plane of the molecule, pointing straight up or down.

**Azimuthal quantum number ($l$)**–Describes the subshell in which an electron is found; possible values range from 0 to $n - 1$, with $l = 0$ representing the *s* subshell, $l = 1$ representing *p*, $l = 2$ representing *d*, and $l = 3$ representing *f*.

**$\beta$-lactam**–Four-membered cyclic amides that are more reactive to hydrolysis than linear amides or larger cyclic amides; often used as the backbone for antibiotics.

**$\beta$-state**–A magnetic state seen in NMR spectroscopy in which nuclei have been irradiated with radiofrequency pulses to bring them to a higher-energy state.

**Biotin (vitamin $B_7$)**–A water-soluble vitamin that acts as an essential cofactor for enzymes involved in the metabolism of fats, carbohydrates, and amino acids.

**Bonding orbital**–A lower-energy, more stable orbital that results from the overlap of wave functions with the same sign.

**Carbonyl**–A double bond between a carbon and an oxygen.

**Carboxylic acid**–A functional group that contains a carbonyl and a hydroxyl group on the same carbon (RCOOH).

**Carboxylic acid derivative**–A compound that can be created from a carboxylic acid by nucleophilic acyl substitution; includes anhydrides, esters, amides, and others.

**Chemical properties**–Characteristics of compounds that change chemical composition during a reaction; determine how a molecule will react with other molecules.

**Chemical shift ($\delta$)**–An arbitrary variable used to plot NMR spectra; measured in parts per million (ppm).

**Chemoselectivity**–A reaction's preference for one location over another within a molecule.

**Chiral**–A molecule or carbon atom bonded to four different groups and without a plane of symmetry; thus, it is not superimposable on its mirror image and has an enantiomer.

**Chiral center**–Atoms that are chiral within a molecule.

**Chromatography**–A tool used to separate compounds based on how strongly they adhere to a stationary phase or travel with a mobile phase.

***Cis***–A molecule in which the two substituents are on the same side of an immovable bond.

***Cis–trans* isomers**–Diastereomers with different arrangements of substituents around an immovable bond.

**Column chromatography**–A type of chromatography that uses a column filled with silica or alumina beads as an adsorbent, allowing for separation; uses gravity to move the solvent and compounds down the column.

**Condensation reaction**–A reaction that combines two molecules into one, with the loss of a small molecule.

**Configuration**–The spatial arrangement of the atoms or groups in a molecule.

**Configurational isomers**–Isomers that can only interconvert by breaking bonds; include enantiomers, diastereomers, and *cis–trans* isomers.

**Conformational isomers**–Isomers that are the same molecule, just at different points in their natural rotation about a $\sigma$ bond.

**Conjugation**–Alternating single and multiple bonds that create a system of parallel unhybridized *p*-orbitals; thus, electrons can be shared between these orbitals, forming electron clouds above and below the plane of the molecule and stabilizing the molecule.

**Constitutional isomers**–Molecules that have the same molecular formulas but different connectivity; also called structural isomers.

**Coordinate covalent bond**–A covalent bond in which both electrons in the bond come from the same starting atom.

**Coupling**–In NMR spectroscopy, a phenomenon that occurs when there are protons in such close proximity to each other that their magnetic moments affect each other's appearance in the NMR spectrum by subdividing the peak into subpeaks; also called splitting.

**Coupling constant (*J*)**–The magnitude of splitting in NMR spectroscopy, measured in hertz.

**Covalent**–One of two types of chemical bonds in which electrons are shared between atoms.

**Cyanohydrin**–A functional group containing a nitrile ($-C{\equiv}N$) and a hydroxyl group.

***d*-orbital**–An atomic orbital that is composed of four symmetrical lobes and contains two nodes.

**Decarboxylation**–The complete loss of a carboxyl group as carbon dioxide.

**Deprotection**–Reversion of a protecting group to its original functional group.

**Deprotonation**–The removal of a hydrogen cation ($H^+$) from a molecule.

**Deshielding**–The phenomenon of atoms pulling electron density away from surrounding atoms; in NMR spectroscopy, pulls a group further downfield on the spectrum.

**Developing chamber**–A beaker with a lid or wide-mouthed jar used in thin-layer chromatography.

**Dialcohols**–Alcohols with two hydroxyl groups that are commonly used as protecting groups for aldehyde or ketone carbonyls; also called diols.

**Diastereomers**–Non-mirror-image configurational isomers that differ at at least one–but not all–chiral carbons; have different chemical and physical properties.

**Distillate**–The liquid evaporated, condensed, and collected during distillation.

**Distillation**–A separation and purification technique that takes advantage of differences in boiling point to separate two liquids by vaporization and condensation.

**Doublet**–Two peaks of identical intensity in an NMR spectrum that are equally spaced around the true chemical shift of a group of protons; it results from splitting by another hydrogen.

**Downfield**–Movement toward the left in an NMR spectrum.

**Electron-donating**–Describes groups that push additional electron density toward another atom; stabilizes positive charges and destabilizes negative charges while decreasing acidity.

**Electron-withdrawing**–Describes groups that pull electron density away from another atom; stabilizes negative charges and destabilizes positive charges while increasing acidity.

**Electrophile**–"Electron-loving" atoms with a positive charge or positive polarization that can accept an electron pair when forming new bonds with a nucleophile.

**Eluent**–The solvent used in chromatography, after it has passed through the stationary phase.

**Elute**–To displace with solvent, as in thin-layer chromatography.

**Enantiomers**–Nonsuperimposable mirror images of a chiral molecule; have all the same physical and chemical properties except for rotation of plane-polarized light and reactions in a chiral environment.

**Enol**–The resonance form of a carbonyl that has a carbon–carbon double bond (*ene*) and an alcohol (*–ol*).

**Equatorial**–Describes groups on a cyclic molecule that are in the plane of the molecule.

**Ester**–A functional group containing a carbonyl and an alkoxy group (RCOOR).

**Extraction**–The transfer of a dissolved compound from a starting solvent into a solvent in which the product is more soluble.

**Fingerprint region**–In an IR spectrum, the region of 1500 to 400 $cm^{-1}$ where more complex vibration patterns, caused by the motion of the molecule as a whole, can be seen; it is characteristic of each individual molecule.

**Fischer esterification**–The formation of an ester from a carboxylic acid and an alcohol in acidic conditions.

**Fischer projection**–A system to represent three-dimensional molecules in which horizontal lines indicate bonds that project out from the plane of the page (wedges) and vertical lines indicate bonds going into the plane of the page (dashes); points of intersection represent carbon atoms.

**Flash column chromatography**–A technique that speeds up column chromatography by forcing the solvent through the column by increasing pressure with a nonreactive gas.

**Fractional distillation**–A modified form of distillation used to separate two liquids with similar boiling points (less than 25°C apart); uses a fractionation column, which contains inert materials onto which the liquids can condense and reflux back into the reaction vial, allowing more refined separation.

**Fraction**–A volume of eluted fluid from column chromatography; each fraction contains different compounds that are collected as they leave the column.

**Gabriel (malonic-ester) synthesis**–A method of synthesizing amino acids that uses potassium phthalimide and diethyl bromomalonate followed by an alkyl halide; two substitution reactions are followed by hydrolysis and decarboxylation.

**Gas chromatography (GC)**–A type of chromatography used to separate vaporizable compounds; the stationary phase is a crushed metal or polymer, and the mobile phase is a nonreactive gas.

***Gauche* conformation**–A type of staggered conformation in which the two largest groups are 60° apart.

**Geminal diol**–A functional group with two hydroxyl groups on the same carbon; also called a hydrate.

**Glycerol**–A simple triol compound with a three-carbon backbone, which serves as the structural foundation for all lipids known as glycerides, including triglycerides.

**Heme**–A porphyrin ring in hemoglobin that contains $Fe^{2+}$.

**Hemiacetal**–A functional group that contains a carbon atom bonded to one –OR group, one –OH group, an alkyl chain, and a hydrogen atom.

**Hemiketal**–A functional group that contains a carbon atom bonded to one –OR group, one –OH group, and two alkyl chains.

**Heterolysis**–Cleavage of a bond in which both electrons are given to the same atom.

**High-performance liquid chromatography (HPLC)**–A form of chromatography in which a small sample is put into a column that can be manipulated with sophisticated solvent gradients to allow very refined separation and characterization; formerly called high-pressure liquid chromatography.

**Highest occupied molecular orbital (HOMO)**–The highest-energy molecular orbital containing electrons; in UV spectroscopy, electrons are excited from the HOMO to the LUMO.

**Hydride reagent**–Reducing reagents containing hydride anions ($H^-$).

**Hydrogen bonding**–An intermolecular force that results from the extreme polarity of the bonds when hydrogen atoms are attached to highly electronegative atoms (N, O, or F).

**Hydrolysis**–The breaking of a molecule using water.

**Hydroxyl group**–An -OH group; seen in alcohols, hemiacetals and hemiketals, carboxylic acids, water, and other compounds.

**Hydroxyquinone**–A compound containing a quinone (conjugated ring with carbonyls) and a hydroxyl group.

**Imidazole**–A five-membered ring with 2 N atoms that is found in the amino acid histidine.

**Imine**–A double bond between a carbon and a nitrogen.

**Immiscible**–Describes two solvents that will not mix with or dissolve each other.

**Indole**–A bicyclic compound containing a benzene and pyrrole. The aromatic amino acid tryptophan and the neurotransmitter serotonin both contain an indole group.

**Induction**–The pull of electron density across sigma bonds.

**Infrared (IR) spectroscopy**–A technique that measures molecular vibrations at different frequencies, from which specific bonds can be determined; functional groups can be inferred based on this information.

**Inorganic phosphate ($P_i$)**–Derived from phosphoric acid, the molecule that forms high-energy bonds for energy transfer in nucleotide triphosphates like ATP; also used for enzyme regulation.

**Ion-exchange chromatography**–A special type of column chromatography in which the beads in the column are coated with charged substances so that they attract or bind compounds with an opposite charge.

**Ionic**–One of two types of chemical bonds in which electrons are transferred from one atom to another.

**Isoalloxazine**–A tricyclic organic molecule composed of carbon, hydrogen, nitrogen, and oxygen.

**Isomers**–Molecules with the same molecular formula but different chemical structures.

**Jones oxidation**–An oxidation reaction in which primary alcohols are oxidized to carboxylic acids and secondary alcohols are oxidized to ketones; requires $CrO_3$ dissolved with dilute sulfuric acid in acetone.

**Ketal**–A functional group that contains a carbon atom bonded to two $-OR$ groups and two alkyl chains.

**Ketone**–A functional group containing a carbonyl with two alkyl groups (RCOR); always found within a chain.

**Lactam**–A cyclic amide; named according to the Greek letter of the carbon closing the ring.

**Lactone**–A cyclic ester; named according to the Greek letter of the carbon closing the ring and for the straight-chain form of the compound.

**Leaving group**–The molecular fragment that retains electrons after heterolysis; must be stable in solution.

**Lewis acid**–An electron acceptor in the formation of a covalent bond.

**Lewis base**–An electron donor in the formation of a covalent bond.

**Lowest unoccupied molecular orbital (LUMO)**–The lowest-energy molecular orbital that does not contain electrons; in UV spectroscopy, electrons are excited from the HOMO to the LUMO.

**Magnetic quantum number ($m_l$)**–Describes the orbital in which an electron is found; possible values range from $-l$ to $+l$.

***Meso* compound**–A molecule that has chiral centers but is not optically active because it has an internal plane of symmetry.

**Mesylate**–A compound containing the functional group $-SO_3CH_3$, derived from methanesulfonic acid.

**Michael addition**–A reaction in which a carbanion attacks an $\alpha,\beta$-unsaturated carbonyl.

**Mobile phase**–A liquid (or a gas in gas chromatography) that is run through the stationary phase in chromatography.

**Molecular orbital**–The resulting electron structure when two atomic orbitals combine.

**Multiplet**–Peaks that have more than four shifts in NMR spectroscopy.

**Newman projection**–A method of visualizing a compound in which the line of sight is down a carbon–carbon bond axis.

**Node**–In orbital structure, an area where the probability of finding an electron is zero.

**Nonbonded strain**–Increased energy that results when nonadjacent atoms or groups compete for the same space; also called steric strain.

**Nuclear magnetic resonance (NMR) spectroscopy**–A technique that measures the alignment of magnetic moments from certain molecular nuclei with an external magnetic field; can be used to determine the connectivity and functional groups in a molecule.

**Nucleophiles**–"Nucleus-loving" atoms with either lone pairs or $\pi$ bonds that can be used to form new bonds with electrophiles.

**Nucleophilic acyl substitution**–The substitution of a nucleophile for the leaving group of a carboxylic acid or carboxylic acid derivative.

**Optical isomers**–A type of configurational isomers that have different spatial arrangements of substituents, which affect the rotation of plane-polarized light.

**Organic phosphates**–Organic molecules–usually nucleotides–that have a variable number of phosphate groups attached.

**Oxidation**–Loss of electrons causing an increase in oxidation state; increasing bonds to oxygen or other heteroatoms in a molecule.

**Oxidation state**–An indication of the hypothetical charge that an atom would have if all of its bonds were completely ionic.

**Oxidizing agent**–An element or compound that accepts an electron from another species, thereby being reduced in the process.

***p*-orbital**–An atomic orbital that is composed of two lobes located symmetrically about the nucleus and contains a node.

**Paper chromatography**–A type of chromatography that uses paper as the stationary phase.

**Partitioning**–When components in a sample adhere differentially to the mobile and stationary phases of a chromatographic setup; this causes the different substances to migrate at different speeds through the stationary phase.

**Peptide bond**–An amide bond formed between two amino acids through a condensation (nucleophilic acyl substitution) reaction.

**Phenol**–An alcohol with an aromatic ring, which has slightly more acidic hydroxyl hydrogens than other alcohols.

**Phosphodiester bond**–The type of bond linking the sugar moieties of adjacent nucleotides in DNA.

**Physical properties**–Characteristics of compounds that do not change chemical composition, such as melting point, boiling point, solubility, odor, color, and density.

**Pi ($\pi$) bond**–The bonding molecular orbital formed when two parallel *p*-orbitals share electrons; exists as electrons clouds above and below the sigma ($\sigma$) bond between the two nuclei.

**Polarity**–An uneven distribution of charge caused by atoms in the same molecule having different electronegativities.

**Polypeptide**–A molecule formed from multiple amino acids connected by peptide bonds.

**Porphyrin**–A large, ring-shaped organic molecule that is essential for life, forming the core of critical biological pigments like heme and chlorophyll.

**Preparative thin-layer chromatography**–Large-scale use of thin-layer chromatography (TLC) as a means of purification; as the large plate develops, the larger spot of sample splits into bands of individual compounds, which can then be scraped off and washed to yield pure compounds.

**Principal quantum number (*n*)**–Describes the shell in which an electron is found; values range from 1 to $\infty$.

**Protonation**–The addition of a hydrogen cation ($H^+$) to a molecule.

**Purine**–A bicyclic structure with a six-membered ring fused to a five-membered ring. The purines include adenine (A) and guanine (G), both of which are in DNA and RNA.

**Pyridine**–A six-membered ring with 1 N atom. An example can be observed in the structure of NAD+.

**Pyrimidine**–A single six-membered ring structure; includes cytosine (C) and thymine (T), both found in DNA, and uracil (U), found in RNA.

**Pyrophosphate ($PP_i$)**–The ester dimer of phosphate $\left(P_2O_7^{4-}\right)$; released when a new nucleotide is joined to a growing strand of DNA by DNA polymerase.

**Pyrrole–**A five-membered ring with 1 N atom. Five Pyrroles make a porphyrin ring.

**Quinone**–A compound produced by the oxidation of a phenol containing a conjugated ring with ketones.

**R group**–In general, an alkyl chain; in amino acid chemistry, the variable side chain on the $\alpha$-carbon.

**Racemic mixture**–A mixture where both (+) and (−) enantiomers are present in equal concentrations.

**Reduction**–Gain of electrons causing a decrease in oxidation state; decreasing bonds to oxygen or other hetero-atoms in a molecule.

**Relative configuration**–The spatial arrangement of groups in a chiral molecule compared to another chiral molecule.

**Resonance**–Delocalization of $\pi$ electrons, which increases stability of a molecule.

**Resonance structure**–A possible arrangement of $\pi$ electrons in a molecule; the actual electronic structure of a molecule is the weighted average of resonance structures, based on their stability.

**Retardation factor ($R_f$)**–A ratio used in thin-layer chromatography to identify a compound; calculated as how far the compound traveled relative to how far the solvent front traveled.

**Retro-aldol reaction**–The reverse of an aldol condensation reaction, in which a carbon–carbon bond is cleaved with heat and base, yielding two aldehydes, two ketones, or one of each.

**Reverse-phase chromatography**–The opposite of traditional thin-layer chromatography, in which the stationary phase is nonpolar and the mobile phase is polar.

**Riboflavin (vitamin $B_2$)**–The core chemical structure of FAD ($FADH_2$) that contains a tricyclic isoalloxazine structure.

**Ring strain**–Energy created in a cyclic molecule by angle strain, torsional strain, and nonbonded strain; determines if a ring is stable enough to stay intact.

***s*-orbital**–An atomic orbital that is spherical and symmetrical, centered on the nucleus.

**Saponification**–The process by which fats are hydrolyzed under basic conditions to produce soap.

**Separatory funnel**–A piece of laboratory equipment used in extraction; immiscible solvents are separated by gravity, causing the denser layer to sink to the bottom, where it can be removed by turning the stopcock at the bottom.

**Shielding**–The phenomenon of atoms pushing electron density toward surrounding atoms; in NMR spectroscopy, pulls a group further upfield on the spectrum.

**Sigma ($\sigma$) bond**–The bonding molecular orbital formed by head-to-head or tail-to-tail overlap of atomic orbitals; all single bonds are sigma bonds.

**Simple distillation**–Distillation without any special features; can be used to separate liquids that boil below 150°C and that have at least a 25°C difference in boiling points.

**Size-exclusion chromatography**–A special type of column chromatography in which the beads in the column contain tiny pores of varying sizes, slowing down small compounds that enter the beads.

***sp***–A hybrid orbital with 50% *s*-character and 50% *p*-character.

***sp*²**–A hybrid orbital with 33% *s*-character and 67% *p*-character.

***sp*³**–A hybrid orbital with 25% *s*-character and 75% *p*-character.

**Specific rotation ($[\alpha]$)**–A standardized measure of a compound's ability to rotate plane-polarized light.

**Spectroscopy**–Laboratory technique that relies on measurement of the energy differences between the possible states of a molecular system by determining the frequencies of electromagnetic radiation (light) absorbed by the molecules or response to a magnetic field.

**Spin quantum number ($m_s$)**–Describes the intrinsic spin of the two electrons in an orbital by arbitrarily assigning one of the electrons a spin of $+\frac{1}{2}$ and the other a spin of $-\frac{1}{2}$.

**Spotting**–In thin-layer chromatography, placing the sample directly onto the adsorbent as a small, well-defined spot.

**Staggered conformation**–When a molecule has no overlapping substituents along the line of sight between two carbons, as in a Newman projection.

**Stationary phase**–A solid medium onto which a sample is placed for chromatography; also called the adsorbent.

**Stereogenic**–Describes a chiral center in a molecule.

**Stereoisomers**–Isomers that have the same chemical formula and the same atomic connectivity, but differ in how atoms are arranged in space; any isomer that is not a structural isomer is a stereoisomer.

**Stereoselective**–A reaction that forms an unequal distribution of isomer products that is determined by stability of those products.

**Stereospecific**–A reaction that preferentially yields a specific conformation of product, such as $S_N2$ reactions.

**Steric hindrance**–The prevention of a reaction at a particular location in a molecule by substituent groups around the reactive site.

**Steric protection**–The prevention of the formation of alternative products using a protecting group.

**Strecker synthesis**–A method of synthesizing amino acids that uses condensation between an aldehyde and hydrogen cyanide, followed by hydrolysis.

**Structural isomers**–Molecules that have the same molecular formulas but different connectivity; also called constitutional isomers.

**Substituent**–Any functional group that is not part of the parent chain.

**Tautomer**–An isomer that differs from another by the placement of a proton and a double bond.

**Tetramethylsilane (TMS)**–The calibration standard that marks 0 ppm when plotting an NMR spectrum.

**Thin-layer chromatography (TLC)**–A type of chromatography that uses silica gel or alumina on a card as the medium for the stationary phase.

**Torsional strain**–Increased energy that results when molecules assume eclipsed or *gauche* staggered conformations.

**Tosylate**–A compound containing the functional group $-SO_3C_6H_4CH_3$, derived from toluenesulfonic acid.

**Totally eclipsed conformation**–A type of conformation in which the two largest groups are 0° apart; the most energetically unfavorable conformation.

***Trans***–A molecule in which the two substituents are on opposite sides of an immovable bond.

**Transesterification**–The process that transforms one ester to another when an alcohol acts as a nucleophile and displaces the alkoxy group on an ester.

**Triacylglycerols**–Esters of long-chain carboxylic acids (fatty acids) and glycerol (1,2,3-propanetriol); used as a storage form of energy.

**Triplet**–Three peaks with an area ratio of 1:2:1 in an NMR spectrum that are centered around the true chemical shift of a group of protons; results from splitting by two equivalent hydrogens.

**Ubiquinol**–The reduced, active form of ubiquinone that is an essential electron carrier in the electron transport chain and protects cells from oxidative damage.

**Ubiquinone**–A biologically active quinone that is a vital electron carrier in the electron transport chain; also called coenzyme Q.

**Ultraviolet (UV) spectroscopy**–A technique that measures absorbance of ultraviolet light of various wavelengths passing through a sample.

**Upfield**–Movement to the right in an NMR spectrum.

**Vacuum distillation**–A modified form of distillation used to separate two liquids with boiling points over 150°C; lowers the pressure to decrease the temperature at which a liquid will boil.

**Vicinal diol**–A dialcohol with hydroxyl groups on adjacent carbons.

**Wash**–The reverse of extraction, in which a small amount of solvent is poured over the compound of interest to dissolve and remove impurities.

**Wavenumber**–An analog of frequency used for infrared spectra instead of wavelength.

**Zwitterion**–A compound that contains charges but is overall neutral.

# INDEX

## Symbols



## A

# INDEX

# ART CREDITS

Chapter 2 Cover—Image credited to Vladyslav Starozhylov. From Shutterstock.

Chapter 3 Cover—Image credited to FikMik. From Shutterstock.

Chapter 4 Cover—Image credited to Andrea Danti. From Shutterstock.

Chapter 5 Cover—Image credited to Wollertz. From Shutterstock.

Chapter 7 Cover—Image credited to Science Photo Library – Inti St Clair. From Getty Images.

Chapter 8 Cover—Image credited to Quayside. From Shutterstock.

Chapter 9 Cover—Image credited to Mike Laptev. From Shutterstock.

Chapter 11 Cover—Image credited to Oliver Sved. From Shutterstock.

Figure 11.8 (MRI) Source: Krishna Rao, Uniformed Services University (Illustration) Image adapted from source: sdbs.db.aist.go.jp (National Institute of Advanced Industrial Science and Technology)

Chapter 12 Cover—Image credited to luchschen. From Shutterstock.

# Notes

# Notes

## Notes

## Notes

## Notes

# Notes

## Notes

## Notes

# Notes